Wright & Leahey's

Nurses *and* Families

A Guide to Family Assessment and Intervention

SEVENTH EDITION

Wright & Leahey's

Nurses *and* Families

A Guide to Family Assessment and Intervention

SEVENTH EDITION

Zahra Shajani, RN, MPH, EdD (c), CCHN (c),
Canadian Certified Nurse Educator (CCNE)
Senior Instructor, Associate Dean of Undergraduate Practice Education
Faculty of Nursing
University of Calgary
Calgary, Alberta, Canada

Diana Snell, MN, RN
Instructor
Faculty of Nursing
University of Calgary
Calgary, Alberta, Canada

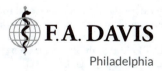

F.A. DAVIS

Philadelphia

F. A. Davis Company
1915 Arch Street
Philadelphia, PA 19103
www.fadavis.com

Printed in the United States of America

Last digit indicates print number: 10 9 8 7 6 5 4 3 2 1

Acquisitions Editor: Jacalyn Sharp
Associate Content Project Manager: Sean West
Manager of Design and Illustration: Carolyn O'Brien

As new scientific information becomes available through basic and clinical research, recommended treatments and drug therapies undergo changes. The author(s) and publisher have done everything possible to make this book accurate, up to date, and in accord with accepted standards at the time of publication. The author(s), editors, and publisher are not responsible for errors or omissions or for consequences from application of the book, and make no warranty, expressed or implied, in regard to the contents of the book. Any practice described in this book should be applied by the reader in accordance with professional standards of care used in regard to the unique circumstances that may apply in each situation. The reader is advised always to check product information (package inserts) for changes and new information regarding dose and contraindications before administering any drug. Caution is especially urged when using new or infrequently ordered drugs.

Library of Congress Cataloging-in-Publication Data

Names: Shajani, Zahra, RN, author. | Snell, Diana, author. | Preceded by
(work): Wright, Lorraine M., 1944- Nurses and families.
Title: Wright & Leahey's nurses and families : a guide to family assessment
and intervention / Zahra Shajani, Diana Snell.
Other titles: Wright and Leahey's nurses and families | Nurses and families
Description: Edition 7. | Philadelphia : F.A. Davis Company, [2019] |
Preceded by: Nurses and families / Lorraine M. Wright and Maureen Leahey.
6th ed. c2013. | Includes bibliographical references and index.
Identifiers: LCCN 2018053870 (print) | LCCN 2018055096 (ebook) | ISBN
9780803699038 | ISBN 9780803669628 (pbk. : alk. paper)
Subjects: | MESH: Family Nursing—methods | Nursing Assessment | Family
Health | Interviews as Topic—methods | Models, Nursing
Classification: LCC RT120.F34 (ebook) | LCC RT120.F34 (print) | NLM WY 159.5
| DDC 616.07/5—dc23
LC record available at https://lccn.loc.gov/2018053870

Our experiences as registered nurses working with families in a variety of settings over the past 20 years have inspired us significantly and encouraged us to write about their stories and experiences and the impact nurses can make. *Nurses and Families,* seventh edition, has been a journey for us, filled with stimulating conversations and discussions rooted in our passion for family nursing. We dedicate this edition to each other, and we thank all those who have been a part of this journey: patients and clients, colleagues, mentors, and our families—you know who you are!

Zahra Shajani & Diana Snell

Reviewers

Amanda Alonzo, PhD, RN, BSN, CNE
Adjunct Faculty
Oklahoma Wesleyan University School
of Nursing
Chanute, Kansas

Beverley Jones, RN, MScN, MPA
Faculty
St. Clair College
West Windsor, Ontario, Canada

Victoria Kyarsgaard, DNP, PHN,
RNC, CNE
Associate Professor of Nursing
Crown College
Saint Bonifacius, Minnesota

M. Star Mahara, RN, MSN
Associate Professor
Thompson Rivers University
Kamloops, British Columbia, Canada

Barbara McClaskey, PhD, APRN,
RNC
Professor, School of Nursing
Pittsburg State University
Pittsburg, Kansas

Verna C. Pangman, RN, MEd, MN
Senior Scholar, Rady Faculty of Health
Science
College of Nursing, University of
Manitoba
Winnipeg, Manitoba, Canada

Meredith Scannel, PhD, MSN, MPH,
CNM, SANE, CEN
Institute of Health Professions MGH
Nursing Faculty
Boston, Massachusetts

Joy Shewchuk, RN, BSc, BSN, MSN
Professor
Humber College
Toronto, Ontario, Canada

Wendy Wheeler, MN, RN
Instructor
Red Deer College
Red Deer, Alberta, Canada

Acknowledgments

We are grateful to Lorraine Wright and Maureen Leahey, who have inspired us as nurses and educators working with families. Their dedication to and passion for family nursing have been instrumental in shaping our journey. Our first exposure to *Nurses and Families* during our own undergraduate education has been foundational to the way in which we have interacted with families over the years. We have had the privilege to implement the concepts of the Calgary Family Assessment Model (CFAM) and the Calgary Family Intervention Model (CFIM) in both our clinical practices with families and with undergraduate nursing students as educators.

We are especially grateful to

- Susan Rhyner, Senior Acquisitions Editor, F. A. Davis, for her guidance, leadership, unfailing support, and belief in us as emerging authors.
- Sean West, Associate Content Project Manager, F. A. Davis, for keeping us on track, keeping the momentum going, and ensuring the success of the seventh edition.
- Lynda Hatch, Development Editor, for her attention to detail, for always supporting our continuously evolving ideas, and for her excellent suggestions.
- Jacalyn Sharp, Acquisitions Editor, F. A. Davis, for her support in ensuring our vision for the seventh edition.

Finally, we are grateful to our families, who have listened to us, supported us, and reminded us of the importance of family. To our husbands, Nizam and Logan, for their encouraging words and ongoing support. To our children, Shaheena, Rahmaan, Cameron, and Aiden, who continually amaze us and inspired us to believe in ourselves during this journey. To our parents, for their unconditional love, support, and guidance.
Thank you!

Zahra Shajani & Diana Snell

Contents

Introduction

REFLECTIONS ON THE FIRST TO SEVENTH EDITIONS

We welcome you to the seventh edition of *Wright and Leahey's Nurses and Families: A Guide to Family Assessment and Intervention*. Whether you are a nursing student, a practicing nurse, a nurse educator, and/or a nurse researcher, this book is for you. Research evidence, whether evidence-based or practice-based, and the clinical narratives of families experiencing illness make it a mandatory and moral imperative for nurses to include families with compassion and competence in whatever nursing context they find themselves. The development and evolution of family nursing have moved beyond the debate of whether families should be included in health care to a more important focus and emphasis on *how to* involve families. Therefore, the main emphasis or thrust of the seventh edition is once again to offer ideas on *how to* include families in nursing practice, along with the specific knowledge and skills to accomplish that. Yes, this is a "how-to" book.

We published the first edition of *Nurses and Families* in 1984, the second in 1994, the third in 2000, the fourth in 2005, the fifth in 2009, and the sixth in 2013. Now the seventh edition in 2019 is under the authorship of Zahra Shajani and Diana Snell. They have retained the majority of our original text and added case scenarios with useful reflective and critical thinking questions, additional tables, and a new chapter. Learning objectives and key concepts have been added to increase the user-friendliness of the text.

Evolution of *Nurses and Families*

In 1994 *Nurse and Families: A Guide to Family Assessment and Intervention*, our second edition, was awarded the American Journal of Nursing Book of the Year Award. Some of the changes and developments in family nursing plus the influence of larger societal differences in the past 35 years are obvious and apparent to us and are discussed in the text, whereas others are more subtle and perhaps tenuous.

One example of the palpable globalization of family nursing is that *Nurses and Families* has been translated into French, German, Icelandic,

Japanese, Korean, Portuguese, Spanish, and Swedish. Another example is the development of our website *www.familynursingresources.com* for educational resources and the production of our eight "how-to" family nursing videos.

Further tangible evidence of the expansion of family nursing is the worldwide development and adoption of family assessment models. We are gratified how our Calgary Family Assessment Model (CFAM) has substantially contributed to family nursing knowledge. We introduced the CFAM in the first edition in 1984, and it continues to be widely adopted in undergraduate and graduate nursing curricula, by practicing nurses, and in nursing research. The CFAM is utilized in nursing curricula in over 26 countries, including Australia, Brazil, Canada, Chile, China, Denmark, England, Finland, Germany, Hong Kong, Iceland, Japan, Korea, Norway, Portugal, Qatar, Scotland, Singapore, Spain, Sweden, Switzerland, Taiwan, Thailand, the United States, and Vietnam. The International Council of Nurses published a significant document entitled "The Family Nurse" and recognized the CFAM as one of the four leading family assessment models in the world (Schober & Affara, 2001).

With this global expansion, we have had to revisit and revise our thinking about the CFAM in order to acknowledge, recognize, and embrace the evolving importance of certain dimensions of family life that influence health and illness, such as class, gender, ethnicity, race, family development, and beliefs. The social determinants of health are compelling pertinent factors that we have increasingly addressed.

A significant amplification in our text was the development of a framework and model for interventions, namely, the Calgary Family Intervention Model (CFIM), which was introduced in the second edition. This was done in recognition of the need to give as much emphasis to intervention as there had been on assessment of families and to provide a framework within which to capture family interventions. This change was clearly influenced by the advances in family nursing research, education, and practice from a primary emphasis on assessment to an expanding and equal emphasis on intervention.

In the family nursing literature, particularly the *Journal of Family Nursing,* there have been numerous publications discussing the application, implementation, and usefulness and/or effectiveness of the CFAM, the CFIM, and the 15-minute family interview. In 2015, a bibliography was developed to identify any and all known English-language books, articles, and media productions that reference the CFAM/CFIM (see http://www.familynursingresources.com/bibliography.htm). Of course, there may also be references to the CFAM/CFIM that we are not familiar within non-English journals. Currently, there are six books, 54 conceptual articles, 56 data-based research reports, two book reviews, two research instruments, eight media productions (DVDs), and 21 articles on pedagogy in family nursing that identify and apply the CFAM/CFIM (see http://www.familynursingresources.com/bibliography.htm).

In considering how widespread the models have become, several questions arise. First, what is the essence of these models? What differentiates the CFAM and CFIM from other practice models for family assessment and intervention within nursing? Our answer is that the conceptualization of the CFAM and CFIM has emerged directly from our own actual clinical practice and the observation and supervision of colleagues and nursing students. We refer to this phenomenon as the clinical scholarship of practice (Bell, 2003). To us, clinical practice has always been an intense experience where we engage with families, learn about their illness beliefs and illness suffering, and discover what they find most helpful that enables and promotes family healing (practice-based evidence). Also, we have conducted practice-based research examining live and videotaped family interviews to learn what it is that nurses actually do that softens illness suffering. We also offer ideas and interventions to families that we have gleaned from our own and others' research with families (evidence-based practice) and note whether these are useful in particular situations. We find the circular process intriguing and enhancing.

Why is it important that our clinical models have evolved from actual practice with families? It is significant because these models link theory to practice in an easy-to-understand manner. Over the years, colleagues and learners have offered us feedback that the models are straightforward, comprehensible, and easy to apply. The International Family Nursing Association (IFNA) *Position Statement on Generalist Family Nursing Practice* lists many skills that are useful and helpful aspirations for learners (IFNA, 2015). In addition, the IFNA has developed the *Position Statement on Advanced Practice Competencies for Family Nursing* (IFNA, 2017). However, lists of skills and competencies often fly out the window when a nurse is in an actual clinical situation with a live family. When nurses possess a thorough grounding in conceptual practice models, they can then practice these competencies and skills more easily to assist families. They can progress from lip service to actual practice. As Benner (2001) argues, practice is a way of knowing; it is situated knowledge use.

A third question arising from a perusal of the existing CFAM/CFIM literature pertains to popularity. What is the most popular aspect of the CFAM and CFIM that is applied in practice settings? It has definitely been the adoption and implementation of the 15-minute family interview, introduced in the third edition, which integrates and distills the most important aspects of both clinical models. And why? The 15-minute (or less) family interview is most easily translatable and transferable to clinical settings. It fits nurses' practice in a wide variety of contexts.

With massive restructuring in North American health-care institutions and community clinics and budgetary constraints, many nurses feel they cannot afford the opportunity to get involved in or attend to the needs of families in health-care settings. Nurses, particularly those in acute-care hospital settings, have expressed their frustration about the substantially reduced time to address and attend to families' needs and concerns because of increased caseloads, heightened acuity of patients, and short-term stays. It was for this reason—to respect and respond to the massive changes in the North American health-care systems—that we developed practice ideas for how to conduct a 15-minute (or less) family interview.

We have been very gratified by how our family nursing conceptualizations of clinical practice have been enthusiastically accepted, both in our text and when presenting these ideas at nursing and health-care workshops and/or conferences. More importantly, based on anecdotal and research reports, the implementation of our models and clinical practice ideas has shown great promise. We have been encouraged by nurses' reports of softened illness suffering by family members and enhanced health promotion and healing with families in their care. Equally gratifying are reports of increased job satisfaction by practicing nurses when collaborating with families, even if only for 15 minutes or less (Sigurdadottir, Svavarsdottir, & Juliusdottir, 2015).

The majority of nursing students and even some practicing nurses comment that they have never seen a family interview. Therefore, they often feel anxious about meeting with a family and sometimes will mask their apprehensions by commenting that they do not have enough time to involve families in their nursing practice. But once practicing nurses embrace the belief that "illness is a family affair," they realize they can make a profound difference to softening suffering in just 15 minutes or less. When they observe actual family interviews, they challenge their constraining belief of not having enough time and realize, instead, that it was not having the clinical and/or relationship skills that was inhibiting them from involving families in their care rather than a lack of time.

Opportunities to observe actual demonstration family interviews either live or on DVDs enable learners to increase their confidence and competence in conducting actual family meetings. Our DVD entitled *How to Conduct a 15-Minute Family Interview* (Wright & Leahey, 2000) has been the most sought-after of our eight educational programs applying the CFAM/CFIM (Wright & Leahey, 2000, 2001, 2002, 2003, 2006, 2010a, 2010b, 2010c). Another very interesting observation is that of all the ideas utilized in the CFAM, the two assessment tools, the genogram and ecomap, have been the most frequently integrated into actual everyday clinical practice. The most utilized family nursing interventions from the CFIM have been the offering of commendations and the asking of particular kinds of therapeutic questions.

Perhaps a more subtle but equally significant development is our ever-changing and evolving relationship with the families with whom we work. This change is reflected in our choice of language to describe the nurse-family relationship that we deem most desirable. Our preferred stance/posture with families has evolved into a more collaborative, consultative, relational, and nonhierarchical relationship over the past 35 years. When we adopt this stance, we notice greater equality, respectfulness, and status given to the family's expertise with their experience of illness, loss, and/or disability. Therefore, the combined expertise of both the nurse and the family form a new and effective synergy in the context of therapeutic conversations that otherwise did not and could not exist.

Another subtle development evolving throughout the seven editions has been the movement toward a postmodernist worldview. We embrace the notion that there are multiple realities in and of "the world" and that each family member and nurse sees a world that he or she brings forth through interacting with him- or herself and with others through language. We encourage an openness in ourselves, our students, and the families with whom we work to the many "worlds," differences, and diversity between and among family members and among health-care providers.

We consider it a great privilege to collaborate and consult with families for health promotion and/or to diminish or soften emotional, physical, or spiritual suffering from illness. We are also grateful for opportunities to teach professional nurses and undergraduate and graduate nursing students about involving, caring for, and learning from families in health care. Through our own clinical practice and teaching of health professionals for over 40 years and personal family experiences with illness, we recognize the extreme importance of nurses' possessing sound family assessment and intervention knowledge, skills, and compassion in order to assist families. We also acknowledge the profound influence that families have upon our own lives and relationships (Leahey & Wright, 2016).

A SNAPSHOT OF 35 YEARS OF PROGRESS AND PARADIGM EVENTS IN FAMILY NURSING

Over the 35 years since the publication of the first edition of *Nurses and Families*, there have been paradigm events in family nursing very worthy of celebration. There has been progress, and yet there are other areas where we still need to put "our shoulders to the wheel." We believe one of the most far-reaching paradigm events in family nursing has been the publication of the *Journal of Family Nursing* in 1995. Since its inception, it has been under the very able and competent editorship of Dr. Janice M. Bell. The establishment provided a central place, for the first time, for the uniting of family nurses and the dissemination of family nursing knowledge. Another paradigm event was the offering, without any formal organization or association, of the First International Family Nursing Conference in 1988, in Calgary, Canada. Since then, 13 International Family Nursing Conferences (IFNCs) have been held in Canada and the United States, South America (Chile), Asia (Thailand, Japan), and Europe (Iceland, Denmark, Spain). Conferences being held internationally have enabled a further appreciation of family nursing's global expansion and the contributions in other countries beyond the boundaries of North America. The 14th IFNC returns to North America in 2019 and will be held in Washington, D.C.

With each IFNC, there is confirmation of clear, steady progress in the development, knowledge translation, and expansion of family nursing. It is evident and visible in the presentations, workshops, and keynotes offering an observable advancement of knowledge in theory, research, assessment, and interventions in family work. The community of family nurses has expanded to truly be a global force and phenomenon with enduring colleagueships and friendships.

Another momentous development occurred at the ninth IFNC in Iceland in 2009 when the International Family Nursing Association (IFNA) was created. With a formal organization, even more opportunities are now available for nurses to network and share knowledge and expertise outside of the conference format (see http://www.internationalfamilynursing.org). Webinars, chat groups, and Twitter are now available for connecting.

The face of families has dramatically changed over the past 35 years as our demographics in North America indicate an ever-increasing aging population as baby boomers have moved into retirement with significantly reduced numbers of Generation Xers to care for them. Marriages are being delayed or omitted entirely in committed relationships, and various family forms have proliferated. Diversity in North American populations is clearly evident, with increased numbers of refugees, immigrants, and undocumented persons/families. Respect for a wider array of cultural, religious, and sexual orientation differences in our health-care system is required. Increased globalization invites the possibility for better health-care practices worldwide but also allows for the universal transmission of diseases, making it much more difficult for health-care providers to isolate, control, and segregate the origins of disease.

Amidst all the changes in demographics, technology, health-care delivery, and diversity, there are also profound changes occurring in our worldviews, from modernism to postmodernism, from secularism to spiritualism. Family nursing has not been immune to these changes, nor have we.

Numerous other paradigm events have influenced families and the development of family nursing. Massive health-care restructuring and downsizing in North America have directly and indirectly placed more responsibility on the backs of families for the care of their ill family members. There is an expanded consumer movement, and there is more collaboration with families about their health-care needs. The explosion of health-related websites and the increasingly pervasive use of technology, such as messenger, Skype, Facetime, e-mail, texting, and digital phones, have significantly influenced the transmission of health information. The increased number of health-care apps for monitoring heart rates to footsteps is also an invitation for individuals and families to be more directly involved in their own health care. Social networking, such as blogs, Twitter, Facebook, and YouTube, enables family members to be more proactive and knowledgeable about their health issues and share possible coping strategies. Internet health sites and social media open doors never before possible for families to obtain current knowledge about their health problems, options for treatments, and traditional and alternative health-care resources.

It is so very gratifying and rewarding to learn and witness how we as nurses can make such a remarkable and profound difference in the softening of illness suffering and the improvement in the quality of life with the families we are privileged to encounter. We wish you, Zahra and Diana, well in your important and meaningful work with families experiencing health-care issues.

Lorraine M. Wright, RN, PhD, and Maureen Leahey, RN, PhD

August 3, 2018

THE SEVENTH EDITION: WHAT IT IS, WHAT IS NEW

The seventh edition of *Nurses and Families* continues to be a "how-to" basic text for undergraduate, graduate, and practicing nurses. This practical how-to guide for clinical work offers the opportunity for nursing students, practitioners, and educators to deliver better health care to families in all practice areas. Nurse educators who currently teach a family-centered approach and/or those who will be introducing the concept of the "family as the client" will find it a valuable resource, and educators involved in continuing or advanced education courses or programs will be able to use this book to update and substantially enhance nurses' clinical knowledge and skills in family-centered care.

This book provides specific guidelines and skills for nurses to consider when preparing for and conducting family meetings, from the first interview through to discharge or termination. Clinical case examples are given throughout the book and have been updated to reflect the diversity of families in today's society. Issues in a variety of practice settings, including hospital, primary care, school, community, outpatient, and the home, are addressed.

How to Do a 15-Minute (or Shorter) Family Interview (Chapter 9) remains one of the most popular, well-received, and useful chapters in the book as reported by numerous practicing nurses and nursing students. It assists nurses working in time-pressured environments to offer valuable assistance to families.

Nurses and Families, seventh edition, continues to do the following:

- Provide nurses with a sound theoretical foundation for family assessment and intervention
- Provide nurses with clear, concise, and comprehensive evidence-based family assessment and intervention models, namely, the Calgary Family Assessment and Intervention Models, for current best practice
- Present guidelines for family interviewing skills

- Offer detailed ideas and suggestions with clinical examples of how to prepare, conduct, use questions in, and terminate family interviews
- Provide nurses with an appreciation of the powerful influence of nurse-family collaboration to diminish, soften, or alleviate illness suffering.

NEW ADDITIONS TO *NURSES AND FAMILIES,* SEVENTH EDITION

- A new chapter (Chapter 13) has been added: *Pulling It All Together*. This chapter provides an in-depth clinical case example using the CFAM/CFIM to conduct a family interview with the O'Shannell family. We hope that this chapter will give students and nurses clear, specific examples of how to apply the CFAM/CFIM to enhance their knowledge and skills at all levels.
- Each chapter now begins with **Learning Objectives** that delineate what students will learn after studying the chapter and provide an overview of the chapter topics.
- An at-a-glance list of each chapter's **Key Concepts** in family nursing comes next. Snapshot definitions of the Key Concepts are presented in boxes throughout the chapter and then explained in more detail in the text.
- A **Case Scenario** with reflective questions follows the chapter text and provides the opportunity to apply and reinforce knowledge specific to each chapter's content.
- Every chapter ends with **Critical Thinking Questions** designed to provide opportunities for students to apply their knowledge to their own clinical practice areas.
- All chapters have been thoroughly updated and expanded to include many new references and the most current research and theory. These updates enhance evidence-based nursing practice and provide context to current issues and trends. We hope that this continues to ensure that the CFAM/CFIM is an easy-to-apply, practical, and relevant model for busy nurses working with a wide variety of complex issues and family structures and encountering various developmental stages.

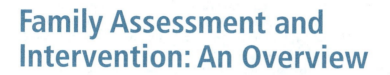

Chapter **1**

Family Assessment and Intervention: An Overview

Learning Objectives

- Understand the evolution of family nursing.
- Identify the difference between nursing interventions and family nursing interventions.
- Describe the indications and contraindications for a family assessment and interventions.
- Identify the Calgary Family Assessment Model (CFAM) and the Calgary Family Intervention Model (CFIM) as frameworks for family systems nursing.

Key Concepts

Calgary Family Assessment Model (CFAM)

Calgary Family Intervention Model (CFIM)

Family nursing interventions

Family systems nursing

Nursing interventions

N urses have an ethical and moral obligation to involve families in their health-care practice. Family has a significant impact on the health and well-being of individual members. Family-centered care is achieved responsibly and respectfully by relational practices consisting of collaborative nurse-family relationships together with sound family assessment and intervention knowledge and skills.

As nurses theorize about, conduct research on, and involve families more in health care, they modify their usual patterns of clinical practice. The implication for this change in practice is that nurses must become competent in assessing and intervening with families through collaborative nurse-family relationships. Nurses who embrace the belief that illness needs to be treated as a family affair can more efficiently learn the knowledge and clinical skills required to conduct family interviews (Wright & Bell, 2009). This belief invites nurses to think interactionally, or reciprocally, about families. The dominant focus of family nursing assessment and intervention must be the reciprocity between health and illness and the family. Providing nurses with a framework for family assessment and the interventions for treating families can facilitate the transition from thinking in an individualistic manner toward thinking interactionally and, thus, thinking "family."

It is most helpful and enlightening for nurses to assess the impact of illness on the family and the influence of family interaction on the cause, course, and cure of illness. Additionally, the reciprocal relationship between nurses and families is also a significant component of both easing suffering and enhancing healing.

Family systems nursing integrates nursing, systems, cybernetics, change, and family therapy theories (Bell, 2009; Wright & Leahey, 1990). It requires familiarity with an extensive body of knowledge: family dynamics, family systems theory, family assessment, family intervention, and family research. It also requires accompanying competence in family interviewing skills. Family systems nursing focuses simultaneously on the family and individual systems (Bell, 2009; Wright & Leahey, 1990). All nurses should be knowledgeable about and competent in involving families in health care across all domains of nursing practice.

KEY CONCEPT DEFINED

Family Systems Nursing

A framework that integrates nursing, systems, cybernetics, change, and family therapy theories and focuses interventions simultaneously on the family and the individual systems.

The language of family nursing has been growing and evolving over the course of many years. Table 1-1 summarizes the terms that name, describe, and communicate aspects of family-centered care and identifies the authors and sources of these vital additions to nursing practice.

EVOLUTION OF THE NURSING OF FAMILIES

Throughout nursing's history, family involvement has always been part of health care, but it has not always been labeled as such. Because nursing originated in patients' homes, family involvement and family-centered care were

TABLE 1-1	Common Terms Used in Family-Centered Care and Their Sources
TERMS	**SOURCE**
Family interviewing	Wright and Leahey, 2013
Family health promotion nursing	Bomar, 2004
Family health-care nursing	Hanson, 2001; Hanson and Boyd, 1996; Kaakinen, Coehlo, Steele, Tabacco, and Hanson, 2018
Family nursing	Bell, Watson, and Wright, 1990; Friedman, Bowden, and Jones, 2003; Gilliss, 1991; Gilliss, Highly, Roberts, and Martinson,1989; Svavarsdottir and Jonsdottir, 2011; Wegner and Alexander, 1993; Wright and Leahey, 1990
Family nursing practice Family systems nursing	Bell, 2009; Wright and Leahey, 1990; Wright, Watson, and Bell, 1990
Nursing of families	Feetham, Meister, Bell, and Gilliss, 1993
Family nursing as relational inquiry	Doane and Varcoe, 2005

natural occurrences. With the transition of nursing practice from homes to hospitals during the Great Depression and World War II, families became excluded not only from involvement in caring for ill members but also from major family events such as birth and death. After having undergone all these developmental changes, the practice of nursing has now come full circle, with an obligation to invite families once again to participate in their own health care. However, this invitation is being made with much more knowledge, research evidence, respect, and collaboration than at any other time in nursing history.

The history, evolution, and theory development of the nursing of families in North America have been discussed in depth in the literature (Anderson, 2000; Doane, 2003; Duhamel, 2015; Feetham, Meister, Bell & Gilliss, 1993; Ford-Gilboe, 2002; Friedman, Bowden, & Jones, 2003; Gilliss, 1991; Gilliss, Highly, Roberts, & Martinson,1989; Hartrick, 2000; Kaakinen, Coehlo, Steele, Tabacco, & Hanson, 2018; Kobayashi, 2011). These authors have made significant contributions to the advancement of family nursing knowledge. Table 1-2 summarizes the evolution of family nursing.

The evolution, development, and practice of family nursing are well established and are being documented in many countries outside North America (see Table 1-3).

Numerous disciplines have attempted to define and conceptualize the concept of *family*. Each discipline has its own point of view or frame of

TABLE 1-2	Timeline of the Evolution of Family Nursing
YEAR	**EVOLUTION OF FAMILY NURSING**
1970–Present	Institute for the Family, Family Therapy Services, Department of Psychiatry, University of Rochester, Rochester, New York, is begun.
1973–Present	Calgary Family Therapy Centre, Calgary, AB, Canada, is begun.
1982–2007	Family Nursing Unit, University of Calgary, Calgary, AB, Canada, is opened.
1984	First edition of *Nurses and Families* is published (Wright & Leahey).
1985–2010	Family Therapy Training Program, Calgary, AB, Canada, is begun.
1988	First International Family Nursing Conference, Calgary, AB, Canada, was held.
1990–1998	Family Nursing Center, University of Wisconsin–Eau Claire, is in operation.
1991–Present	Chicago Center for Family Health, affiliate of the University of Chicago, Chicago, Illinois, is opened.
1993–2017	Denise Latourelle Family Nursing Unit, University of Montreal, Quebec, Canada, is opened.
1995	*Journal of Family Nursing* is started.
2000	Family Health Nurse—Context, Conceptual Framework and Curriculum (World Health Organization, 2000) is developed.
2001	World Health Organization Family Health Nurse Multinational study begins.
2001	International Council of Nurses (ICN) document entitled "The Family Nurse: Frameworks for Practice" is published.
2001–Present	Family Stress and Illness Program, Behavioral Health Center, the Children's Hospital of Philadelphia, Pennsylvania, is opened.
2002	International Council of Nurses (ICN) Nurses Day theme: Family Nursing Nine Star Family Nursing is identified.
2007–2011	Landspitali University Hospital Family Nursing Implementation Project is operational.
2008	Glen Taylor Nursing Institute for Family and Society, Minnesota State University, Mankato, Minnesota, is established.
2009	International Family Nursing Association (IFNA) is established.
2013	International Family Nursing Association (IFNA) "IFNA Position Statement on Pre-Licensure Family Nursing Education" is published.
2015	International Family Nursing Association (IFNA) "IFNA Position Statement on Generalist Competencies for Family Nursing Practice" is published
2017	International Family Nursing Association (IFNA) "IFNA Position Statement on Advanced Practice Competencies for Family Nursing" is published.

TABLE 1-3	Documented Family Nursing Research and Practice Outside of North America
COUNTRY	**AUTHORS**
Brazil	Angelo, 2008
Denmark	Voltelen, Konradsen, and Østergaard, 2016
Finland	Astedt-Kurki, 2010; Astedt-Kurki and Kaunonen, 2011
Hong Kong	Simpson et al, 2006
Iceland	Svavarsdottir, 2008; Svavarsdottir and Sigurdardottir, 2011
Japan	Bell, 1999; Moriyama, 2008; Sugishita, 1999
Nigeria	Irinoye, Ogunfowokan, and Olaogun, 2006
Nordic countries	Svavarsdottir, 2006
Scotland	O'Sullivan Buchard, Claveirole, Mitchell, Walford, and Whyte, 2004
Sweden	Saveman, 2010; Saveman and Benzein, 2001
Thailand	Wacharasin and Theinpichet, 2008

reference for viewing the family, and all have an ever-increasing appreciation of diversity issues, for example:

- Economists are concerned with how the family works together to meet material needs.
- Sociologists are concerned with the family as a specific group in society.
- Psychologists are concerned with the emotional ties within a family.

It is helpful for nurses to be aware of the many models offered by various disciplines and the distinct variables emphasized in each model because no one assessment model explains all family phenomena. In any clinical practice setting, nurses benefit from adopting a clear conceptual framework, or map, of the family. This framework encourages the synthesis of data so that family strengths and problems can be identified and a useful nursing plan devised. When no conceptual framework exists, it is extremely difficult for the nurse to group disparate data or to examine the relationships among the multiple variables that affect the family. Use of a family assessment framework helps to organize this massive amount of seemingly different information. It also provides a focus for intervention.

NURSING PRACTICE LEVELS WITH FAMILIES: GENERALIST AND SPECIALIST

Schober and Affara (2001) emphasize that nursing practice with families is directed by whether the concept of the family is defined as *family as context* or *family as client*. One way to alleviate potential confusion of practice levels is to clearly distinguish two levels of expertise in nursing with regard to clinical work with families: generalists and specialists. Typically, generalists are nurses at the baccalaureate level who predominantly use the concept of the family as context (Wright & Leahey, 1990), although upper-level baccalaureate students begin to conceptualize the family as the unit of care. Specialists, on the other hand, are nurses at the graduate (master's or doctoral) level who predominantly use the concept of family as the unit of care. This requires specialization in family systems nursing (Wright & Leahey, 1990). Family systems nursing specialization requires that "the focus is always on interaction and reciprocity. It is not 'either/or' but rather 'both/and'" (Wright & Leahey, 1990, p. 149). However, these boundaries can become blurred, with upper-level baccalaureate students recognizing the importance of focusing on interaction and reciprocity. These students often develop nursing competence and are able to deal with individual and family systems simultaneously.

CALGARY FAMILY ASSESSMENT MODEL: AN INTEGRATED FRAMEWORK

The Calgary Family Assessment Model (CFAM) is a multidimensional framework consisting of three major categories: structural, developmental, and functional (see Chapter 3). The model is based on a theory foundation involving systems, cybernetics, communication, and change. It was adapted from Tomm and Sanders's (1983) family assessment model and has been substantially embellished since the first edition of *Nurses and Families* in 1984. The model is also embedded within larger worldviews of postmodernism, feminism, and the biology of cognition. Diversity issues are also emphasized and appreciated within this model.

> **KEY CONCEPT DEFINED**
>
> ### Calgary Family Assessment Model (CFAM)
>
> A multidimensional framework consisting of three major categories—structural, developmental, and functional—based on a theory foundation involving systems, cybernetics, communication, and change.

Of course, any model is useful only if it can be comprehended by nurses and then transferred into their generalist practice with families.

There has been recent research conducted to validate the usefulness of the CFAM/Calgary Family Intervention Model (CFIM) such as the following:

- Perceived level of knowledge and difficulty in applying family assessment among senior undergraduate nursing students (Lee, Leung, Chan, & Chung, 2010)
- Psychometric development of the Iceland-Family Perceived Support Questionnaire (ICE-FPSQ; Sveinbjarnardottir, Svavarsdottir, & Hrafnkelsson, 2012a)
- Psychometric development of the Iceland-Expressive Family Functioning Questionnaire (ICE-EFFQ; Sveinbjarnardottir, Svavarsdottir, & Hrafnkelsson, 2012b)

INDICATIONS AND CONTRAINDICATIONS FOR A FAMILY ASSESSMENT

It is important to identify guidelines for determining which families will automatically be considered for family assessment. Because families now tend to have increased health-care awareness and knowledge, nurses are encountering families who present themselves as a unit for assistance with family health and illness issues. Frequently, however, families believe the illness involves only one family member. Therefore, with each illness situation, a judgment must be made about whether that particular illness or problem should be approached within a family context. Box 1-1 lists the indications for family assessment.

Conducting and completing a family assessment does not absolve nurses from assessing serious risks, such as suicide and homicide, or serious illnesses in individual family members. Family assessment is neither a panacea nor a substitute for an individual assessment. Contraindications for family assessment are shown in Box 1-2.

During the engagement process, nurses must explicitly present the rationale for a family assessment. (Refer to Chapters 6 and 7.) A nurse's decision to conduct a family assessment should be guided by sound clinical principles and judgment. The nurse can take advantage of opportunities to consult with peers and supervisors if questions exist about the suitability of such an assessment.

After completing the family assessment, the nurse must decide whether to intervene with the family. In the next section, general ideas about intervention are discussed. Specific ideas for nurses to consider when making clinical decisions about interventions with particular families are presented in Chapters 4, 8, and 9.

Box 1-1 Indications for Family Assessment

- A family is experiencing emotional, physical, or spiritual suffering or disruption caused by a family crisis (e.g., acute or chronic illness, injury, or death).
- A family is experiencing emotional, physical, or spiritual suffering or disruption caused by a developmental milestone (e.g., birth, marriage, youngest child leaving home).
- A family defines an illness or problem as a family issue, and a motivation for family assessment is present.
- A child or adolescent is identified by the family as having difficulties (e.g., cyberbullying, fear of cancer treatment).
- The family is experiencing issues that jeopardize family relationships (e.g., end-of-life illness, addictions).
- An adult family member is being admitted to the hospital.
- A child is being admitted to the hospital.

KEY CONCEPT DEFINED

Calgary Family Intervention Model (CFIM)

An organizing framework conceptualizing the intersection between a particular domain—cognitive, affective, or behavioral—of family functioning and a specific intervention offered by health-care professionals; a companion to the CFAM.

Box 1-2 Contraindications for Family Assessment

- Family assessment compromises the individuation of a family member (e.g., if a young adult has recently left home, a family interview may not be desirable).
- The context of a family situation permits little or no leverage (e.g., the family might have a constraining belief that the nurse is working as an agent of some other institution, such as the court).

CALGARY FAMILY INTERVENTION MODEL: AN ORGANIZING FRAMEWORK

The Calgary Family Intervention Model (CFIM) is an organizing framework for conceptualizing the relationship between families and nurses that helps change to occur and healing to begin. Specifically, the model highlights the family-nurse relationship by focusing on the intersection between family member functioning and interventions offered by nurses (see Chapter 4). It is at this intersection that healing can take place. The CFIM is a resilience- and strength-based, collaborative, nonhierarchical model that recognizes the expertise of family members experiencing illness and the expertise of nurses in managing illness and promoting health. The model is rooted in notions from postmodernism and the biology of cognition. It can be applied and used with patients and families from diverse cultures because it emphasizes the "fit" of particular interventions from a particular cultural viewpoint. To the best of our knowledge, it remains the only family nursing intervention model that is currently documented.

NURSING INTERVENTIONS: A GENERAL DISCUSSION

Numerous terms are used to distinguish and label the treatment portion of nursing practice, including *intervention, treatment, therapeutics, action, activity, moves,* and *micromoves* (Bell & Wright, 2011; Bulechek & McCloskey, 1992). This textbook prefers the designation *intervention*. The most rigorous effort to standardize the language for nursing interventions is the work of McCloskey and Bulechek (1992) and their colleagues at the University of Iowa who developed the Nursing Interventions Classification (NIC), which is a comprehensive, research-based, standardized classification of nursing interventions on nurses' reports of their practices (Butcher, Bulechek, McCloskey, Dochterman, & Wagner, 2018).

> **KEY CONCEPT DEFINED**
>
> **Nursing Interventions**
>
> Any action or response of the nurse, including the clinician's overt therapeutic actions and internal cognitive-affective responses, that occurs in the context of a nurse-client relationship; actions offered to effect and enhance individual, family, or community functioning for which the clinician is accountable.

Family nursing practice differs in that a list of strengths and problems is generated rather than diagnoses. We conceptualize the list as one observer's perspective, not as the "truth" about a family. The list presents problems or concerns that nurses can address. It has been our experience that nursing diagnoses have become too rigid and do not include enough consideration of the determinants of health. We prefer to identify the strengths of a family and list them alongside the problems. The advantage of this type of listing is that it gives a balanced view of a family. It also asks the nurse not to be blinded by a family's problems or diagnosis but to realize that every family has strengths and resources, even in the face of potential or actual health problems.

Definition of a Nursing Intervention

Butcher et al (2018) define nursing interventions as "any treatment based upon clinical judgment that a nurse performs to enhance patient/client outcomes" (p. 2). Nursing interventions include both direct and indirect care aimed at individuals, families, and the community. These interventions include physiological and psychological approaches, illness treatment and prevention, and health promotion (Butcher et al, 2018, p. 2). Wright and Bell (2009) offer an alternate definition: "any action or response of the clinician, which includes the clinician's overt therapeutic actions and internal cognitive-affective responses, that occurs in the context of a clinician-client relationship offered to effect individual, family, or community functioning for which the clinician is accountable" (p. 140). Wright and Bell (2009) expand on their definition of intervention by suggesting that clinical interventions are actualized only in a *relationship* between the clinician and the family members" (p. 140). Interventions are normally purposeful and conscious and usually involve observable behaviors of the nurse.

Context of a Nursing Intervention

Nursing interventions should focus on the nurse's behavior and the family's response followed by the nurse's response to the family and so forth. We believe that nurse behaviors and client behaviors are contextualized in the nurse-client relationship and are therefore interactional. This differs from nursing diagnoses and nursing outcomes, which focus on client behavior and are not usually interactional in nature (Butcher et al, 2018). An interactional phenomenon occurs whereby the responses of a nurse (interventions) are invited by the responses of clients/family members (outcome) that are, in turn, invited by the responses of a nurse. To focus on only client behaviors or nurse behaviors does not take into account the relationship between nurses and clients. All of our nursing interventions are interactional—that is, not doing to or for the patient but *with* the patient. Nursing interventions are actualized only in a relationship.

However, some nurses do find the classification of nursing interventions to be helpful in providing a language to describe and conceptualize specific treatment efforts (Butcher et al, 2018).

Intent of Nursing Interventions

The intent or aim of any nursing intervention is to effect change, whether to decrease a high temperature of a patient or improve family functioning when caring for a young boy with chronic illness and his family. Therefore, effective nursing interventions are those to which clients and families respond because of the "fit," or meshing between the intervention offered by the nurse and the biopsychosocial-spiritual structure of family members. In relational practice with families, there is no predetermined, standardized intervention to use across a number of families. Rather, the nurse, in collaboration with a specific family, determines what interventions are most useful for a family experiencing a particular illness.

NURSING INTERVENTIONS FOR FAMILIES: A SPECIFIC DISCUSSION

Nurses can intervene with families in numerous ways, depending on the compassion, competence, skills, and even imagination of each nurse and, most importantly, depending on the nurse's relationship with each family (Bell, 2011).

Wright and Leahey (2013) identified factors that contribute to the slower pace of developing nursing interventions with families, which have negatively influenced the implementation of family nursing (Leahey & Harper-Jaques, 2010):

- Lack of appreciation for the interactional aspect of families and illness
- Shortage of nurse educators who are also skilled family clinicians
- Shortage of administrative support for implementation of family nursing
- Minimal ongoing educational support of family interventions in clinical settings

Because interventions related to the family are independent nursing actions for which nurses are accountable, nurse educators and researchers need to name, specify, explore, understand, and test interventions related to the family. There are encouraging signs, with more literature being published not only in nursing journals but a wide variety of multidisciplinary journals. In addition, discussions of family interventions are being presented at conferences worldwide. More nurses are committed to increasing knowledge of family nursing interventions through describing and examining their effectiveness in actual clinical practice and through quantitative and qualitative studies; however, we believe that nurses' contributions must increase in order for family nursing interventions to be implemented in clinical settings. "There is a critical need for more research methods and research evidence about how to best move family nursing knowledge into action" (Duhamel, 2017, p. 461). Nurses in direct clinical contact with families perceive family interventions differently than nurses who predominantly conduct research or engage in theory development. Nurse educators and researchers need to understand more about the challenges, successes, and difficulties of implementing family nursing in practice settings.

KEY CONCEPT DEFINED

Family Nursing Interventions

Actions based on clinical judgment and knowledge that are used when nurses work with families; they focus on changing the cognitive, affective, or behavioral domains of family functioning.

For example, Duhamel, Dupuis, and Wright (2009) implemented a clinical project in which nurses were found to have difficulty integrating the theoretical aspects of family systems nursing into their practice and therefore desired to acquire additional clinical skills. Specifically, the nurses stated their most pressing need was to develop their abilities to deal with relational issues such as conflict between families and health professionals and family-communication problems. However, they frequently labeled families as "demanding" or "complaining," which was perceived as separate from the relational aspect of care. One of the conclusions was that nurses' beliefs about families often led them to label families' responses to illness as being "dysfunctional" or members being in "denial" rather than more benevolent responses such as family members suffering, being under stress, or experiencing anxiety. This project led these nursing educators to further study three methods of training in family systems nursing (FSN) for successful knowledge transfer into practice (Duhamel, et al, 2009). This study called attention to the need for more educational support in the clinical setting to promote utilization of FSN knowledge in addition to the provision of administrative support. These various studies make clear that a circular, interactional process between education, research, and practice needs to be adhered to and respected (Duhamel & Dupuis, 2011).

More recently, Eggenberger and Sanders (2016) conducted a pilot project to examine the influence of educational interventions on nurses' attitudes toward and confidence in providing family care. Findings indicated that educational interventions increased nurses' understanding of family illness experiences and related knowledge and skills (p. 221). Svavarsdottir et al (2015) reinforce the idea of providing meaningful clinical family nursing education to support nurses in applying family systems nursing in clinical practice.

In a participatory action designed study by Duhamel and Talbot (2004), nurses indicated that they gained a better understanding of the illness's impact on the family members' relationships, acquired an appreciation of the importance of active listening, practiced a humanistic and personalized approach that centered on family members' specific concerns and helped to reduce their anxiety, and integrated new family systems nursing interventions into their practice.

Interventions With Families

Notions about reality gleaned from postmodernism and social constructionism are helpful when conceptualizing ideas about interventions. It is unwise to attempt to ascertain what is "really" going on with a particular family or what the "real" problem or suffering is. Rather, nurses should recognize that what is "real" to them as nurses is always a consequence of the nurse's construction of the world. Maturana (1988) presents an intriguing notion of reality by submitting that individuals (living systems) bring forth reality—they do not construct it, and it does not exist independent of them. This concept has implications for nurses' clinical work with families—specifically, what nurses perceive about particular situations with families is influenced by how nurses behave (i.e., their interventions), and how they behave depends on what they perceive. (Refer to Chapter 2 for more understanding of Maturana's biology of cognition.)

Therefore, one way to change the "reality" that family members have constructed is to assist them with developing new ways of interacting in the family. The interventions that we use in this endeavor focus on changing the cognitive, affective, or behavioral domains of family functioning. As family members' perceptions or beliefs about each other and the illness in their family change, so do their behaviors.

Nurses need to keep the element of time in mind with regard to interventions. Interventions are an integral part of family interviewing, spanning engagement to termination. Normally, interventions used during family interviews are influenced by the nurse's and family's experiences of dealing with problems or illnesses or other forms of suffering.

If engagement and assessment have been adequate, the interventions are generally more effective. For example, if a nurse working with a family perpetually addresses certain family members first, the family may disengage, and the opportunity to further intervene may be eliminated. The nurse must possess family interviewing skills and must be sensitive to family function before embarking on specific goal-oriented interventions.

Family nurse clinicians are grounded in the everyday complexities and uniqueness of each family they serve. Although clinicians may benefit from the research literature that offers a description of family responses in health and illness, they are intimately involved in doing intervention and consequently find themselves wanting to know about the specific practices offered to families. We have found it encouraging to learn about the increased examples of intervention programs to assist families.

Family Interactions

There is research being conducted to uncover family interventions with families experiencing physical illness, particularly regarding the usefulness of family interventions that target family interactions and examine the influence of each family member's illness experiences on other family members (Duhamel & Dupuis, 2004; Duhamel & Talbot, 2004; Eg, Frederiksen, Vamosi, & Lorentzen, 2017; Noiseux & Duhamel, 2003; O'Farrell, Murray, & Hotz, 2000). Chesla (2010) reviewed a meta-analysis of randomized control trials of family intervention research and found that family interventions improve health in persons with chronic illness and their family members across the life span. Her results were encouraging in that the review of family intervention studies with adults indicated there were beneficial effects for family member health and for patient mental health. There was also reasonable evidence that a family-centered approach for children with type 1 diabetes was helpful. Nurses were involved in one-quarter to one-third of the research studies that were reviewed.

Home Visits

Crossman, Warfield, Kotelchuck, Hauser-Cram, and Parish (2018) conducted a study to examine the relationship between the importance of home visitation in early intervention and positive family relationships for parenting a child with a developmental disability. Early intervention home visits provided the opportunity to identify mothers who were challenged, thus providing the development of family strength-based partnerships to foster competency and resiliency.

An example of nurses taking the initiative to promote family health with children with attention deficit-hyperactivity disorder (ADHD) is an in-home intervention called Parents and Children Together (PACT; Kendall & Tabacco, 2011). Recognizing that families with children with ADHD have more interpersonal conflict and negativity in their family and social lives, a program was designed to provide both assessment and resources. This is an impressive effort to empower families, particularly mothers, in the daily management of their children.

Therapeutic Conversations

There is an abundant amount of literature discussing the significance and outcomes of therapeutic conversations as intervention (Bell, Moules & Wright, 2009; Gisladottir & Svavarsdottir 2017; Limacher & Wright, 2006; Marklund, Eriksson, Lindh & Saveman, 2018; McLeod & Wright, 2008; Moules, 2009; Ragnarsdóttir & Svavarsdottir, 2014; Robinson & Wright, 1995; Sveinbjarnardottir, Svavarsdottir, & Wright, 2013; Voltelen, Konradsen & Ostergaard, 2016; Wright, 2015). One example is the work of Gisladottir, Treasure, and Svavarsdottir (2017), who evaluated the effectiveness of therapeutic conversation interventions in group and caregiver sessions on the supporting role of caregivers of people with eating disorders using the CFAM and CFIM as theoretical frameworks. Therapeutic conversations as a family intervention with caregivers in both group and private sessions were found to be beneficial.

Psychosocial/Psychoeducational Interventions

Hirschman and Hodgson (2018) conducted a review of the literature on interventions targeting transitions in care for persons living with dementia and their caregivers. Results identified that "successful interventions were those that included five key elements: (a) educating the individual and caregiver about likely transitions in care and ways to delay or avoid the transition; (b) providing timely communication of information among everyone involved, including the individual, caregiver and care team; (c) involving the individual and caregiver in establishing goals of care (person-centered); (d) comprising a strong collaborative interprofessional team; and (e) implementing evidence-based models of practice" (p. s135).

Konradsdottir and Svavarsdottir (2011) conducted a quasi-experimental study of families with adolescents who had diabetes. Following their educational and support intervention with these families utilizing CFAM and CFIM, there was a significant improvement in the parents' coping patterns compared with before the intervention.

Web-Based Interventions

Increasing use of Web-based interventions because of their low cost, flexibility, time requirements, and accessibility for families is revealed in recent literature (Kaltenbaugh et al., 2015; Wasilewski, Stinson & Cameron, 2017). Blanton, Dunbar, and Clark (2018) evaluated a caregiver-focused Web-based intervention to improve stroke survivor physical function and reduce caregiver negative outcomes. Results supported content validity and user satisfaction of the Web-based intervention and identified this as an important beginning step towards testing the efficacy of the intervention in a large clinical trial.

Barbabella et al (2016) conducted a Web-based psychosocial intervention for family caregivers of older adults in three European countries. The findings indicated that the intervention improved family caregivers' awareness, efficacy, and empowerment, which led to better recognition of their own needs and improved efforts for developing and accessing coping resources.

Another innovative intervention program promoting family health is a Web-based asthma education project (Garwick, Seppelt, & Belew, 2011). This program addresses the cultural and literacy backgrounds of families and involved family members in the actual needs assessment and in the development of the Web site.

Family Health Promotion

Efforts to develop and identify intervention strategies for family health promotion are also being made, although little documentation of their effectiveness is evident. We believe this to be due to the fact that researchers are focused on family interventions as treatment rather than as health promotion. Family health promotion is an area of family nursing in which there are tremendous opportunities for the development and testing of family interventions.

Family Responses to Interventions

The previous discussion of interventions in family nursing practice primarily focused on the nurse's behaviors. However, interventions are actualized only in a relationship. Therefore, it is equally important to ascertain the responses of family members to interventions that are offered. Bell and Wright (2007) challenge the predominant belief within "good science" that before intervention research can be designed and conducted, there first must be a thorough understanding of the phenomena (i.e., an in-depth knowledge of what the variables are that mediate families' response to health and illness). They offer an alternate view that in daily nursing practice, nurses encounter families suffering in a variety of clinical settings that require immediate care and intervention. Therefore, family nursing practice as it occurs in the daily life of nurses needs to be described, explored, and evaluated to gain an understanding of what is working in the moment. What are nurses actually doing and saying that is helpful to families in their experience of illness?

Robinson and Wright (1995) identified what nurses do that makes a positive difference to families. They found that families who experienced difficulty managing a member's chronic condition and sought assistance in an outpatient nursing clinic could readily identify interventions that alleviated or eased their suffering. The nursing interventions that made a difference for these families fell within two stages of the therapeutic change process:

- Creating circumstances for change
  - Bringing the family together to engage in new and different conversations
  - Establishing a therapeutic relationship between the nurse and family, particularly in the areas of providing comfort and demonstrating trust
- Moving beyond and overcoming problems
  - Inviting meaningful conversation
  - Noticing and distinguishing family and individual strengths and resources
  - Paying careful attention to and exploring concerns
  - Putting illness problems in their place

Families are increasingly expressing the importance of having opportunities to examine with nurses the influence of each family member's illness experiences on other family members, noting that these interventions are significant for them (Benzein, Olin & Persson, 2015; Eggenberger & Sanders, 2016; O'Farrell, Murray, & Hotz, 2000; Svavardottir et al, 2015). Literature unpacking the interventions of therapeutic conversations (Benzies,

2016; Ostlund, Backstrom, Saveman, Lindh, & Sundin, 2016), commendations (Benzies, 2016; Houger Limacher & Wright, 2003, 2006), and therapeutic letters (Moules, 2002, 2003, 2009) have enhanced our understanding of how, when, and why these interventions are healing for families. Duhamel and Talbot (2004) also identify that family members described the "humanistic attitude of the nurse, constructing a genogram, interventive questioning, offering educational information, normalization, and exploring the illness experience in the presence of other family members" as the most useful interventions (p. 21).

INDICATIONS AND CONTRAINDICATIONS FOR FAMILY INTERVENTIONS

After a family assessment, a nurse must decide whether to intervene with a family. Considerations should include the family's level of functioning, the nurse's own skill level, and the resources available. Indications for family interventions are described in Box 1-3.

After the nurse and family have decided that intervention is indicated, they must then collaboratively decide on the duration and intensity of the family sessions. If sessions occur too frequently, the family may have insufficient time to recalibrate and process the change. The optimal number of days, weeks, or months between sessions is difficult to state categorically. We recommend that nurses ask family members when they would like to have another meeting, particularly if the family meetings are occurring on an outpatient basis. Families are much better judges than nurses of how frequently they need to be seen to resolve a particular problem.

Furthermore, nurses should be aware that the duration and intensity of sessions depend on the context in which the family is seen. For example, if a hospital nurse is working with a family, the nurse may have the opportunity for only one or two meetings before the patient is discharged, whereas a community health nurse may be able to schedule a series of meetings. The context in which the nurse encounters a family commonly dictates the frequency and number of family meetings. Additionally, whether a nurse has 1 or 10 meetings with a family for assessment or intervention, there are important considerations for terminating with a family. An in-depth discussion of termination is provided in Chapter 12.

Family intervention is not always required, and contraindications for family intervention exist. These contraindications are generally evident to the nurse immediately after the family assessment. Sometimes during the course of intervention, however, families indicate a desire to stop treatment (see Chapter 12). Box 1-4 lists possible contraindications for family interventions.

Nurses working with patients and families in a variety of health-care settings need to have a good understanding of when family involvement

Box 1-3 Indications for Family Interventions

A family member presents with an illness that has an obvious detrimental impact on other family members.

- A grandfather's Alzheimer disease may cause his grandchildren to be afraid of him.
- A young child's cyberbullying behavior may be related to his mother's deterioration from multiple sclerosis.

A family member contributes to another family member's symptoms or problems.

- Lack of visitation from adult children exacerbates physical or psychological symptoms in an elderly parent.
- One family member's improvement leads to symptoms or deterioration in another family member.
- Decreased asthma symptoms in one child correlate with increased abdominal pain in a sibling.

A child or an adolescent develops an emotional, behavioral, or physical problem in the context of a family member's illness.

- An adolescent with diabetes suddenly requests that his mother administer his daily insulin injections even though he has been injecting himself for the past 6 months.

Illness is first diagnosed in a family member.

- If family members have no previous knowledge of or experience with a particular illness, they require information and may also require reassurance and support.

A family member's condition deteriorates markedly.

- Whenever deterioration occurs, family patterns may need restructuring, and intervention is indicated.

A chronically ill family member moves from a hospital or rehabilitation center back into the community.

- A young adult returns home after being hospitalized for 6 months at a drug rehabilitation center.

An important individual or family developmental milestone is missed or delayed.

- An adolescent is unable to move out of the home at the anticipated time.

A chronically ill patient dies.

- Although the patient's death may be a relief, the family might feel a tremendous void when the caregiving role is lost.

Box 1-4 Contraindications for Family Interventions

- All family members state that they do not wish to pursue family meetings or treatment even though it is recommended.
- Family members state that they agree with the recommendation for family meetings or treatment but would prefer to work with another professional.

---

is indicated and when it is contraindicated. Not only for their own benefit but also for each family's benefit, nurses should distinguish between family assessment and family intervention. Families are often willing to come for an assessment when they can see the nurse face-to-face and make their own assessment of the nurse's competence. When a nurse does a careful, credible assessment, the nurse has an easier time initiating family interventions.

CRITICAL THINKING QUESTIONS

1. In your clinical practice, why would it be important for you to use the CFAM/CFIM?
2. Consider your own clinical practice:
   a. What family nursing interventions do you currently use? How do you know if they are effective?
   b. What family nursing interventions could you implement in your practice, and how would you know if they were effective?

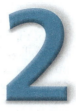
Theoretical Foundations of the Calgary Family Assessment and Intervention Models

Learning Objectives

- Describe the theoretical foundations and worldviews that inform the Calgary Family Assessment Model (CFAM).
- Summarize the theoretical foundations and worldviews that inform the Calgary Family Intervention Model (CFIM).
- Discuss the main concepts of postmodernism, systems theory, cybernetics, communication theory, change theory, and the biology of cognition.

Key Concepts

Biology of cognition	Cybernetics	Symmetry and complementarity
Change theory	Pluralism	Systems theory
Communication theory	Postmodernism	

M odels are useful ways to bring clusters of ideas, notions, and concepts into awareness. However, models cannot stand alone. For example, nursing practice models are built on a foundation of many worldviews, theories, beliefs, premises, and assumptions. These models are more comprehensible and meaningful if the underlying theories, assumptions, and premises are explained. Therefore, to comprehend and use the Calgary Family Assessment Model (CFAM) (see Chapter 3) and the Calgary Family Intervention Model (CFIM) (see Chapter 4) in nursing practice with individuals, couples, and families, nurses must understand the theoretical assumptions underlying these models.

Family structures, functions, and processes are complex, and no single theory, model, or conceptual framework sufficiently describes the relationships between them. This complexity requires nurses to have a broad understanding of a variety of theoretical perspectives to guide their assessments and interventions with families. Therefore, no single theoretical perspective is more correct than another (Kaakinen & Hanson, 2014, p. 67). We believe no one overall model or theory of family nursing exists and concur with Kaakinen and Hanson.

The six theoretical foundations and worldviews that inform the CFAM and CFIM are as follows:

- Postmodernism
- Systems theory
- Cybernetics
- Communication theory
- Change theory
- Biology of cognition

Each theory or worldview and some of its distinguishing concepts are presented in this chapter and related to clinical practice with individuals, couples, and families.

POSTMODERNISM

Humans seem to delight in rethinking, reexamining, reconstructing, and deconstructing their history and culture. One popular way to do this is through the lens of postmodernism. Postmodernism is a philosophical movement that emphasizes "multiplicity: multiple views, multiple possibilities, and multiple lives" (Dickerson, 2010, p. 354). Anything before the present "enlightened" worldview is considered modernist and therefore less desirable to those who rigidly hold postmodernist beliefs. Consequently, the influence of the ideas, conditions, and beliefs of postmodernism have been demonstrated in art, literature, architecture, science, culture, religion, philosophy, and, more recently, in family therapy and nursing, particularly family nursing (Becvar & Becvar, 2003; Glazer, 2001; Kermode & Brown, 1996; Moules, 2000; Salladay, 2011; Tapp & Wright, 1996; Watson, 1999). Within the context of family, postmodern approaches endeavor to create collaborative relationships and joint exploration with clients in which partnerships are formed in clinical practice (Anderson, 2012).

KEY CONCEPT DEFINED

Postmodernism

A philosophical movement that emphasizes multiplicity: multiple views, multiple possibilities, and multiple lives; one of the theoretical foundations that informs the Calgary Family Assessment Model (CFAM).

We, too, have been influenced by and have embraced many of the notions of postmodernism. These ideas have proved useful in our clinical nursing practice with families. However, we do not wish to imply that we have been able to successfully distance ourselves from all modernist ideas, nor would we want to. We concur with Glazer (2001), who criticizes the postmodern movement for abandoning the biological underpinnings of nursing. We cannot deny our history and culture and how they have influenced who we were and are. Therefore, we acknowledge the previous and continuing influences of both modernist and postmodernist paradigms on our lives and our practice of relational family nursing.

The following two concepts about postmodernism will be discussed:

- Pluralism is a key focus of postmodernism.
- Postmodernism is a debate about knowledge.

CONCEPT 1

Pluralism is a key focus of postmodernism.

Postmodernism offers the end of a single worldview, a resistance to single explanations, and a respect for difference. One of the major notions of postmodern thinking is the idea of *pluralism,* or a belief in multiplicity. Pluralism can be defined as a theory that there is more than one or more than two kinds of ultimate realities, a theory that reality is composed of a plurality of entities ("Pluralism," 2018). In essence, there are as many ways to understand and experience the world as there are people who experience it (Moules, 2000; Watson, 1999; Wright & Bell, 2009). In family nursing practice, this idea becomes operational by recognizing that there are as many ways to understand and experience illness as there are families experiencing it. In an ethical and relational family nursing practice, it becomes operational by acknowledging the multiplicity of cultural, ethnic, and religious beliefs and their influences on various complex family structures.

KEY CONCEPT DEFINED

Pluralism

A theory that there is more than one or more than two kinds of ultimate realities, that reality is composed of a plurality of entities.

CONCEPT 2

Postmodernism is a debate about knowledge.

Postmodernism is partly a reaction to the modernist claim that knowledge emerges primarily from science and technology (Glazer, 2001). The belief that progressive technology necessarily leads to a better world has become open to reexamination, questioning, and doubt (Tapp & Wright, 1996). Therefore, an intense critique is being made of the grand belief systems that have formed the foundation of many scientific, religious, and political movements and institutions. As they are questioned, opportunities arise to deconstruct or uncover certain beliefs and practices that are taken for granted, to hear voices of marginalized groups, and to value knowledge from a variety of domains heretofore not legitimized (Tapp & Wright, 1996; Watson, 1999).

In encounters with families experiencing illness, much more emphasis is now given to the illness narratives and experiences of family members within their particular cultural context rather than to medical narratives. Honoring the voices of families about their illness narratives has profound implications for nursing practice with families. It invites collaboration and consultation between nurses and families to honor the knowledge and expertise of both nurses and family members. These practices are the cornerstone of relational nursing. Inviting the illness narratives of families also enhances the possibilities for healing as their stories are heard, understood, and witnessed.

Some offshoots of postmodernism include constructivism, social constructivism, and the biology of cognition (also called *bring forthism*) (Bell & Wright, 2011; Maturana & Varela, 1992; Moules, 2000; Wright & Bell, 2009). The biology of cognition is the offshoot we have found most useful in our clinical work, and we discuss it in more detail later in this chapter.

The postmodernist movement has been strongly critiqued by feminists, who claim that women's voices continue to be diminished or ignored because of patriarchy and oppression (Kermode & Brown, 1996). This has not been our experience in working with families. Evidence for the importance of acknowledging women's voices and their illness burden in family systems nursing practice can be found in Robinson's 1998 study. She discovered that women in families experiencing chronic illness are vulnerable to the demands of illness's responsibility, work, and problems. As a more equitable balance of illness demands was sought by the nurse and family members, the women in this study found better lives for themselves and were able to live beyond illness and the problems they experienced. They also took on new views of their situations and thus behaved differently. More recently, Robinson's 2017 study focusing on the healing processes of families living well with chronic illness builds on her previous work and further emphasizes the importance of being sensitive to the potential vulnerability of women caregivers. These studies' recognition of women's voices as distinct and different from a collective "family voice" seems in keeping with the best that the postmodernist movement has to offer.

> **KEY CONCEPT DEFINED**
>
> ## Biology of Cognition
>
> An emerging science that regards natural cognition as a biological function in which humans bring forth different views to their understanding of events and experiences in their lives; one of the theoretical foundations that informs the Calgary Family Assessment Model (CFAM).

SYSTEMS THEORY

For a number of years, health professionals have applied general systems theory, introduced orally in the 1930s by von Bertalanffy, and later published after World War II in various publications, to their understanding of families. In addition to the original writings on systems theory by von Bertalanffy (1968, 1972, 1974), numerous articles and chapters in books have been written on this subject and its concepts. The proliferation of systems information is also evident within nursing literature (Johnson, 1990; Neuman & Fawcett, 2011; Smith & Parker, 2015). We agree with Kaakinen and Hanson (2014) in their belief that "family systems theory has been the most influential of all the family social science frameworks" (p. 76).

> **KEY CONCEPT DEFINED**
>
> ## Systems Theory
>
> A theoretical approach to the study of systems with the goal of discovering patterns and changing the conceptual focus from parts to wholes; one of the theoretical foundations that informs the Calgary Family Assessment Model (CFAM).

One of the most useful analogies that highlights systems concepts as applied to families is offered by Allmond, Buckman, and Gofman (1979). They suggest that, when thinking of the family as a system, it is useful to compare it to a mobile:

> Visualize a mobile with four or five pieces suspended from the ceiling, gently moving in the air. The whole is in balance, steady yet moving. Some pieces are moving rapidly; others are almost stationary. Some are heavier and appear to carry more weight in the ultimate direction of the mobile's movement; others seem to go along for the ride. A breeze catching only one segment of the mobile immediately influences movement of every piece, some more than others, and the pace picks up with some pieces unbalancing themselves and moving chaotically about for a time. Gradually the whole exerts its influence in the errant part(s) and balance is reestablished but not before a decided change in direction of the whole may have taken place. You will also notice

the changeability regarding closeness and distance among pieces, the impact of actual contact one with another, and the importance of vertical hierarchy. Coalitions of movement may be observed between two pieces. Or one piece may persistently appear isolated from the others; yet its position of isolation is essential to the balancing of the entire system. (Allmond et al, 1979, p. 16)

Keeping the analogy of the mobile in mind, some of the most useful concepts of systems theory, which have frequent application in clinical practice with families, are highlighted in the following paragraphs. These systems concepts provide a theoretical foundation for understanding the family as a system. A system can be defined as a "set of things working together as parts of mechanisms or an interconnecting network; a complex whole" ("System," 2018). When this definition is applied to families, it allows us to view the family as a unit and thus focus on observing the interaction among family members and between the family and the illness or problem rather than studying family members individually. However, remember that each family member is both a subsystem and a system in his or her own right. An individual system is both a part and a whole, as is a family.

The following five concepts about systems theory will be discussed:

- A family system is part of a larger suprasystem and is composed of many subsystems.
- The family as a whole is greater than the sum of its parts.
- A change in one family member affects all family members.
- The family is able to create a balance between change and stability.
- Family members' behaviors are best understood from a view of circular rather than linear causality.

CONCEPT 1

A family system is part of a larger suprasystem and is composed of many subsystems.

The concept of hierarchy of systems is very useful when applied to families. It is especially helpful for nurses struggling with how to conceptualize complex family situations. A family is composed of many subsystems, such as parent-child, marital, and sibling subsystems. These subsystems are also composed of subsystems of individuals. Individuals are extremely complex systems composed of various subsystems, some of which are physical (e.g., the cardiovascular and reproductive systems) or psychological (e.g., cognitive, affective, and behavioral systems). At the same time, the family is just one unit nested in larger suprasystems, such as neighborhoods, organizations, or religious communities. Drawing a large circle and placing elements, parts, or variables inside the circle can be a helpful way to visualize a system. Inside the circle, lines can be drawn among the component parts to represent relationships between elements. Outside the circle is the larger context, where all other factors impinging on the system can be placed. Thus, a nurse can draw a circle to visualize a family and then place the individual family members within it (Figure 2-1).

Systems are arbitrarily defined by their boundaries, which aid in specifying what is inside or outside the system. Normally, boundaries associated with living systems are physical in nature, such as the number of people in a family. It is also possible to construct a boundary and therefore create a system around ideas, beliefs, expectations, or roles. For example, a person may have a system of multiple roles, such as daughter, partner, colleague, wife, sister, nurse, mother, and grandmother. However, from time to time, it may be useful to draw an imaginary boundary and create, for example, a system of parental beliefs about the use of nonmedical drugs by their children.

When working with families, nurses should initially consider the following:

- Who is in this family system?
- What are some of the important subsystems?
- What are some of the significant suprasystems to which the family belongs?

In addition, within family systems and their subsystems, nurses should assess the permeability of the boundaries (see Chapters 3 and 13 for further understanding and examples about boundaries when conducting a family assessment). In family systems, the boundaries must be both permeable and limiting. If the family boundary is too permeable, the system loses identity and integrity (e.g., members may be too open to input from the outside

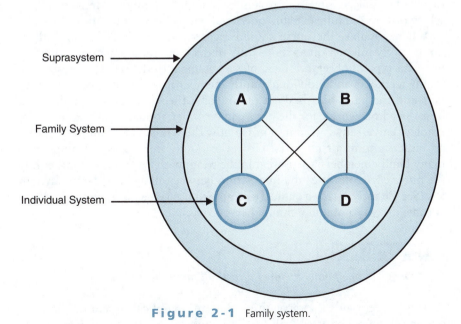

Figure 2-1 Family system.

environment, such as extended family, friends, or health professionals) and therefore does not allow the family to use its own resources in decision making. However, if the boundary is too closed or impermeable, necessary interaction with the larger world is shut off (e.g., an immigrant family that relocates to Canada or the United States may inadvertently remain closed initially because of great differences in language and culture). With increased use of mobile phones; the Internet; personal digital assistants; e-mail; e-Books; blogs; Skype; chat rooms; and social networking sites such as Facebook, Twitter, and YouTube, the permeability of boundaries has changed dramatically in the last decade.

Hierarchy of systems and the boundaries that create systems are useful concepts to apply when working with and attempting to conceptualize the uniqueness of each particular family. Among certain ethnic or cultural groups, for example, honoring hierarchies and boundaries is essential.

CONCEPT 2

The family as a whole is greater than the sum of its parts.

When applied to families, this concept of systems theory emphasizes that the family's "wholeness" is more than simply the addition of each family member. It also emphasizes that individuals are best understood within their larger context, which is normally the family. To study individual family members separately does not equate to studying the family as a unit. By studying the whole family, it is possible to observe interactions among family members, which often more fully explain individual family member functioning.

When possible, the nurse should meet with the whole family and observe family interaction to more fully understand family member functioning. This type of observation enables assessment of the relationships among family members and individual family member functioning. You cannot understand the parts of a body, a family, or a theory unless you understand how the whole works, for the parts can be understood only in relation to the whole. Conversely, you cannot grasp how the whole works unless you have an understanding of its parts. However, family nursing is not about how many family members are present in the room with the nurse but rather how the nurse conceptualizes the interaction between illness and family dynamics. (See Chapter 10 for a clinical example of interviewing an individual with chronic illness to obtain a family perspective.)

CONCEPT 3

A change in one family member affects all family members.

This concept aids the recognition that any significant event or change in one family member affects all family members to varying degrees, as was illustrated in the analogy of the mobile. It can be most useful to nurses considering the impact of illness on families.

> *Example:* The father of a family experienced a myocardial infarction. This event affected all family members and various family relationships. The father and mother were unable to continue their joint participation in sports, and the mother increased her employment from part-time to full-time to supplement the substantially reduced income during the father's convalescence. The eldest daughter, who had been isolated from the family since her marriage, began visiting her father more often. The youngest daughter provided emotional support and so became closer to her mother. Thus, all family members were affected, and the organization and functioning of the family changed.

This concept can also be used to understand how a nurse can change the family system by implementing family interventions—that is, if one family member changes, other family members cannot respond as they previously did because the individual family member now behaves differently (see Chapter 13 for additional examples).

CONCEPT 4

The family is able to create a balance between change and stability.

Over the past years, there has been a shift away from the belief that families tend toward maintaining equilibrium. Instead, the popular belief now is that families are really in constant states of flux and are always changing. The pendulum has now swung to the other end of the continuum. However, von Bertalanffy (1968) warned many years ago to avoid this polarized view of families. He suggested that systems, in this case family systems, can achieve balance among the forces operating within them and on them and that change and stability can coexist in living systems (see the "Change Theory" section later in this chapter).

When change occurs in a family, however, the disturbance can cause a shift to a new position of balance. The family reorganizes in a way that is different from any previous organization. For example, if a family member is diagnosed with a long-term chronic illness, such as multiple sclerosis, the entire family must reorganize itself in ways that are totally different from the ways it was organized before the diagnosis. The balance between change and stability constantly shifts during periods of illness remission and exacerbation; however, a balance between change and stability is most common.

The concept of change and stability coexisting is perhaps one of the most difficult concepts of systems theory for nurses to understand. This is partly because, in actual clinical practice, families frequently present themselves as being either in rigid equilibrium or in constant change rather than manifesting an observable balance between the two. However, the more experienced one becomes in family nursing, the greater appreciation one has for the complexity of families. In many cases, when families are "stuck" or experiencing severe difficulties, they are polarized in maintaining rigid equilibrium or are in a phase of too much change. Eventually, the family needs to find ways to obtain a more equal balance between the phenomena of stability and change. In our own practice, we have noticed how military families and other families directly affected by terrorism and war have developed creative solutions to cope with the fluctuations of stability and change.

CONCEPT 5

Family members' behaviors are best understood from a view of circular rather than linear causality.

One method of dealing with the massive amounts of data presented in a family interview is to observe for patterns. Tomm (1981) offers a useful discussion of the differences between linear and circular patterns:

> One major difference between linear and circular patterns lies in the overall structure of the connections between elements of the pattern. Linear patterns are limited to sequences (e.g., A → B → C) whereas circular patterns form a closed loop and are recursive (e.g., A → B → C → A → ... or A → B, B → C, C → A). A less obvious but more significant difference lies in the relative importance usually given to time and meaning when making the connections or links in the pattern. Linearity is heavily rooted in a framework of a continuous progression of time ... Circularity ... is more heavily dependent on a framework of reciprocal relationships based on meaning. (p. 85)

Linear causality, defined as a relationship in which one event causes another, can serve as a useful and helpful function for individuals and families. For example, when the clock strikes 6:00, a family routinely eats supper. This is an example of linear causality because event A (the clock striking 6:00) is seen as the cause of event B (the eating of supper), or A → B, whereas event B does not affect event A.

However, circular causality occurs when event B does affect event A. For example, if a husband takes an interest in his wife's ostomy care (event A) and the wife responds by explaining the daily procedures (event B), then it is likely to result in the husband continuing to take an interest in and offering support regarding his wife's ostomy care and his wife continuing to feel supported; thus, the cycle continues (A → B → A). Each individual's behavior has an effect on and influences the other individual's behavior. A method for diagramming these very useful circular interactional patterns is discussed in Chapter 3.

The application of these concepts in clinical practice affects the nurse's style of questioning during a family interview (Wright & Leahey, 2013).

Linear questions explore descriptive characteristics:

"Is the father fearful of another heart attack?"

Circular questions explore interactional characteristics, such as the following:

Difference questions:
   "Who is most worried about Sunil having another heart attack?"
Behavioral effect questions:
   "What do you do, Amal, when your wife's pain becomes unbearable for you?"
Hypothetical or future-oriented questions:
   "What might you do in the future to prevent your elderly father from falling?"
Triadic questions:
   "When your dad shows support to your sister Manisha, how does your mom feel?"

Bateson (1979) offers the idea that "information consists of differences that make a difference" (p. 99). Tomm (1981) connects the idea of "differences" to relationships:

Differences between perceptions, objects, events, ideas, etc. are regarded as the basic source of all information and consequent knowledge. On closer examination, one can see that such relationships are always reciprocal or circular. If she is shorter than he, then he is taller than she. If she is dominant, then he is submissive. If one member of the family is defined as being bad, then the others are being defined as being good. Even at a very simple level, a circular orientation allows implicit information to become more explicit and offers alternative points of view. A linear orientation on the other hand is narrow and restrictive and tends to mask important data. (p. 93)

Various types of assessment and interventive questions that could be asked during a family interview are highlighted in Chapters 3, 4, and 6 through 10.

With regard to family member interaction, the assumption is made that each person contributes to adaptive and maladaptive interaction. For example, in geriatric health-care facilities, it is common for elderly parents to complain that their adult children do not visit enough and therefore withdraw; on the other hand, the adult children complain that their elderly parents constantly nag them when they visit (see Chapter 10 for a clinical example). Each family member is "correct" in the perception of the other, but neither recognizes how his or her own behavior influences the behavior of the other family member.

Normally, families and their individual members need help to move from a linear perspective of their situation to a more interactional, reciprocal, and systemic view. This shift is possible only if the nurse avoids linear thinking when attempting to understand family dynamics.

The five concepts discussed in this section are by no means inclusive of all systems concepts, but they reflect those that are deemed most significant and important to the theoretical foundation for working with families.

CYBERNETICS

Cybernetics is the science of communication and control theory. The term *cybernetics* was originally coined by the mathematician Norbert Weiner. It is important to differentiate between general systems theory and cybernetics. We do not use the terms synonymously, although some people regard each as a branch of the other. Systems theory is primarily concerned with changing the conceptual focus from parts to wholes, whereas cybernetics is concerned with changing focus from substance to form.

KEY CONCEPT DEFINED

Cybernetics

The science of communication and control theory; one of the theoretical foundations that informs the Calgary Family Assessment Model (CFAM).

The following two concepts about cybernetics will be discussed:

- Family systems possess self-regulating ability.
- Feedback processes can simultaneously occur at several systems levels with families.

CONCEPT 1

Family systems possess self-regulating ability.

Interpersonal systems, particularly family systems, "may be viewed as feedback loops, since the behavior of each person affects and is affected by the behavior of each other person" (Watzlawick, Beavin, & Jackson, 1967, p. 31). We have found this idea to be very useful in family work because recognizing that each family member's behavior affects other family members and, in turn, that each person is affected by other family members' behavior removes any tendency or impulse a nurse may have to blame one person in a family for the difficulties that an entire family is facing. For any substantial change to occur in a relationship, the regulatory limits must be adjusted so that a new range of behaviors is possible or an entirely new pattern can emerge (transformation). Tomm (1980) offers a useful method of applying cybernetic regulatory concepts to actual clinical interviewing. His method of diagramming circular patterns of communication is discussed in Chapter 3.

CONCEPT 2

Feedback processes can simultaneously occur at several systems levels with families.

Initially, the application of cybernetic concepts in family work began by observations of simple phenomena (e.g., a wife criticizes, and the husband withdraws); this is generally referred to as *simple cybernetics*. However, as cyberneticians began examining more complex orders of phenomena, they recognized different orders of feedback (such as feedback of feedback and change of change). Maturana and Varela (1980) suggest a higher-order cybernetics that links the organization of living process and cognition.

Therefore, the simple feedback phenomenon observed in the interactional pattern of criticizing wife—withdrawing husband may also be understood to be part of a larger feedback loop involving the couple's relationship to their families of origin, which may recalibrate the lower-order loop of the couple's interaction. This concept can be especially helpful to nurses working with complex family situations. Thus, cybernetics of cybernetics moves into a larger context that includes both the observer and the observed.

COMMUNICATION THEORY

The study of communication focuses on how individuals interact with one another. Within families, the function of communication is to assist family members in clarifying family rules regarding behavior, to help them learn about their environment, to explicate how conflict is resolved, to nurture and develop self-esteem for all members, and to model expressions of feeling states constructively within the family as a unit. One of the most significant contributions to the understanding of interpersonal processes is the classic book *Pragmatics of Human Communication* (1967) by Watzlawick, Beavin, and Jackson. The concepts presented here are primarily drawn from this important book on communication and have been updated by the research studies of Dr. Janet Beavin Bavelas conducted in 1992.

KEY CONCEPT DEFINED

Communication Theory

The branch of knowledge dealing with the principles and methods by which information is conveyed; one of the theoretical foundations that informs the Calgary Family Assessment Model (CFAM).

The following four concepts about communication theory will be discussed:

- All nonverbal communication is meaningful.
- All communication has two major channels for transmission: digital and analog.
- A dyadic relationship has varying degrees of symmetry and complementarity.
- All communication has two levels: content and relationship.

KEY CONCEPT DEFINED

Symmetry and Complementarity

A symmetrical relationship is one between two people who behave as if they have equal status. A complementary relationship consists of one individual giving and the other receiving.

CONCEPT 1

All nonverbal communication is meaningful.

This concept helps us to realize that there is no such thing as not communicating because all nonverbal communication by a person carries a message in the presence of another (Watzlawick, Beavin, & Jackson, 1967). In personal communications and in her 1992 publication, Dr. Beavin Bavelas states that she now distinguishes between nonverbal behavior (NVB) and nonverbal communication (NVC). NVC is viewed as a subset of NVB. NVB involves an "inference-making observer," whereas NVC involves a "communicating person" (encoder). In the original text by Watzlawick, Beavin, and Jackson, the concept was presented that all NVB is meaningful.

A significant component of this concept is context. Behavior is relevant and meaningful only when the immediate context is considered.

> *Example:* A mother complains to a community health nurse (CHN) that she has been experiencing insomnia for 2 months and finds herself irritable because of the prolonged sleep deprivation. The mother's behavior must be understood in her immediate context, and on further exploration, the nurse discovers that this mother has a child on an apnea monitor and that the father sleeps soundly. Also, the family apartment is close to a noisy subway station. With this additional context information, the mother's insomnia can be more fully understood and treated by the CHN.

CONCEPT 2

All communication has two major channels for transmission: digital and analog.

Digital communication is commonly referred to as *verbal communication*. It consists of the actual content of the message, or the brute facts. Analogical communication consists not only of the usual types of NVC, such as body posture, facial expression, and tone, but also of music, poetry, and painting.

> *Example:* A man might proudly say, "I lost 15 pounds this past month," or a 10-year-old girl might say, "I can now give myself my own insulin." However, when the analogical communication is also taken into account, the meaning of these statements may change dramatically. A man who is obese and proudly states that he lost 15 pounds in a month sends a more positive message, both digitally and analogically, than a man who is emaciated and states that he lost 15 pounds.

When discrepancies exist between analogical and digital communication, then the analogical message is considered more pertinent to the nurse's observing eye.

> *Example:* A teenager who has been placed in a cumbersome cast for a fractured femur might state, "It doesn't bother me," but her eyes are filled with tears. In this situation, the nurse must recognize the importance of the analogical message. To the teenager's boyfriend, the digital communication may be the most relevant. He may not perceive the significance of the analogical communication.

More suggestions for operationalizing this concept are included in the CFAM in Chapter 3.

CONCEPT 3

A dyadic relationship has varying degrees of symmetry and complementarity.

The terms *symmetry* and *complementarity* are useful in identifying typical family interaction patterns. Jackson (1973) defined these terms:

A complementary relationship consists of one individual giving and the other receiving. In a complementary relationship, the two people are of unequal status in the sense that one appears to be in the superior position, meaning that he initiates action and the other appears to follow that action. Thus the two individuals fit together or complement each other. The most obvious and basic complementary relationship would be the mother and infant. A symmetrical relationship is one between two people who behave as if they have equal status. Each person exhibits the right to initiate action, criticize the other, offer advice and so on. This type of relationship tends to become competitive; if one person mentions that he has succeeded in some endeavor, the other person mentions that he has succeeded in an equally important endeavor. The individuals in such a relationship emphasize their equality or their symmetry with each other. The most obvious symmetrical relationship is a pre-adolescent peer relationship. (p. 189)

Both complementary and symmetrical relationships are appropriate and healthy in certain situations. In family relationships, predominance of either complementary or symmetrical behavior usually results in problems. However, some cultural groups may prefer one style over another. Couples need to balance symmetry and complementarity in their various experiences. Parent-child relationships, however, typically gradually shift from a predominantly complementary relationship to a more symmetrical, egalitarian relationship as the child moves into the teenage and young adult years.

CONCEPT 4

All communication has two levels: content and relationship.

Communication consists of what is being said (content) and information that defines the nature of the relationship between those interacting.

> *Example:* The following statements are similar in content, but each implies a very different relationship:
>
> - A father might say to his son, *"Come over here, son. I want to tell you something."*
>   - This statement could be viewed as part of a loving relationship.
> - A father might say to his son, *"Get over here. I've got something to tell you!"*
>   - This statement implies a conflictual relationship.

In this instance, it is the tone of the content that gives evidence to a particular kind of relationship. Therefore, "family communication not only reveals a message about 'who is saying what and when,' it also conveys a message about the structure and functions of family relationships in relation to the power base, decision-making processes, affection, trust, and coalitions" (Crawford & Tarko, 2004, p. 162).

CHANGE THEORY

The process of change is a fascinating phenomenon, and researchers and clinicians have a variety of ideas about what constitutes change in family systems and how it occurs. In the discussion of change theory that follows, the most profound and salient points from an extensive review of the literature are synthesized and presented along with our own beliefs about change and the conditions that affect the change process.

KEY CONCEPT DEFINED

Change Theory

A comprehensive description or illustration of how and why a desired change is expected to happen in a desired context; one of the theoretical foundations that informs the Calgary Family Assessment Model (CFAM).

Systems of relationships appear to possess a tendency toward progressive change. However, a French proverb states, "The more something changes, the more it remains the same." This paradox beautifully highlights the dilemma frequently faced in working with families. The nurse must learn to accept the challenge of the paradoxical relationship between persistence (stability) and change. Maturana (1978) explains the recursiveness of change and stability in this way: Change is an alteration in the family's structure that occurs as compensation for perturbations and has the purpose of maintaining structure and stability. Change itself is experienced as a perturbation to the system, so change generates further change and stability. A change in state is exhibited as behavior; therefore, differences in family interactional patterns must be explored. Changes in behavior may or may not be accompanied by insight. However, "the most profound and sustaining change will be that which occurs within the family's belief system (cognition)" (Bell & Wright, 2011; Wright & Bell, 2009).

Watzlawick, Weakland, and Fisch (1974) were the first to suggest that persistence and change must be considered together despite their opposing natures. These researchers offer a widely accepted notion of change and suggest that two different types or levels of change exist: first-order change and second-order change.

First-Order Change

- Change occurs within a given system that remains unchanged itself.
- The system itself remains unchanged, but its elements or parts undergo some type of change.
- It is a change in quantity, not quality.

- It involves using the same problem-solving strategies over and over again; each new problem is approached mechanically. If a solution to the problem is difficult to find, more old strategies are used and are usually more vigorously applied.

  > *Example:* Learning of a new behavioral strategy to deal with a child's excessive computer use. A parent who formerly disciplined his child by restricting the child's access to the computer is said to have undergone first-order change when he then limits the child's spending money.

Second-Order Change

- It changes the system—thus, a "change of change."
- For second-order change to occur, actual changes in the rules governing the system must occur, and therefore the system is structurally transformed.
- It is often in the nature of a discontinuity or jump and can be sudden and radical.
- At other times, it occurs in a logical sequence, with the person almost seemingly unaware of the change until it is noted by others.
- It represents a quantum jump in the system to a different level of functioning. Second-order change can be said to occur.

  > *Example:* A family now spends more time together and is able to raise conflictual issues with one another as a result of resolving their teenager's refusal to eat with the family.

Watzlawick, Weakland, and Fisch (1974) also refer to the most obvious type of change, spontaneous change. In spontaneous change, problem resolution occurs in daily living without the input of professionals or sophisticated theories.

  > *Example:*
  > - An anorexic young woman suddenly and apparently spontaneously begins to eat regularly after 2 years of not doing so.
  > - A man suffering from shingles (herpes zoster) reports that his chronic pain disappeared overnight.

Bateson (1979) offers a most thought-provoking statement with regard to change when he proposes that people are almost always unaware of changes. He suggests that changes in social interactions and in the environment are dramatically and constantly occurring but that people become accustomed to the "new state of affairs before our senses can tell us that it is new" (p. 98). Bateson also offers the idea that, with regard to the perception of change, the mind can receive only news of difference. Therefore, as

Bateson states, change can be observed as "difference which occurs across time" (p. 452). These ideas concur with those of Maturana and Varela (1992), who offer the idea that change occurs in humans from moment to moment. This change is either triggered by interactions or perturbations from the environment in which the system (family member) exists or is a result of the system's (family member's) own internal dynamics.

Our own view of change in family work is a combination of the work of the authors previously discussed and insights from our clinical experience in working with families. We believe the following:

- Change is constantly evolving in families.
- People are frequently unaware of change.
- Continuous or spontaneous change occurs with everyday living and progression through individual and family stages of development.
- Change may or may not occur with professional input.

Major transformations of an entire family system can occur and can be precipitated by major life events, such as the following:

- Serious illness
- Disability
- Divorce
- Unemployment
- Addictions
- Terrorism
- Displacement from home as a result of natural and man-made disasters: terrorism, war, floods, hurricanes, or tsunamis
- Death of a family member
- Interventions offered by nurses

Change within a family can occur within the cognitive, affective, or behavioral domains, but change in any one domain impacts the other domains. Therefore, family-nursing interventions can be aimed at any domain or all three domains. Interventions are discussed further in Chapter 4, in which the CFIM is presented. We believe that directly correlating interventions with resulting changes is impossible; therefore, predicting outcomes or the types of change that will occur within families is also impossible.

An important role for nurses (operating from a systems perspective) is to carefully observe the connections between systems. To effect change within the original system (the individual), it is necessary to intervene at a higher systems level or at the metalevel (the family system [see Figure 2-1]). In other words, if nurses wish to effect change within family systems, they need to be able to maintain a metaposition to each family. They must simultaneously conceptualize both the family system interactions and their own interactions with the family. However, if a problem arises between a nurse and a family, this problem must be resolved at a higher level than the nurse-family system, preferably by a supervisor, who can examine the problem from a higher metaposition.

The following nine concepts about change theory will be discussed:

- Change is dependent on the perception of the problem.
- Change is determined by structure.
- Change is dependent on context.
- Change is dependent on co-evolving goals for treatment.
- Understanding alone does not lead to change.
- Change does not necessarily occur equally in all family members.
- Facilitating change is the nurse's responsibility.
- Change occurs by means of a "fit" or meshing between the therapeutic offerings (interventions) of the nurse and the biopsychosocial-spiritual structures of family members.
- Change can be the result of a myriad of causes or reasons.

CONCEPT 1

Change is dependent on the perception of the problem.

In a now-famous statement, Alfred Korzybski proclaimed that "the map is not the territory." In other words, the name is different from the thing named, and the description is different from what is described. In applying this concept to family interviewing, the "mapping" of a particular situation or a nurse's perception of a problem follows from how that nurse chooses to see it. How a nurse perceives a particular problem has profound implications for how the nurse will intervene and therefore how change will occur and whether it will be effective.

One of the most common traps for nurses working with families is the acceptance of one family member's perception or perspective as the "truth" about the family. There is no one "truth" or "reality" about family functioning, or perhaps it is more accurate to say that there are as many "truths" or "realities" as there are members of the family (Maturana & Varela, 1992). The error of taking sides in relational family nursing is discussed in Chapter 11. The important task for the nurse is to accept all family members' perceptions, perspectives, and beliefs and offer the family another view of their health concerns, illness, or problems. Individual family members construct their own realities of a situation based on their history of interactions with people throughout their lives and their genetic history (Maturana & Varela, 1992). Maturana, in an interview with Simon (1985), offers an even more radical idea with regard to different family members' perceptions:

> Systems theory first enabled us to recognize that all the different views presented by the different members of a family had some validity. But, systems theory implied that these were different views of the same system. What I am saying is different. I am not saying that the different descriptions that the members of a family make are different views of the same system. I am saying that there is no one way which the system is; that there

is no absolute, objective family. I am saying that for each member there is a different family; and that each of these is absolutely valid. (p. 36)

Maturana and Varela (1992) emphasize that human systems "bring forth" reality, in language and living with others. Problems can be perceived in very different, yet valid, ways. However, nurses are part of a larger societal system and thus are bound by moral, legal, cultural, and societal norms that require them to act in accordance with these norms regarding illegal or dangerous behaviors (Wright & Bell, 2009).

If a nurse does not conceptualize human problems from a systems or cybernetics perspective, the nurse's perceptions of the family and their illness, problems, and concerns will be based on a completely different conception of "reality" based on different theoretical assumptions. This text emphasizes different theoretical assumptions as opposed to more correct or "right" views of problems.

CONCEPT 2

Change is determined by structure.

Changes that occur in living systems (i.e., human systems) are governed by the present structure of that system. The concept of structural determinism (Maturana & Varela, 1992) offers the notion that each individual's biopsychosocial-spiritual structure is unique and is a product of that person's genetic history (phylogeny) and his or her history of interactions over time (ontogeny).

The implication for nursing practice is that an individual's present structure determines the interpersonal, intrapersonal, and environmental influences that are experienced as perturbations (i.e., that trigger structural changes). Therefore, we cannot say beforehand which family nursing interventions will be useful in promoting change for this particular family member at this time and which will not. Consequently, individuals are selectively perturbed by the interventions that are offered by nurses according to what does or does not "fit" their unique biopsychosocial-spiritual structures. We cannot predict which family nursing interventions will fit for a particular person and which will disturb that person's structure. This theoretical assumption is why we prefer that interventions be tailored to each family rather than utilizing standardized interventions for particular kinds of problems.

A deep respect and awe for and curiosity about family members develop in nurses who are cognizant of the notion of structural determinism. When structural determinism is applied to clinical work with families, Wright and Levac (1992) suggest that the description of families as noncompliant, resistant, or unmotivated is not only "an epistemological error but a biological impossibility" (p. 913). This concept has made a dramatic difference in the way in which we think about families and the interventions that we offer.

CONCEPT 3

Change is dependent on context.

Efforts to promote change in a family system must always take into account the important variable of context. Interventions must be planned with sufficient knowledge of the contextual constraints and resources. This is particularly important considering the emphasis in the health-care industry on accountability, cost-effectiveness, efficiency, and time-effective intervention. Nurses need to be aware of their position in the health-care delivery system in regard to the family. The following questions can help to clarify this:

- Are other professionals involved with the family, and if so, what are their roles with the family?
- How do these roles differ from the nurse's role?
- How are the nurse and family influenced by and influential on the context in which they find themselves, be it a hospital, a primary care clinic, or an extended-care facility?

It is particularly useful to underscore the positive contributions each health-care stakeholder can make to the family's care rather than attributing or assuming self-serving motives to stakeholders who have different vested interests in family care (such as limiting costs).

Larger systems (e.g., schools, mental health agencies, hospitals, public service delivery systems) frequently impose certain "rules" on families that ultimately serve to maintain the larger system's stability and impede change (Imber-Black, 1991; Imber Coppersmith, 1983). An example of this is the *rule of linear blame*: Institutions tend to blame families for difficulties (e.g., lack of motivation) and tend to make referrals for family treatment in order to "cure" or "fix" the family. This process is similar to the one that families use to refer another family member to be "cured."

Because members of some larger systems, particularly nursing staff, become intensely involved in a patient's or family member's life, they commonly tend to go beyond the immediate concerns. The end result is that patients in hospitals and their families find themselves inundated with services that commonly usurp the family's own resources. This then places the family in a "one-down" position in terms of articulating what they perceive their present needs to be. When a nurse is asked to complete a family assessment, the nurse may become one more irritant in the family's life and can be hamstrung before even beginning because of the number of professionals involved. This is another reason why nurses should carefully assess the larger context in which the family and the staff find themselves. In some cases, the more serious problem is at the interface of the family with other professionals rather than within the family itself. Thus, interventions aimed at the family-professional system would need to occur before addressing problems at the family system level.

Another situation that can arise is unclear expertise and leadership. Families may find themselves in a larger system, such as an outpatient drug assessment and treatment clinic. They may receive different ideas on how to deal with a particular problem (e.g., cocaine addiction), depending on whether they are seen at the clinic, at home, or in a class. This usually occurs because no one clinic or educational program offered within a hospital setting has more decision-making power than another regarding a particular family's treatment plan.

Conflicts can also occur between larger systems or between families and larger systems. Unacknowledged or unresolved conflicts commonly result in triads, which inhibit healthy behavior.

> *Example:* Parents wish to send their adolescent son to a drug rehabilitation center, but the nurse and rehabilitation director are in conflict over rehabilitation policies. This places the family in a situation in which pressure from the larger system (nurse-rehabilitation director system) will lead them to align or take sides with either the nurse or the rehabilitation director.

How the family is being influenced by and is exerting influence on their involvement with these suprasystems is important information. Change within a family can be thwarted, sabotaged, or impossible if the issue of context is not addressed.

CONCEPT 4

Change is dependent on co-evolving goals for treatment.

Change requires that goals between nurses and families co-evolve within a realistic time frame. In many cases, the main reason for failure in working with families is either the nurse or family setting unrealistic or inappropriate goals. Frank and open discussions with family members regarding treatment goals can help avoid misunderstandings and disappointments on both sides.

Because one of the primary goals of family intervention is to alter the family's views or beliefs of the problem or illness and alleviate suffering (Wright & Bell, 2009), nurses should help family members to search for alternative behavioral, cognitive, and affective responses to problems. Therefore, one of the nurse's goals is to help the family discover or reclaim its own solutions to problems.

The task of setting specific goals for treatment is accomplished in collaboration with the family. Part of the assessment process is to identify the current suffering or problems with which the family is most concerned and the changes they would like to see. This provides a baseline for the goals of family interviews and becomes the therapeutic contract.

Contracts with families can be either verbal or written. In our clinical practice and in the practice of our nursing students, we typically make verbal contracts with families that state which problems will be tackled during what specified period of time or number of sessions. At the end of that period, progress is evaluated, and either contact with the family is terminated or a new contract is made if further therapeutic work is required.

In most instances, clear goals (in the form of a contract) can be set with families with verbal commitments by family members to work on the problems outlined. On conclusion of the contract, evaluation should consist of assessing changes in the family system and in the identified patient.

Family assessment and intervention are often more effective and successful if they are based on clear therapeutic goals. However, families rarely come to family interviews with the understanding or desire that family change is required. Therefore, in addition to goal setting, the nurse must help the family to obtain a different view of their problems. First, the nurse needs to engage the family; this can most easily be accomplished by first focusing on understanding and exploring their current suffering, the presenting problems and concerns, and the changes the family desires in relation to them. More detailed information and examples about goal setting, contracts, and termination is given in Chapters 7, 10, 12, and 13.

CONCEPT 5

Understanding alone does not lead to change.

Changes in family work rarely occur by increasing a family's understanding of problems but rather through effecting changes in their beliefs and/or behavior. Too often, health professionals engaged in family work assume that understanding a problem brings about a solution by the family. From a systems perspective, however, solutions to problems occur as beliefs about health and illness, problems, and patterns change, regardless of whether this is accompanied by insight (Wright & Bell, 2009).

There has been a tendency in nursing to believe that one must understand "why" in order to solve a problem. Thus, nurses with good intentions spend many hours attempting to obtain masses of data (usually historical) in order to understand the "why" of a problem. In many cases, patients and families encourage the nurse in this quest and participate in it.

> *Example:* Patients might ask, "*Why did I have my heart attack?*" or "*Why won't my son give up crack?*" or "*Why did my wife have to die so young?*"

We strongly discourage searching for the answers because we do not believe this is a precondition for change; rather, it steers one away from effective efforts at change. The prerequisite or precondition for change is not understanding the "why" of a situation but rather understanding the "what." Therefore, we recommend that nurses ask what.

> *Example:* A nurse might ask, "*What is the effect of the father's heart attack on him and his family?*" and "*What are the implications of the father's heart attack on his employment?*"

These questions serve a much more useful purpose in paving the way for possible interventions than do those focusing on the "why" of the situation.

"Why" questions seem to be entrenched in psychoanalytic roots that bring forth psychopathologies. These perspectives are not congruent with a systems or cybernetic foundation of understanding family dynamics that focuses on human problems such as the experience of illness, loss, or disability as interpersonal crises or dilemmas. Even if the "why" of a problem is occasionally understood, it rarely contributes to a solution. Therefore, it is more useful to explore what is being done in the here and now that perpetuates the problem and what can be done in the here and now to effect a change. The search for causes should be avoided because it inadvertently can invite family members to view problems from a linear rather than a systemic or interactional perspective. In other words, we prefer to believe that most problems reside between persons rather than within persons—that is, they are relational.

CONCEPT 6

Change does not necessarily occur equally in all family members.

Recall the analogy of the mobile previously presented in this chapter. Imagine the mobile after a wind has passed it. Some pieces turn or react more rapidly or energetically than do others. This is similar to change in family systems in that one family member may begin to respond or change more rapidly than others and, by this very process, set up an opportunity for change throughout the rest of the family. This occurs because other family members cannot respond in the same way to the family member who is changing, so a ripple effect of change occurs through the system. We have observed this phenomenon in practice with military families when a spouse returns home from a war or a peacekeeping mission. The desire for family members to "return to normal" (i.e., their pre-posting functioning) often conflicts with the returning member's experience of change. This event typically precipitates a time of intense adjustment for all family members.

Robinson's (1998) research also highlighted the concept that when families experience chronic illness, all family members are affected but not necessarily equally. In her study, women suffered more emotionally than other family members, whether the illness was their own, their spouse's, or their child's.

Change depends on the recursive (cybernetic) nature of a family system. Therefore, a small intervention can lead to a variety of reactions, with some family members changing more dramatically or quickly than others.

CONCEPT 7

Facilitating change is the nurse's responsibility.

We believe that it is the nurse's responsibility to facilitate change in collaboration with each family. Facilitating change does not imply that a nurse can predict the outcome, and a nurse should not be invested in a particular outcome. However, there is a distinct difference between facilitating change, directing change, being an expert in resolving family problems, and assuming what must change. We believe families possess expertise about their experiences of their health, illness, and disabilities, whereas nurses have expertise in ideas about health promotion and management of serious illness and disability. It is also crucial for nurses to avoid making value judgments about how families should function. Otherwise, the changes or outcomes in a family system may not be satisfying to the nurse if they are incongruent with how the nurse perceives a family should function. It is more important that the family be satisfied with their new level of functioning than that the nurse be satisfied.

From time to time, nurses must evaluate the level or degree of responsibility they feel for treatment. The level of responsibility is out of proportion if a nurse feels more concerned, worried, or responsible for family problems than the families feel themselves. In the opposite response, sometimes nurses experience a detachment or a lack of concern, compassion, or responsibility for facilitating change within families. Both of these extreme responses indicate the need to obtain clinical supervision.

How much change nurses should expect to facilitate in family work depends on their competence, their capacity for compassion, the context of family treatment, and the family's response. Nurses need to be cognizant that they are not change agents; they cannot and do not change anyone (Bell & Wright, 2011; Wright & Bell, 2009; Wright & Levac, 1992). For some nurses, not being a change agent is counterintuitive to their desire and manner of being helpful. But when nurses can let go of the notion of being a change agent and instead become a facilitator of change, they can move into a truly relational and collaborative relationship with families entrusted in their care.

Ultimate and sustained changes in family members are determined by each member's biopsychosocial-spiritual structures, not by the nurse

(Maturana & Varela, 1992). Therefore, it is the nurse's responsibility to facilitate a context for change. Paying attention to windows of opportunity for facilitating change is one idea put forth by Robinson, Bottorff, and Torchalla (2011). Their findings support the idea that at the time of a diagnosis of lung cancer, families may be more open to addressing smoking-cessation strategies.

CONCEPT 8

Change occurs by means of a "fit" or meshing between the therapeutic offerings (interventions) of the nurse and the biopsychosocial-spiritual structures of family members.

The concept of "fit" or "meshing" arises from the notion of structural determinism (Maturana & Varela, 1992). That is, the family member's structure, not the nurse's therapeutic offering, determines whether the intervention is experienced as a perturbation that triggers, facilitates, or stimulates change. This concept is aligned with the guiding principle that the nurse is not a change agent (Wright & Levac, 1992) but rather one who, among other things, creates a context for change (Bell & Wright, 2011; Wright & Bell, 2009). In our clinical experience, family members who respond to particular therapeutic offerings do so because of a fit, or meshing, between their current biopsychosocial-spiritual structures and the family nursing intervention offered. (For more information on this, see Chapter 4 and the discussion of the CFIM.) This includes the nurse's sensitivity to the family's race, ethnicity, sexual orientation, and socioeconomic level.

The concept of "fit" allows nurses to be nonblaming of patients and themselves when nonfit—and consequently nonadherence and non-follow-through—occurs (Bell & Wright, 2011; Wright & Bell, 2009; Wright & Levac, 1992). Nurses operating from a therapeutic stance who appreciate fit can be highly curious about ways to increase the suitability of interventions for particular family members at a specific time. When the concept of fit is overlooked, neglected, or not appreciated, nurses operate with more lecturing, prescribing behaviors, and often labeling family members as non-compliant, not ready for change, or defiant of the professional system.

CONCEPT 9

Change can be the result of a myriad of causes or reasons.

Change is influenced by so many different variables that, in most cases, knowing specifically what precipitated, stimulated, or triggered the change is difficult. Change is not always a result of well-thought-out intervention. Commonly, it can be the result of a collaborative relationship between the nurse and family and/or the method of inquiry into family problems.

Asking interventive questions (see Chapter 4 for an in-depth discussion about the nurse-family relationship and questions within the CFIM, and see Chapters 8 and 9 for how to use questions in family interviewing) may in and of itself promote change. It is more important for nurses to attribute change to families than to concern themselves with what they did to create change (see Chapter 12 for more information on concluding meetings with families). To search for or take undue credit for change is inappropriate at this stage of our knowledge of the change process in families.

BIOLOGY OF COGNITION

The biology of cognition has been described and articulated by two neuro-biologists, Maturana and Varela (1992), in their landmark publication *The Tree of Knowledge: The Biological Roots of Human Understanding*. They offer the idea that humans bring forth different views to their understanding of events and experiences in their lives. This idea is not new, but Maturana and Varela's perspective on how humans make and claim observations is much more radical: It is based on biology and physiology, not philosophy (Bell & Wright, 2011; Wright & Bell, 2009; Wright & Levac, 1992). If a nurse adopts a particular view of reality, it then follows that the nurse now encompasses a particular view of people and their functioning, relationships, and illnesses.

The following two concepts about the biology of cognition will be discussed:

- Two possible avenues for explaining our world are objectivity and objectivity-in-parentheses (Maturana & Varela, 1992; Wright & Bell, 2009; Wright & Levac, 1992; Wright, Watson, & Bell, 1990).
- We bring forth our realities through interacting with the world, ourselves, and others through language.

CONCEPT 1

Two possible avenues for explaining our world are objectivity and objectivity-in-parentheses.

The view of objectivity assumes that one ultimate domain of reference exists for explaining the world. Within this domain, entities are assumed to exist independent of the observer. Such entities are as numerous and broad as imagination might allow and may be explicitly or implicitly identified as mind, knowledge, truth, and so on. Within this avenue of explanation, people come to believe they have access to a true and correct view of the world and its events, an objective reality. From this "objectivist" view, "a system and its components have a constancy and a stability that is independent of the observer that brings them forth" (Mendez, Coddou, & Maturana, 1988,

p. 154). Nursing diagnoses, emotional conflict, pride, and politics are all products of an "objective" view of reality.

When objectivity is "placed in parentheses," people recognize that objects do exist but that they are not independent of the living system that brings them forth. The only "truths" that exist are those brought forth by observers, such as nurses and family members. Each person's view is not a distortion of some presumably correct interpretation. Instead of one objective universe waiting to be discovered or correctly described, Maturana has proposed a "multiverse," where many observer "verses" coexist, each valid in its own right. To increase options and possibilities for families to cope with illness using a variety of strategies or to improve their well-being, nurses need to help family members drift toward objectivity-in-parentheses. When nurses are able to maintain an objective stance, they are increasingly able to invite family members to resist the "sin of certainty"—that is, to resist the notion that there is only one true or correct way to manage health or illness, loss, or disability.

CONCEPT 2

We bring forth our realities through interacting with the world, ourselves, and others through language.

We propose that reality does not reside "out there" to be absorbed; rather, people exist in many domains of the realities that they bring forth to explain their experiences (Maturana & Varela, 1992). The ability to bring forth personal meaning and to respond to and interact with the world and with each other, but always with reference to a set of internal coherences, can be seen as the essential quality of living. Maturana and Varela (1980) assert that this statement applies to all organisms, with or without a nervous system. They further suggest that it is best to think of cognition as a continual interaction between what people expect to see (owing to unconscious premises or beliefs) and what they bring forth. In a telephone interview, Maturana (1988) embellished this notion of reality as follows:

> We exist in many domains of realities that we bring forth ... What I'm saying in the long-run is that there is no possibility of saying absolutely anything about anything independent from us. So whatever we do is always our total responsibility in the sense that it depends completely on us, and all domains of reality that we bring forth are equally legitimate although they are not equally desirable or pleasant to live in. But they are always brought forth by us, in our coexistence with other human beings. So if we bring forth a community in which there is misery, well, this is it. If we bring forth a community in which there is well-being, this is it. But it is us always in coexistence with others that ... are bringing forth reality. Reality is indeed an explanation of the world that we live [in] with others.

In sum, the world everyone sees is not the world but a world that they bring forth with others (Maturana & Varela, 1992). When nurses adopt this particular ethical stance, they find themselves more curious about the world each family member brings forth and how this world influences the person's ability or inability to cope with or manage his or her illness.

CRITICAL THINKING QUESTIONS

1. Consider your own clinical practice:
   a. How do the hierarchy of systems and the boundaries that create systems apply when working with families?
2. In what way can nurses continue to conduct family research-based practice and family practice-based research to enhance the understanding of theories that inform family nursing assessment and interventions?
3. Within your own clinical practice, how could you promote family research-based practice? What are the challenges?

Chapter **3**

The Calgary Family Assessment Model

Learning Objectives

- Describe the three major categories of the Calgary Family Assessment Model (CFAM), structural, developmental, and functional, and their associated subcategories.
- Define terms used in the CFAM.
- Identify questions to ask families to obtain information and how they apply to each category of the CFAM.

Key Concepts

Circular communication

Circular pattern diagrams (CPDs)

Developmental assessment

Ecomap

Family development

Family life cycle

Functional assessment

Genogram

Structural assessment

The Calgary Family Assessment Model (CFAM) is an integrated, multidimensional framework based on the foundations of systems, cybernetics, communication, and change theory and influenced by postmodernism and the biology of cognition. This text includes a discussion of the distinction between using the CFAM to assess a family and using the CFAM as an organizing framework, or template, for working with families to help them resolve health-related problems or other issues.

The CFAM has received wide recognition since the first edition of this book in 1984. It has been adopted by many faculties, schools of nursing, and other health science disciplines. It has been referenced frequently in the literature, especially the *Journal of Family Nursing*. In addition, the International Council of Nurses has recognized it as one of the four leading family assessment models in the world (Schober & Affara, 2001). Originally adapted from a family assessment framework developed by Tomm and Sanders (1983), the CFAM was substantially revised in 1994, 2000, and 2005.

The CFAM consists of three major categories:

1. Structural
2. Developmental
3. Functional

Each category contains several subcategories. It is important for *each* nurse to decide which subcategories are relevant and appropriate to explore and assess with *each* family at *each* point in time. That is, not all subcategories need to be assessed at the first meeting with a family, and some subcategories need never be assessed. If too many subcategories are used, the nurse may become overwhelmed by all the data. If the nurse and the family discuss too few subcategories, each may have a distorted view of the family's strengths or problems and the family situation.

It is useful to conceptualize these three assessment categories and their many subcategories as a branching diagram (Figure 3-1). As the nurse uses the subcategories on the right of the branching diagram, the nurse collects more and more microscopic data. It is important for nurses to be able to move back and forth on the diagram in order to draw together all of the relevant information into an integrated assessment. This process of synthesizing data helps nurses working with complex family situations.

It is also important for a nurse to recognize that a family assessment is based on the nurse's personal and professional life experiences, beliefs, and relationships with those being interviewed. It is useful for nurses to determine whether they are using CFAM as a model to assess a family or as an organizing framework for clinical work with a specific family to help the family address a health issue. When learning the CFAM, students and practicing nurses new to family work will likely find the model helpful for directly assessing families. Similarly, researchers seeking to assess families will find the model useful. This use of the model involves asking the family questions about themselves for the express purpose of gaining a snapshot of the family's structure, development, and functioning at a particular point in time.

However, how we have used the CFAM is not in a research manner but rather in a clinical manner. Once nurses become experienced with the categories and subcategories of the CFAM, they can use the CFAM as a clinical organizing framework to help families solve problems or issues.

For example, a single-parent family in the developmental stage of families with adolescents will have many positive experiences from earlier

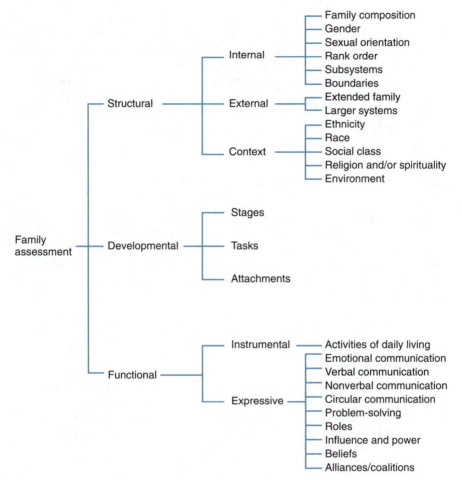

Figure 3-1 Branching diagram of the CFAM.

developmental stages to draw from in coping with the teenager's unexpected illness. The nurse, being reminded of family developmental stages by using the CFAM, will draw forth those resiliencies. The nurse will ask questions and collaboratively develop interventions with the family to enhance their functioning during this health-care episode.

Families do not generally present to health-care professionals to be "assessed." Rather, they present themselves or are encountered by nurses while coping with an illness or seeking assistance to improve their quality of life. The CFAM helps guide nurses in helping families.

In this chapter, each assessment category is discussed separately. Terms are defined, and sample questions relevant to each CFAM category are proposed for the nurse to ask family members. We do not suggest that nurses ask these questions in a disembodied way. Rather, real-life clinical examples are provided in Chapters 4, 7, 8, 9, and 10 to further describe how to use the sample questions and apply the CFAM. The use of assessment and interventive questions will be discussed in Chapter 4 (The Calgary Family Intervention Model [CFIM]). We wish to emphasize that not all questions about various subcategories of the model need to be asked in the first interview, and questions about each subcategory are not appropriate for every family. Families are obviously composed of individuals, but the focus of a family assessment is less on the individual and more on the interaction *among* all of the individuals within the family.

STRUCTURAL ASSESSMENT

In assessing a family, the nurse needs to examine its structure—that is, who is in the family, the connections among family members vis-à-vis those outside the family, and the family's context. Three aspects of family structure can most readily be examined: internal structure, external structure, and context. Each of these dimensions of family structural assessment is addressed separately.

KEY CONCEPT DEFINED

Structural Assessment

One of the categories of the Calgary Family Assessment Model (CFAM) that nurses use to identify who is in the family, the connections among family members in regard to those outside the family, and the family's context.

Internal Structure

Internal structure includes six subcategories:

1. Family composition
2. Gender
3. Sexual orientation
4. Rank order
5. Subsystems
6. Boundaries

Family Composition

The subcategory *family composition* has many meanings because of the many definitions given to family. Wright and Bell (2009) define family as "a group of individuals who are bound by strong emotional ties, a sense of belonging, and a passion for being involved in one another's lives" (p. 46).

There are five critical attributes to the concept of family:

1. The family is a system or unit.
2. Its members may or may not be related and may or may not live together.
3. The unit may or may not contain children.
4. There are commitment and attachment among unit members that include future obligation.
5. The unit caregiving functions consist of protection, nourishment, and socialization of its members.

Using these ideas, the nurse can include the various family forms that are prevalent in society today, such as the biological family of procreation, the nuclear family (family of origin), the sole-parent family, the stepfamily, the communal family, and the lesbian, gay, bisexual, queer, intersex, transgender, or twin-spirited (LGBQITT) couple or family. Designating a group of people with a term such as "couple," "nuclear family," or "single-parent family" specifies attributes of membership, but these distinctions of grouping are not more or less "families" by reason of labeling. Rather, attributes of affection, strong emotional ties, a sense of belonging, and durability of membership determine family composition.

Nurses need to find a definition of family that moves beyond the traditional boundaries that limit membership using the criteria of blood, adoption, and marriage. We have found the following definition of family to be most useful in our clinical work: *the family is who they say they are* (Wright & Leahey, 2013). With this definition, nurses can honor individual family members' ideas about which relationships are significant to them and their experiences of health and illness.

Although we recognize the dominant North American type of separately housed nuclear families, our definition allows us to address the emotional past, present, and anticipated future relationships within the family system. It is important to note that our definition of family is based on the family's conception of family rather than who lives in the household. Family configurations continue to evolve in society, for example, LGBQITT families, adoptive and foster families, stepfamilies, multigenerational families, and sole-parent families.

Changes in family composition are important to note. These changes could be permanent, such as the loss of a family member or the addition of a new person into the family home, such as a new baby, a nanny, a boarder, or an elderly parent who can no longer live independently. Changes in family composition can also be transient. For example, stepfamilies commonly have different family compositions on weekends or during vacation periods when children from previous relationships cohabit. Families with a child in placement or those experiencing homelessness often temporarily live with other relatives and then move on.

Losses tend to be more severe depending on how recently they have occurred, the younger some of the family members are when the loss occurs, the smaller the family, the greater the numerical imbalance between male and female members of the family resulting from the loss, the greater the number of losses, and the greater the number of prior losses. The circumstances surrounding the loss may be of exquisite concern for the nurse. For example, some parents of severely mentally ill children have reported that they were encouraged to give up custody of their children to foster care as a way of securing intense health-care treatment for them.

Serious illness or death of a family member, violence or war, and natural disasters can lead to profound disruption in the family and have long-term impacts. These situations often result in aunts and uncles raising nieces and nephews, or grandparents raising grandchildren, or friends or faith-based communities raising children and are often overlooked in regard to family structural arrangement. The extent of the impact of a member's death on the family depends on the social and cultural meaning of death, the history of previous losses, the timing of the death in the life cycle, and the nature of the death (Becvar, 2001, 2003).

Every family touched by tragedy faces the task of making sense of what happened, why it happened, and how to adjust to the changed landscape. Families can find inspiration from many sources to cope with unprecedented tragedy.

The position and function of the person who died in the family system and the openness of the family system must also be considered. We have found it useful to note the family's losses and deaths during the structural assessment process, but not necessarily to make an immediate assumption that these losses are of major significance to the family. By taking this stance, we disagree with the position taken by some clinicians who assert that it is important to track patterns of adaptation to loss as a routine part of family assessment even when it is not initially presented as relevant to the chief complaints.

In our clinical practice with families, we have found it useful to ask ourselves these questions to determine the composition of families:

- "Who is in this family?"
- "Who does this family consider to be 'family'?"

Questions to Ask the Family.

- "Could you tell me who is in your family?"
- "Does anyone else live with you, for example, grandparents, boarders?"
- "Has anyone recently moved out?"
- "Is there anyone else you think of as family who does not live with you? Anyone not related biologically?"

Gender

The subcategory of *gender* is a basic construct, a fundamental organizing principle. We believe in the constructivist "both/and" position—that is, we view gender as both a universal "reality" operational in hierarchy and power and as a reality constructed by ourselves from our particular frame of reference. We recognize gender as both a fundamental basis for all human beings and as an individual premise. Gender is important for nurses to consider because the difference in how men and women experience the world is at the heart of the therapeutic conversation. We can help families by assuming that the differences between women and men can be changed, discarding unhelpful cultural scripts for women and men, and recognizing and attending to hidden power issues. However, nurses need to consider that not all couples want to equalize the imbalance of power and that some may prefer traditional roles.

In couple relationships, the problems described by men and women commonly include unspoken conflicts between their perceptions of gender—that is, how their family and society or culture tell them that men and women should feel, think, or behave—and their own experiences.

We argue on behalf of the integration of male and female attributes in each person. Human development is a process of increasingly complex forms of relatedness and integration rather than a progression from attachment to separation. Gender is, in our view, a set of beliefs about or expectations of male and female behaviors and experiences. These beliefs have been developed by cultural, religious, and familial influences as well as by socioeconomic status and sexual orientation.

It's important to understand the difference between gender and sex. Sex is defined as the physiological difference between the male and female, whereas gender references social and cultural distinctions, such as social relationships and their symbolic meaning. Gender identity is related to how one identifies oneself as being masculine or feminine (McDowell, 2018).

According to the World Health Organization (WHO, 2015), gender is increasingly being recognized as an important determinant of health, and issues such as gender inequality and lack of understanding of gender norms and roles can lead to poor health outcomes. Sharma, Chakrabarti, and Grover (2016) reviewed recent studies on gender difference in caregiving among families with mental illness and found that women are predominately the caregivers and, as a result, experience physical burdens and higher levels of psychological distress. The authors found that women tended to have multiple roles, such as wives, daughters, sisters, mothers, and employees, which increased pressure on them and caused role strain and conflict. These role strains and conflicts had major adverse effects on families, including fatigue and burnout, leading to emotional disturbance and depression.

Levac, Wright, and Leahey (2002) recommend that assessment of the influence of gender in the family is especially important when societal, cultural, or family beliefs about male and female roles are creating family tension. In this situation, couples may desire to establish more equal relationships, with characteristics such as the following:

- Partners hold equal status (e.g., equal entitlement to personal goals, needs, and wishes).
- Accommodation in the relationship is mutual (e.g., schedules are organized equally around each partner's needs).
- Attention to the other in the relationship is mutual (e.g., equal displays of interest in the other's needs and desires by both partners).
- Enhancement of the well-being of each partner is mutual (e.g., the relationship supports the psychological health of each equally).

In our clinical supervision with nurses doing relational family practice, we have found it useful to have them consider their own ideas about male, female, intersex, twin-spirited, and transgender persons. Bjarnadottir, Bockting, and Dowding (2017) conducted an integrative review of patient perspectives when answering questions about sexual orientation and gender identity and found that nurses need to be mindful of heteronormative assumptions. The evidence from this review also identified the patients' willingness to answer questions about sexual orientation and their perceptions of its importance.

Questions to Ask the Family.

- "What effect did your parents' ideas have on your own ideas of masculinity and femininity?"
- "If your arguments with your male children were about how to stay connected rather than how to separate, would your arguments then be different?"
- "If you would show the feelings you keep hidden, Harry, would your wife think more or less of you?"
- "How did it come to be that Mom assumes more responsibility for the dialysis than Dad does?"

Sexual Orientation

The subcategory of *sexual orientation* includes sexual majority and sexual minority populations. According to the American Psychological Association (2015), sexual orientation is "a component of identity that includes a person's sexual and emotional attraction to another person and the behavior and/or social affiliation that may result from this attraction. A person may be attracted to men, women, both, neither, or to people who are genderqueer, androgynous, or have other gender identities. Individuals may identify as lesbian, gay, heterosexual, bisexual, queer, pansexual, or asexual, among others" (p. 6).

Nurses need to reflect critically on attitudes about sexual orientation when working with families. We believe that nurses should be able to support a patient along whatever sexual-orientation path the individual takes and that the patient's sense of integrity and interpersonal relatedness are the most important goals of all. The United Nations (2015) further supports this in identifying that societal discrimination against lesbian, gay, bisexual, and transgender (LGBT) people is a direct threat to their health and well-being. We agree with Yingling, Cotler, and Hughes (2017) that there is a global need for nurses to develop their knowledge and skills in a culturally sensitive manner to appropriately provide care for LGBT people and their families.

Questions to Ask the Family.
- "Elsbeth, at what age did you first engage in sexual activity?"
- "When LaCheir first told your mom that she was lesbian, what effect did it have on your mom's caregiving with her?"
- "When your brother, Lee, announced that he was gay and leaving his marriage, how did your parents respond?"
- "What did your parents tell you, Lilah, about your ambiguous genitals?"

Rank Order

The subcategory *rank order* refers to the position of the children in the family with respect to age and gender. Birth order, gender, and distance in age between siblings are important factors to consider when doing an assessment. Toman (1993) has been a major contributor to research about sibling configuration. In his main thesis, the duplication theorem, he asserts that the more new social relationships resemble earlier intrafamilial social relationships, the more enduring and successful they are. For example, the marriage between an older brother (of a younger sister) and a younger sister (of an older brother) has good potential for success because the relationships are complementary. If the marriage is between two firstborns, a symmetrical competitive relationship might exist, with each one vying for the position of leadership.

The following factors also influence sibling constellation: the timing of each sibling's birth in the family history, the child's characteristics, the family's idealized "program" for the child, and the parental attitudes and biases regarding gender differences. Although we believe that sibling patterns are important to note, we urge nurses to also remember that different child-rearing patterns have emerged as a result of increased use of birth control, the women's movement, the large number of women in the workforce, and the great variety of family configurations. We hold the view that sibling position is an organizing influence on the personality, but it is not a fixed influence. Each new period of life brings a re-evaluation of these influences. An individual transfers or generalizes familial experiences to social settings outside the family, such as kindergarten, schools, and clubs. Given the availability and powerful influence of the Internet, the universe of available relationships and experiences is greatly expanded. As an individual is influenced by the environment, his or her relationships with colleagues, friends, and spouses are also generally affected. With time, multiple influences in addition to sibling constellation can affect personality organization.

Prior to meeting with a family, we encourage nurses to hypothesize about the potential influence of rank order on the reason for the family interview. For example, nurses could ask themselves, *"If this child is the youngest in the family, could this be influencing the parents' reluctance to allow him to give his own insulin injections?"* Nurses could also consider the influence of birth order on motivation, achievement, and vocational choice. For example, is the firstborn child under pressure to achieve academically? If the youngest child is starting school, what influence might this have on the couple's persistent attempts with in vitro fertilization? We urge clinicians not only to consider rank order when children are young but also its relevance when working with siblings in later life. Overlooking the fact that individuals may be influenced by old or ongoing conflicts may lead to missed opportunities for healing.

Questions to Ask the Family.

- "How many children do you have, Amber?"
- "Who is the eldest? How old is he or she?"
- "Who comes next in line?"
- "Have there been any miscarriages or abortions?"
- "If your older sister, Gerda, showed more softness and were less controlling of your mom, might you be willing to talk more with your mom?"
- "Would you be willing to talk about difficult issues, such as her giving up driving because of her macular degeneration?"

Subsystems

Subsystems is a term used to discuss or mark the family system's level of differentiation; a family carries out its functions through its subsystems. Dyads, such as husband-wife, wife-wife, or mother-child, can be seen as subsystems. Subsystems can be delineated by generation, gender, interest, function, or history.

Each person in the family belongs to several different subsystems. In each subsystem, that person has a different level of power and uses different skills. A 65-year-old woman can be a grandmother, mother, wife, and daughter within the same family. An eldest boy is a member of the sibling subsystem, the male subsystem, and the parent-child subsystem. In each of the subsystems, he behaves according to his position. He has to concede the power that he exerts over his younger brothers in the sibling subsystem when he interacts with his stepmother in the parent-child subsystem. An only child living in a single-parent household has different subsystem challenges when she lives on alternate weekends with her mother, her new wife, and their new baby. The ability to adapt to the demands of different subsystem levels is a necessary skill for each family member.

In our clinical practice, we have found it useful to consider whether clear generational boundaries are present in the family. If they are, does the family find them helpful or not? For example, we ask ourselves whether one child behaves like a parent or husband surrogate. Is the child a child, or is there a surrogate-spouse subsystem? By generating these hypotheses before and during the family meeting, we are able to connect isolated bits of data to either confirm or negate a hypothesis.

Questions to Ask the Family.

Some families have special subgroups—for example, those who identify that women do certain things, those who identify that men do certain things, and those who identify that children do certain things.

* "Do different subgroups exist in your family? If so, what effect does this have on your family's stress level?"
* "When Mom and your sister, Nora, stay up at night and talk about Dad's use of crack, what do the boys do?"
* "Who in the family is most affected by Cleve's crack problem, and how does it affect them?"
* "Who gets together in the family to talk about Shabana's self-mutilating behaviors?"

Parent-child:

* "How has your relationship with Caitylin changed since her diagnosis with severe acute respiratory syndrome?"

Marital:

* "How much couple time can you and Simon carve out each month without talking about the children?"

Sibling:

* "On a scale of 1 to 10, with 10 being the most, how scared were you when Alex developed congestive heart failure?"

Boundaries

The subcategory *boundaries* refers to the rule "defining who participates and how" (Minuchin, 1974, p. 53). Family systems and subsystems have boundaries, the function of which is to define or protect the differentiation of the system or subsystem.

For example, the boundary of a family system is defined when a father tells his teenage daughter that her boyfriend cannot move into the household. A parent-child subsystem boundary is made explicit when a mother tells her daughter, "You are not your brother's parent. If he is not taking his medication, I will discuss it with him."

Boundaries can be diffuse, rigid, or permeable. As boundaries become diffuse, the differentiation of the family system decreases. For example, family members may become emotionally close and richly cross-joined. These family members can have a heightened sense of belonging to the family and less individual autonomy. A diffuse subsystem boundary is evident when a child is "parentified," or given adult responsibilities and power in decision making.

When rigid boundaries are present, the subsystems tend to become disengaged. A husband who rigidly believes that only wives should visit the elderly relatives, and whose wife agrees with him, can become disengaged from or peripheral to the senior adult-child subsystem. Clear, permeable boundaries, on the other hand, allow appropriate flexibility. Under these conditions, the rules can be modified. We do not support the pathologizing of coalitions or subsystems just because they exist. In working with families from different cultures, races, and social classes or those from rural settings, we have found that fostering other central ties may be most beneficial for the family.

Boundaries tend to change over time. Boss (2002) suggests that family boundaries become ambiguous during the process of reorganization after the acquisition or the loss of a member. This is particularly evident in families experiencing separation or divorce. As couples make the transition to parenthood, they may experience the desired child as a family member who is psychologically present but physically absent. This is particularly relevant if there is a surrogate mother or a known sperm donor involved during the pregnancy. Other variations include the ambiguity experienced by some families when a family member is in prison, or overseas fighting in a war, or living in a rehab hospital following a tour of duty or some other traumatic event, or when a family member has dementia or is undergoing gender transition. Boss (2016) uses the term *ambiguous loss* "to describe a situation of unclear loss that remains unverified and thus without resolution" (p. 270) and discusses how ambiguous loss leads to boundary ambiguity, that is, not knowing who is within or out of a family system.

Boundary styles can facilitate or constrain family functioning. For example, an immigrant family that moves into a new culture may be very protective of its members until it gradually adapts to the cultural milieu. Its boundaries regarding outside systems may be quite firm and rigid at first but may gradually become more flexible.

The closeness-caregiving dimension of boundaries is another aspect for nurses to consider. The relative sharing of territory can be assessed along aspects of contact time (time together), personal space (physical nearness, touching), emotional space (sharing of affects), informational space (information known about each other), private space (shared private conversations separate from others), and decisional space (extent to which decisions are localized within various individuals or subsystems). The closeness-caregiving dimension of a boundary may be very significant for nurses to assess when dealing with older people with chronic illnesses and their adult children.

In our clinical supervision with nurses, we encourage them to consider how each family differentiates itself from other families in the community and in the city. The nurse considers whether there is a parental subsystem, a marital subsystem, a sibling subsystem, and so forth. The nurse should consider the following questions:

- "Are the boundaries clear, rigid, or diffuse?"
- "Does the boundary style facilitate or constrain the family?"
- "If there are multiple stepfamilies, which boundary predominates?"

Questions to Ask the Family.

- "Is there anyone with whom you can talk to when you feel stressed by your upcoming retirement?" (The nurse can ask family members the same question.)
- "To whom would you go if you felt happy? If you felt sad?"
- "Would there be anyone in your family opposed to your talking with that person?"
- "Who would be most in favor of you talking with that person?"
- "What impact might it have on your mom's ability to deal with your dad's illness if she had more support from your grandparents?"

External Structure

External structure includes two subcategories:

1. Extended family
2. Larger systems

Extended Family

The subcategory of *extended family* includes the family of origin and the family of procreation as well as the present generation and stepfamily members. Multiple loyalty ties to extended family members can be invisible but may be very influential forces in the family structure. Special relationships and support can exist at great geographical distances. Also, conflicted and painful relationships can seem fresh and close at hand despite the extended family living far away or not being in frequent contact. How each member sees himself or herself as a separate individual yet part of the "family ego mass" (Bowen, 1978) is a critical structural area for assessment.

Levac, Wright, and Leahey (2002) recommend assessment of the quantity and type of contact with extended family to provide information about the quality and quantity of support. The importance of social media connections cannot be overemphasized. A young man paralyzed following a sports injury may be connected with many people through Facebook, Twitter, and blogs, which is a helpful way for the family, friends, and colleagues to link to the patient and to each other. Such connective inter-action "does hope," a notion we support and find healing. In our clinical work we consider whether there are many references to the extended family. How significant is the extended family to the functioning of this particular family? Are they available for support in times of need? If so, how? By mobile or land phones, e-mail, webcam, Skype, iChat, and Internet chat groups? Are they in close physical proximity?

Questions to Ask the Family.
- "Where do your parents live?"
- "How often do you have contact with them?"
- "What about your brothers, sisters, and step-relatives?"
- "Which family members do you never see?"
- "Which of your relatives are you closest to?"
- "Who phones whom? With what frequency?"
- "Whom do you ask for help when problems arise in your family?"
- "What kind of help do you ask for?"
- "Would your family in Ireland be available if you needed their help?"
- "Would you feel more comfortable contacting your family by e-mail or in a chat room?"

Larger Systems

The subcategory *larger systems* refers to the larger social agencies and personnel with whom the family has meaningful contact. Larger systems generally include work systems, and for some families, they include public welfare, child welfare, foster care, courts, and outpatient clinics. There are also larger systems designed for special populations, such as agencies mandated to provide services to the mentally or physically handicapped or the frail elderly. For many families, engagement with such larger systems is not problematic and can be life-affirming. We believe that larger professional systems can be an appreciative audience that supports families' narratives of hope and preferred new lives. We encourage nurses to use language carefully in discussing clients with larger-system helpers so as to support family stories of courage, growth, and persistence instead of perpetuating stories of hopelessness and problems.

Some families and larger systems, however, may develop difficult relationships that exert a toll on normative development for family members. Some health-care professionals in larger systems contribute to families being labeled "multiproblem," "resistant," "noncompliant," or "uncooperative." Health-care professionals limit their perspectives by using these labels.

Another larger-system relationship that nurses should consider is the computer network. Electronic bulletin boards, chat rooms, text messaging, and discussion groups are increasing. The Internet can offer families valuable assistance in terms of information, validation, empathy, advice, and encouragement; however, it can also provide inaccurate and misleading information, and thus it is important for nurses to support families to access reliable information. Some have used e-mail to augment, extend, deepen, inform, enrich, and prepare for in-person psychotherapy. However, online dialogues can sometimes be more sustaining than transformative. Vigorous attention should be given to ways that professional expertise and electronic connectivity can be combined. Telenursing is one such example. Nurses need to consider how they can ensure that the voices of *all* family members are part of the discussion between the nurse and the family when using telehealth care. Using videoconferencing to gather all the larger-system helpers in one space with the family to discuss, plan, and evaluate care can be a solution.

In our clinical supervision with nurses, we encourage them to discover whether the *meaningful system* is the family alone or the family *and* its larger-system helpers.

Nurses can ask themselves questions such as the following:

- "Who are the health-care professionals involved?"
- "What is the relationship between the family and the larger system?"
- "How regularly do they interact? Is their relationship symmetrical or complementary?"
- "Are the larger systems overconcerned? Overinvolved? Underconcerned? Underinvolved?"
- "Does the larger system blame the family for its problems?"
- "What do the helpers desire for the family?"
- "Is the nurse being asked to take responsibility for another system's task?"
- "How do the family and helpers define the problem?"

One young woman suffering from metastases from breast cancer, when asked, "Who do you think of like family?" answered, "I have three families: my own family, my church family, and my 'family' at the cancer center."

Questions to Ask the Family.

- "What agency professionals are involved with your family, Mr. Rajwani?"
- "How many agencies regularly interact with you?"
- "Has your family moved from one health-care system to another?"
- "Who most thinks that your family needs to be involved with these systems?"
- "Who most thinks the opposite?"
- "Would there be agreement between your definition of the problem and the system's definition of the problem?"

- "How about between the definitions of the solution?"
- "What has been the best or worst advice you have been given by professionals for this issue, Atul?"
- "How is our working relationship going so far, Laura? If it were not going well, would you tell me?"

Context

Context is explained as the whole situation or background relevant to some event or personality. Each family system is itself nested within broader systems, such as neighborhood, socioeconomic status, region, and country, and is influenced by these systems. The connectivity experienced by persons using the Internet is another context to be considered. Because the context permeates and circumscribes both the individual and the family, its consequences are pervasive. Context includes but is not limited to these five subcategories:

1. Ethnicity
2. Race
3. Social class
4. Spirituality and/or religion
5. Environment

Ethnicity

Ethnicity refers to the concept of a family's "peoplehood" and is derived from a combination of its history, race, social class, and religion. It describes a commonality of overt and subtle processes transmitted by the family over generations and usually reinforced by the surrounding community. Ethnicity is an important factor that influences family interaction. We believe that nurses must be aware of the great variety within as well as among ethnic groups. Some people are second-, third-, or fourth-generation immigrants, with ancestors who were born in a foreign country. Others may be from "recently arrived" immigrant families, either legally arrived or undocumented, of whom some are refugees.

Ethnic differences in family structure and their implications for intervention have often been highlighted in a stereotypical manner. For example, some families may have strong extended family connections and loyalties, others may have flexible family boundaries, and some may include other family members in child-rearing. There may be emotionality between relatives and between generations, whereas other families may have strictly defined boundaries between generations.

We believe our own cultural narratives help us to organize our thinking and anchor our lives, but they can also blind us to the unfamiliar and unrecognizable and can foster injustice. For example, the importance of learning their histories and experiences when caring for refugee immigrant women is invaluable because it provides context and a greater understanding of their situations.

Nurses should sensitize themselves to differences in family beliefs and values and be willing to alter their "ethnic filters." We believe it is important for nurses to recognize their own ethnic blind spots and adjust their interventions accordingly. We are never "expert," "right," or in full possession of the "truth" about a family's ethnicity. Also, if we engage a translator to assist us with family work, we should not assume that the translator is an "expert" on this particular family's ethnicity. Rather, both we and the translator should strive to be informed and curious about ourselves and others' diversity as we collaborate in health care. The importance of participatory models of knowledge transfer and exchange cannot be underestimated.

Questions that we have found useful to ask ourselves include the following:

- "What is the family's ethnicity?"
- "Have the children and parents had periods of separation in their immigration experience? If so, with what impact?"
- "Is their social network from the same ethnic group? Do they find that helpful or not?"
- "If the available economic, educational, health, legal, and recreational services were similar to the family's ethnic values, how would our conversation be different?"
- "Are the assessment and testing instruments we use in our clinic relevant for this ethnic group? Do they match the values and beliefs of this particular family?"

Questions to Ask the Family.

- "Could you tell me about your Japanese cultural practices or traditions regarding illness?"
- "How does being an immigrant from Afghanistan influence your beliefs about when to consult with health professionals?"
- "What does health mean to you?"
- "How would you know that you are healthy? How would I know that you are healthy?"
- "As a second-generation Chilean family, how are your health-care practices similar to or different from those of your grandparents?"
- "Which practices seem most useful to you at this point in your family's life?"

Race

The subcategory of *race* is a basic construct and not an intermediate variable. Race influences core individual and group identification. Race intersects with mediating variables such as class, religion, and ethnicity. Racial attitudes, stereotyping, and discrimination are powerful influences on family interaction and, if left unaddressed, can be negative constraints on the relationship between the family and the nurse.

There is a dearth of literature on potential relationship strengths in intercultural and interracial relationships. We encourage nurses to elicit strengths rather than challenges in working with these couples.

Racial differences, whether intracultural or intercultural, are not problems as such. Rather, prejudice, discrimination, and other types of intercultural aggression based on these differences are problems. For some persons, whether of the majority or minority race, the word "race" is very distasteful because we are all members of the human race. They feel that the word itself implies harsh borders between groups of people in the human race and is therefore not very constructive in binding us together.

It is important for nurses to understand family health beliefs and behaviors influenced by racial identity, privilege, or oppression. In our clinical work with families, we have found it very useful to critically reflect on our own ideas about our race, marginalization, invisible and visible minorities and to vigorously pursue the differences between and within various racial groups. We believe health professionals should be racially and culturally sensitive.

Questions to Ask the Family.

- "What differences do you notice between, for example, your relatives' child-rearing practices and your own?"
- "Could you help me to understand what I need to know to be most helpful to you?"

Social Class

Social class, or socioeconomic status, shapes educational attainment, income, and occupation. Each class, whether upper-upper, lower-upper, upper-middle, lower-middle, upper-lower, or lower-lower, has its own clustering of values, lifestyles, and behaviors that influence family interaction and health-care practices. Social class affects how family members define themselves and are defined; what they cherish; how they organize their day-to-day lives; and how they meet challenges, struggles, and crises. For example, middle-class seniors may be more likely to help their adult children, whereas working-class older adults may be more likely to receive help.

Social class has been referred to as one of the prime molders of the family value and belief system. Much of the sociological and psychological research has been confounded by social class differences among ethnic groups. We believe that, in a racist and classist society, class and race are not inseparable.

Just as nursing has often been presented as intercultural, it has also been presented as interclass and nonpolitical. We believe that many nurses have pursued sickness in families to the exclusion of obtaining the *meaning* people give to events; their day-to-day living standards; and their access to employment, income, and housing. Social class issues have often been considered to be of little consequence to the "serious talk" about illness. This viewpoint has enabled nurses to sidestep many class issues associated with inequality and injustice. However, treatment must take into account the cultural, social, and economic context of the people seeking help. From factory workers to farmers to business executives, families are trying to cope with higher health-care costs and threats of losing insurance coverage. They continually make decisions based on which health care they can afford. With higher prescription drug costs and growth in the aging population, many families are anxious about their long-term care and ability to provide for their loved ones. Economic uncertainty, conflict and war, and fears of terrorism have created increased difficulties for the working poor.

Assessment of social class helps the nurse understand in a new way the family's stressors and resources. Generally speaking, women move down in social class following a divorce, whereas men do not. Recognizing differences in social class beliefs between themselves and families may encourage nurses to utilize new health promotion and intervention strategies. It is important for health-care delivery that nurses be aware of such influences as the "glass ceiling" and part-time temporary work versus full-time permanent work with benefits. In our clinical work we have often asked ourselves how a family's social class might influence their health-care beliefs, values, utilization of services, and interaction with us. Serious illness can intensify financial problems, diminish the capacity to deal with them, and call for solutions at odds with conventional financial wisdom. We have wondered about the intrafamilial differences with respect to class and how these might help or hinder a family coping with, for example, chronic illness.

Questions to Ask the Family.

- "How many times have you moved within the past 5 years?"
- "Have these moves had a positive or negative influence on your ability to deal with your son's HIV?"
- "How many schools has your daughter, Frances, attended?"
- "How does your money situation influence your use of health-care resources?"
- "What impact does Neil's shift work have on your family's stress level?"

Spirituality and/or Religion

Family members' spiritual and religious beliefs, rituals, and practices can have a positive or negative influence on their ability to cope with or manage an illness or health concern. Therefore, nurses must explore this previously neglected area. Emotions such as fear, guilt, anger, peace, and hope can be nurtured or tempered by one's spiritual or religious beliefs. Wright (2017) encourages distinguishing between spirituality and religion for the purposes of assessment and believes that doing so has the potential to invite more openness by family members regarding this potentially sensitive domain of inquiry. *Spirituality* is defined as whatever or whoever gives ultimate meaning and purpose in one's life and invites particular ways of being in the world toward others, oneself, and the universe (Wright, 2017). *Religion* is defined as an affiliation or a membership in a particular faith community that shares a set of beliefs, rituals, morals, and sometimes a health code centered on a defined higher or transcendent power most frequently referred to as God (Wright, 2017).

Levac, Wright, and Leahey (2002) recommend that assessment of the influence of religion is most critical at the time of diagnosis of a chronic or life-threatening illness. Assessment is especially important and relevant when crises have occurred that may cause extreme suffering, such as a traumatic death caused by a motor vehicle accident; sudden death due to illness, violence, or abuse; or a life-threatening diagnosis. In these situations, it is critical that the nurse ascertain what meaning the family gives to their suffering due to these tragic events and ultimately how family members make sense of their suffering (Wright, 2017). We think that beliefs, spirituality, and transcendence are keys to family resilience.

Spirituality and religion also influence family values, size, health care, and socialization practices. For example, individualism can be intricately related to religious ideals and work ethic. Community and family support, on the other hand, can also be evident in certain religions, and this can foster intergenerational and intragenerational support. Folk-healing traditions that combine health and religious practices are quite common in some ethnic groups. In some spiritualistic practices, a medium, or counselor, helps to exorcise the spirits causing illness. Such healers, religious leaders, shamans, and clergy can be invaluable resources for families dealing with crises and with long-term needs such as caregiver support.

Spirituality and religion are hidden and commonly underused resources in family work. We encourage nurses visiting families' homes to note the presence of signs of religious influence in the home—for example, statues, candles, flags, and religious texts, such as the Bible, Torah, or Koran. We have been curious about dietary restrictions and habits as well as traditional or alternative health practices influenced by religious beliefs. We have been cautious, however, not to assume that strong spiritual or religious beliefs enhance marital happiness or interaction, although they may diminish the possibility of divorce.

Our clinical work with families has taught us that the experience of suffering frequently becomes transposed to one of spirituality as family members try to find meaning in their suffering (Wright, 2017). If nurses are to be helpful, they must acknowledge that suffering, and in many cases the senselessness of it, is ultimately a spiritual issue. Therefore, in our clinical work we have asked ourselves about the influence of religion and spirituality on the family's health-care practices.

Questions to Ask the Family.

- "What meaning does spirituality or religion have for you in your everyday life?"
- "Are you involved with a mosque, temple, church, or synagogue?"
- "Would talking with anyone in your church help you cope with Pierre's illness?"
- "Are your spiritual beliefs a source of support for you in coping with your illness? A source of stress for you? For other family members?"
- "Who among your family members would most encourage your use of spiritual beliefs to cope with Perminder's cancer?"
- "What are your sources of hope?"
- "Have you found that prayer or other religious practices help you cope with your son Surinder's schizophrenia? If so, may I ask what you pray for?"
- "Have your prayers been answered?"
- "What does your religion say about gender roles? Ethnicity? Sexual orientation? How have these beliefs affected you, Davinderpal?"

Environment

The subcategory *environment* encompasses aspects of the larger community, the neighborhood, and the home. Environmental factors such as adequacy of space and privacy and accessibility of schools, day care, recreation, and public transportation influence family functioning. These are especially relevant for older adults, who are more likely to remain in a poor environment even if it has become dangerous to live there.

In our clinical work with families, we have asked ourselves and the nurses with whom we work to consider whether the home is adequate for the number of people living there. Does our perception differ from the family's perception? What health and other basic services are available within the home? Within the neighborhood? How accessible, in terms of distance, convenience, and so forth, are transportation and recreation services? How safe is the area? By asking in an open-ended way what other contextual forces may influence the family, it is possible to obtain a much broader range of responses. These can vary from "belief in politics" to "shopping at the mall" to "music."

Questions to Ask the Family.

- "What community services does your family use?"
- "Are there community services you would like to learn about but do not know how to contact?"

- "On a scale of 1 to 10, with 10 being most comfortable, how comfortable are you in your neighborhood?"
- "What would make you more comfortable so that you can continue to function independently at home?"

Structural Assessment Tools

The genogram and the ecomap are two tools that are particularly helpful in outlining a family's internal and external structures. Each is simple to use and requires only a piece of paper and a pen. The genograph designed by Duhamel and Campagna (2000) can also be used to draw the genogram. Alternatively, some computer programs have genograms as a feature.

KEY CONCEPT DEFINED

Genogram

A structural assessment tool that shows a diagram of the family constellation.

The *genogram* is a diagram of the family constellation. The *ecomap,* on the other hand, is a diagram of the family's contact with others outside the immediate family. It pictures the important connections between the family and the world. We are aware of the arbitrariness of the distinction for some cultural groups between a genogram and an ecomap. For example, the standard genogram may be difficult to complete with families who do not solely believe that family is strictly a biological entity. We encourage nurses to develop a fit between these tools to depict specific family compositions.

KEY CONCEPT DEFINED

Ecomap

A structural assessment tool that shows a diagram of the family's contact with others outside the immediate family and illustrates the important connections between the family and the world.

These tools have been developed as family assessment, planning, and intervention devices. They can be used to reframe behaviors, relationships, and time connections within families, as well as to detoxify and normalize families' perceptions of themselves. By pointing to the future as well as to the past and the present, genograms facilitate alternative interpretations of family experience. They can help both the nurse and the family see the larger picture and view problems in both a historical and current context. Genograms can also be used to foster the training of culturally competent clinicians and for nurses to increase their self-awareness.

Darwent, McInnes, and Swanson (2016) adapted the genogram to develop an Infant Feeding Genogram to map the family structure of women who were the first in their families to breastfeed their children. This unique use of a genogram resulted in setting the context for discussions about women's experience of breastfeeding within their family culture by helping to identify strengths and possible deficits in social supports.

We agree with McGoldrick, Gerson, and Petry (2008) that although much can be said about expanding genograms to include issues from larger social contexts (the sexual, cultural, religious, or spiritual genogram), realistically such mapping is extremely difficult to accomplish. Gendergrams have been developed to map gender relationships over the life cycle. At best, we can probably explore only a few dimensions at a time, and we recommend that these dimensions be directly connected to the purpose of the family's encounter with the nurse. For example, a nurse meeting with a couple in a rehabilitation treatment center for sexual addiction might reasonably explore a family's sexual and addiction history on a genogram. This content area would likely not be appropriate for a nurse meeting with a family in an intensive care unit. McGoldrick et al (2008) have outlined important issues that are difficult to capture on genograms:

- Family members involved in family business
- Family members' relationships to the health-care system
- Cultural genogram issues
- Family secrets
- Particular family-relationship nuances, including power, patterns of avoidance, and so forth
- Patterns of friendship
- Relationships with work colleagues
- Spiritual genograms
- Community genograms
- Tracking medical and psychological stressors

Genograms don't typically show the emotional connections among family members, present or past. The complex relationships of those who have warmed our hearts, mentored and nurtured us, aggravated us, or caused us severe trauma generally are not depicted. This is both a limitation of genograms and an asset; genograms tend to be a quick snapshot of the present.

With the help of computers, we can make three-dimensional maps that enable us to track complex genogram patterns. Our caution for practicing nurses is to use the genogram as a clinically relevant tool, not as a map or data-collection sheet. Computerized genograms enable us to explore specific family patterns, resiliencies, and symptom constellations. Gathering, mapping, and tracking family history is much easier using a computer database. We urge nurses to ask themselves: "What is the purpose of collecting vast amounts of information about this family's history, and how will this information be helpful for the purpose of my work with this family?" Using computers and genogram information will provide rich data for family research, but it is unknown how useful this will be for immediate family care. Of course, by using computer genogram software, there will be many more possibilities for depicting family issues at different moments in family history. Clinicians and family members will have the opportunity to choose what aspects of a genogram they want to display for a particular purpose and at the same time create a database of a family's whole history.

Genogram

Genograms convey a great deal of information in the form of a visual gestalt. When one considers the number of words it would take to portray the facts thus represented, it becomes clear how simple and useful these tools are. Genograms, when placed on patients' charts, act as constant visual reminders for nurses to "think family." As an engagement tool, the genogram is helpful to use during the first meeting with the family. It provides rich data about relationships over time and may also include small amounts of data about health, occupation, religion, ethnicity, and migrations. The genogram can be used to elicit information helpful to both the family and the nurse about development and other areas of family functioning. It is a tool that enables clinicians to develop hypotheses for additional evaluation in a family assessment.

The skeleton of the genogram (a blank genogram is shown in Figure 3-2) tends to follow conventional genetic and genealogic charts and depicts the internal family structure:

- It includes at least three generations.
- Family members are placed on horizontal rows that signify generational lines (a marriage or common-law relationship is denoted by a horizontal line).
- Children are denoted by vertical lines.
- Children are rank-ordered from left to right beginning with the eldest child.
- Each individual is represented.

Some authors differ slightly in the symbols they use to denote the details of the genogram. The symbols in Figure 3-3, however, are generally agreed on. With the increased use of computer genograms, symbols and color coding will become standardized.

The person's name and age should be noted inside the square or circle. Outside the symbol, significant data gathered from the family (e.g., "travels a lot," "depressed," "overinvolved in work") should be noted. If

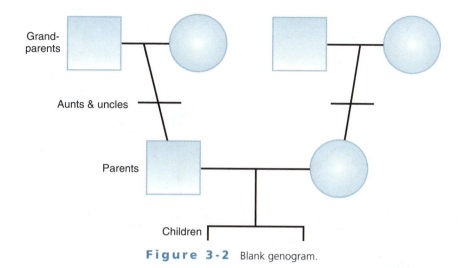

F i g u r e 3 - 2 Blank genogram.

a family member has died, the year of his or her death is indicated above the square or circle. When the symbol for miscarriage is used, the sex of the child should be identified if it is known. A small square is used to denote a sperm donor (McGoldrick et al, 2008). It is helpful to draw a circle around the different households. We find that when children have lived in several contexts (e.g., immediate biological family, foster family, grandparents, adoptive family), separate genograms can help to show the child's multiple families over time.

The following is an example of a nuclear and extended family genogram (Figure 3-4):

The Lamensa Family

- Raffaele, age 47, married to Silvana, age 35, since 2000, lived common-law for 2 years prior to their marriage.
- There are two children: Gemma, age 14, in grade 8, and Antonio, age 7, repeating grade 1.
- Raffaele is employed as a machinist; Silvana refers to him as "an alcoholic."
- Silvana is a homemaker and states that she has been "depressed" for several years.
- Both of Raffaele's parents are deceased; his father died in 2010, and his mother died in 2008 of a stroke.
- Raffaele's older brother Antonio also has a drinking problem; Antonio was named for his grandfather.
- Silvana's mother, Nunziata, age 54, has arthritis and is getting progressively worse since her husband died in 2007.
- Silvana has two older sisters and a brother.

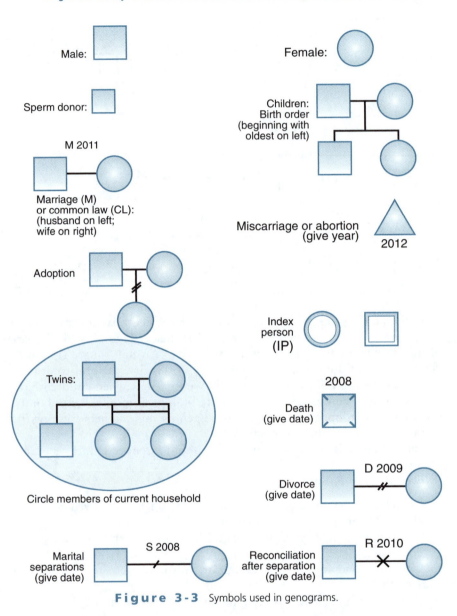

Figure 3-3 Symbols used in genograms.

The following is an example of a family genogram for a lesbian couple with a child born to one of them (Figure 3-5):

Jennifer and Amanda

- Jennifer (age 30) and Amanda (age 28) have lived as a couple since 2016 and have been married since 2018.

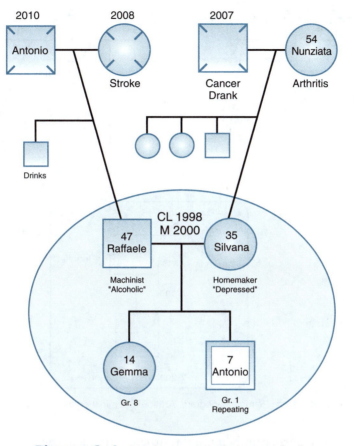

Figure 3-4 Sample genogram: The Lamensa family.

- Jennifer's biological son, Griffin (age 8), was conceived by artificial insemination (the unknown sperm donor is depicted as a small square).
- Jennifer's mother, Adrienne, a retired nurse (age 65), divorced Jennifer's father in 1991; remarried in 1993; had another daughter, Mitzi, by her second husband; and became a widow when he died in 1999.
- Mitzi (age 24) is considering transgender surgery.
- Amanda's parents are separated, and her father is living common-law with Dan, his business partner.
- Amanda has no siblings.
- Jennifer has a younger brother, Spencer (age 28), and a half sister, Mitzi.

How to Use a Genogram At the beginning of the interview, the nurse engages the family by informing them that they will be having a conversation so that the nurse can gain an overview of who is in the family and their

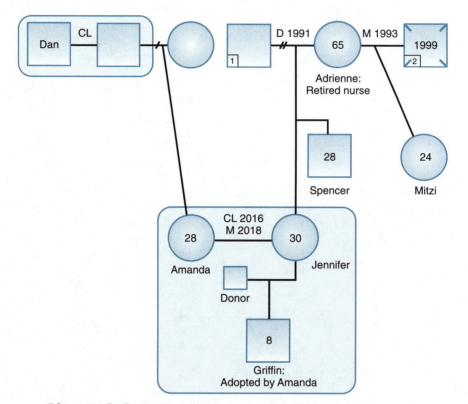

Figure 3-5 Sample genogram: Artificial insemination and lesbian couple.

situation. The nurse can then use the structure of the genogram to discern the family's internal and external structures as well as context. Thus, the nurse gains an understanding of the family's composition and boundaries.

Initially, the nurse starts out with a blank sheet of paper and draws a line or circle for the first person in the family to whom a question is directed.

The following is a sample interview with the Manuyag family:

> *Nurse:* Elena, you said you were 23, and Matias, how old are you?
>
> *Matias:* Thirty-four.
>
> *Nurse:* How long have you been married?
>
> *Matias:* This time or the first time?
>
> *Nurse:* This time. And then the first time.
>
> *Matias:* Just 2 years for Elena and me.
>
> *Nurse:* And the first time?
>
> *Matias:* Ten years for the first one.

Nurse: And, Elena, have you been married before?

Elena: (*Laughs nervously*) I'm only 23.

Nurse: Sure, it's just that many people have lived together in common-law marriages or married when they were very young.

Elena: No. I lived with my parents till I met Matias.

Nurse: Do either of you have children from prior relationships? (*Turns to both Matias and Elena*)

Matias: Yes, I have two sons.

Elena: No.

Nurse: In addition to Teresita here (*Looks at baby on couch*), do the two of you have any other children?

Elena: Yes, there's Manandro.

Matias: Old stinko, you mean.

Nurse: Old stinko?

Matias: He isn't toilet trained yet.

Nurse: Oh, I see. And he's how old?

Elena: He's almost 3. I've been trying to train him since I knew I was pregnant with Teresita, but he just doesn't seem to want to be trained.

Nurse: (*Nods*) Mm.

Matias: Yeah, old stinko!

Nurse: And Teresita is how many weeks now?

Elena: She'll be 21 days tomorrow (*Smiles at baby*).

Nurse: Does anyone else live with you?

Matias: No. Her parents live next door.

The nurse now has a rudimentary genogram of the Manuyag family (Figure 3-6) and has gathered information that may or may not be significant, depending on the way in which the family has responded to various events in the history of their family, such as the following:

- Manandro was conceived before the marriage.
- Manandro is unaffectionately called "old stinko" by his father.
- Elena has been trying to toilet train Manandro since he was 24 months old.
- Elena lived with her family of origin before the marriage; they now live next door.
- Matias has been married before and has two other sons.

After inquiring about the nuclear family, the nurse can continue to inquire about the extended family. It is generally not very important to go into

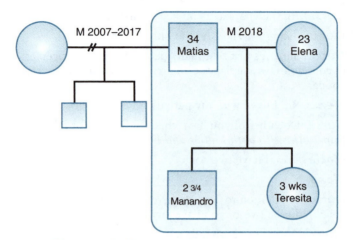

Figure 3-6 Genogram of the Manuyag family.

great detail about these relatives, but clinical judgment should prevail. If, for example, the grandparents are involved in a child's colostomy care, then a three-generational genogram should be constructed. On the other hand, if a child has a sprained wrist or something relatively minor, then a two-generational genogram is sufficient. After asking questions about the husband's parents and siblings, the nurse should then inquire about the wife's family of origin. It is important for the nurse to gain an overview of the family structure without getting sidetracked or inundated by a large volume of information. Box 3-1 contains helpful hints for constructing genograms.

The same question format used for nuclear families is used for stepfamilies, with one exception. It is generally easier to ask one spouse about his or her previous relationships before going on to ask the other spouse the same questions. This idea holds true especially in working with complex family situations involving multiple parenting figures and siblings. Again, it is unnecessary to gather specific information on all extended family members. It is useful to draw a circle around the current family members to distinguish among the various households. Usually it is easiest to indicate the year of a divorce rather than the number of years ago that it happened.

The following is an example of a sample genogram for a stepfamily (Figure 3-7):

- Michael (age 35) and Melanie (age 33) have had a common-law marriage since 2016.
- Melanie is a part-time waitress.
- Melanie has two children by her first marriage, Kathy (age 12) and Jacob (age 11).
- Jacob has attention deficit-hyperactivity disorder (ADHD) and is in a special class in grade 4.

Box 3-1 Helpful Hints for Constructing Genograms

- Determine priorities for genogram construction based on the family situation.
- A three-generational genogram may be useful when the child's health problem (physical or emotional) is influenced by or affects the third generation.
- A brief two-generational genogram is generally most useful initially, especially for a family that has preventive health-care needs (immunizations) or minor health concerns (sports injury). The nurse can always expand to the third generation if needed.
- Invite as many family members to the initial meeting or visit as possible to obtain each family member's view and to observe family interaction.
- Engage the family in an exercise to complete the genogram.
- Use the genogram to "break the ice," provide structure, and introduce purposeful conversation.
- Ask family members how an absent significant family member might answer a question.
- Avoid discussion that is hurtful or blameful, especially of absent family members.
- Take an interest in each family member, and be sensitive to developmental differences.
- Tailor questions to children's developmental stages so that they become active contributors.
- Notice children's nonverbal and verbal comments.
- If some members are shy or seem uninterested in participating directly (such as adolescents), ask other family members about them.
- Begin by asking "easy" questions of individuals, followed by an exploration of subsystems.
- Ask concrete, easy-to-answer questions of individuals (especially children) about ages, occupations, interests, health status, school grades, and teachers to increase their comfort levels.
- Move the discussion about individuals to subsystems to elicit family relational data. Inquire about parent-child or sibling relationships, depending on parenting concerns.
- With stepfamilies, ask questions about contact with the noncustodial parent, custody, the children's satisfaction with visits, and stepfamily relationships.
- Observe family interactions.
- During genogram construction, note the content (what is said) and the process (how it is said).
- Move from the discussion about the present family situation to questions about the extended family if it seems relevant (for example, "Are Ruhi's parents able to help with the baby's tracheostomy care? What about babysitting?").

Continued

Box 3-1 Helpful Hints for Constructing Genograms—cont'd

- When discussing generations, the nurse may find it useful to ask about psychosocial family health history (for example, "Is there a history of alcohol abuse [or violence, learning problems, or mental illness] in your family?"). Questions should be tailored to the family's particular area of concern rather than generic exploration.

Levac, A. M., Wright, L. M., & Leahey, M. (2002). Children and families: Models for assessment and intervention. In J. Fox (Ed.), Primary healthcare of infants, children and adolescents (p. 14). St. Louis, MO: Mosby. Copyright 2002. Adapted with permission.

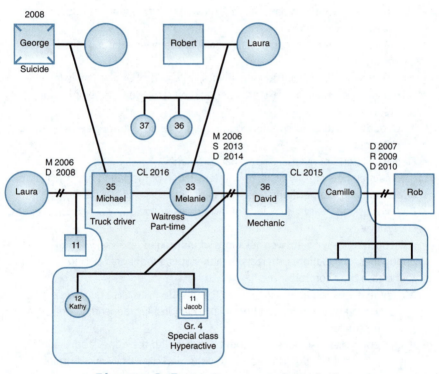

Figure 3-7 Sample genogram of a stepfamily.

- Michael married his first wife, Laura, in 2006 and divorced in 2008.
- Michael and Laura had one son, who is now age 11.
- Michael is an only child; his father committed suicide in 2008; his mother is still alive.
- Melanie is the youngest of three daughters, and both of her parents are living.

- Melanie married David in 2006, separated in 2013, and divorced in 2014.
- David (age 36) is a mechanic who is presently living in a common-law marriage with Camille and her three sons.
- Camille and her first husband, Rob, divorced in 2007, reconciled in 2009, and then divorced in 2010.

There are no specific guidelines for drawing genograms illustrating complex stepfamily situations. Generally, however, what works best is for the nurse to start by gathering information about the immediate household. After this, the nurse draws each family's constellation. Whenever possible, it is best to show children from different marriages in their correct birth order, oldest on the left and youngest on the right. We agree with McGoldrick et al (2008) that the rule of thumb is, when feasible, that different marriages follow in chronological order from left to right. We have sometimes found it helpful to indicate the number of the relationship or marriage in the lower left-hand corner when there have been several relationships. See Figure 3-5, where Adrienne's husbands are indicated as #1 and #2. It can be useful to draw a circle around each separate household. If one member of a couple is involved in an affair, then their relationship is depicted with a dotted rather than a solid line. Additional pertinent information, such as children moving between two households, can be written to the side of the genogram. It is important for the nurse to remember that the purpose of drawing the genogram is to obtain a visual overview of the family. The genogram is not meant to be an exact chart for genetics.

Other problems arise when there are multiple marriages, intermarriages, and remarriages within the family. For example, when cousins or stepsiblings marry, the clinician should use separate pages to clarify intricacies. With complex family situations, the nurse needs to choose between clarity and level of detail. When computers are used to diagram genograms, complexity can be reduced by zooming in on relevant significant information. We advise nurses to let practicality and possibility be their guide.

Develop a genogram that is useful rather than one that is overly inclusive and too confusing. Sometimes the only feasible way for pediatric nurses to clarify where children were raised is to take chronological notes on each child and draw multiple genograms through time to show the various family constellations the child experienced. With software, specific genograms can be created for specific moments in a person's life. When discrepancies exist in information shared by various family members, we advise nurses to note this on the genogram but not to take on an investigative role. There can be multiple truths and recollections of information.

Another example of a stepfamily genogram is depicted in Figure 3-8.

The Faris Family

- David (age 42) is a software designer living common-law since 2015 with Patti (age 40), a part-time retail associate.

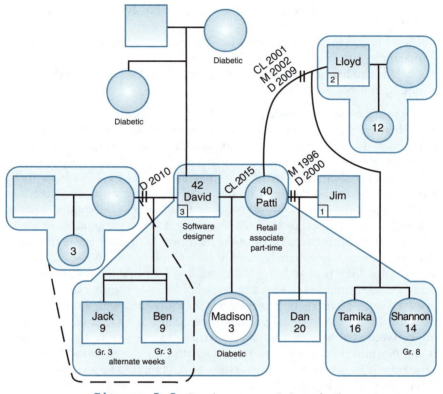

Figure 3-8 Sample genogram: Faris stepfamily.

- David and Patti have a daughter, Madison (age 3), recently diagnosed with juvenile diabetes.
- David's twin sons, Jack and Ben (age 9), spend alternate weeks at their mom's townhouse and at David and Patti's apartment.
- David was divorced in 2010; his former wife has a daughter, age 3.
- Patti has a son, Dan (age 20), by her first husband, Jim, whom she divorced in 2000.
- Dan lives alone and works several part-time jobs in bars.
- Patti has two other daughters: Tamika (age 16), who recently dropped out of school, and Shannon (age 14), in grade 8, from her second marriage, to Lloyd, which ended in divorce in 2009.
- Tamika and Shannon live with their mom and visit Lloyd and his family for 2 weeks most summers.
- The current health concern is Madison's juvenile diabetes.
- The current household consists of David, Patti, the three girls, and on alternate weeks, the twin boys.
- David's mom has diabetes, as does his older sister.

An example of a family in which a child lives with the grandmother and her husband is provided in Figure 3-9:

The Fitzgerald-Kucewicz Family

- Sophia Kucewicz (age 8), lives with her grandmother, Patricia Fitzgerald (age 45); Vincent, Patricia's common-law partner of 10 years; and Sophia's aunt, Susan.
- Patricia was previously married to Steven Fitzgerald for 14 years.
- Patricia and Steven had three children: Susan (age 19), Douglas (age 23), and Joan (age 25), who is Sophia's mother.
- Joan became pregnant with Sophia when she was 16.
- Sophia's father, Michael Kucewicz, and her mother had a brief relationship, through which she was conceived.
- Michael was aware of the pregnancy; he left the city shortly before Sophia was born, never meeting her.
- When Sophia was 2 years old, Joan had another child, Kayla, who subsequently went to live with her natural father when she was 4.
- When Sophia was 3, her mother moved in with Ben, whom Sophia came to know as her father.
- Joan and Ben had difficulty providing a stable environment for Sophia and Kayla and, from time to time, moved in with Patricia and Vincent.

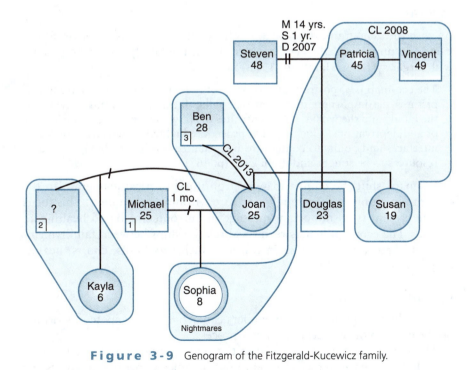

Figure 3-9 Genogram of the Fitzgerald-Kucewicz family.

- Patricia reports that both Joan and Ben used drugs and alcohol and were often unemployed.
- Ben was physically and verbally abusive to Joan, and after a particularly frightening episode between Joan and Ben that took place in the basement of Patricia's home, Joan called the police. The child welfare department became involved, leading Patricia and Vincent to take guardianship of Sophia.
- Joan and Ben moved to a place of their own, agreeing to take Sophia every other weekend.
- The health concern for this family is Sophia's nightmares, especially after returning from visits to Joan and Ben's trailer home.

Most families are extremely receptive to and interested in collaborating with the nurse to complete a genogram. For some, it is the first time that they have ever seen their family life pictured in this manner. Therefore, the nurse needs to be aware that the family may have a reaction to significant events. One family, for example, may express some sensitive material in a very blasé fashion. If divorce is common in their families of origin, they may not hesitate to discuss their several marriages and those of their siblings. On the other hand, a devout Catholic family may be exquisitely sensitive to seeing the nurse write the word "divorce."

Ecomap

As with the genogram, the primary value of the ecomap is in its visual impact. The purpose of the ecomap is to depict the family members' contact with larger systems. Hartman (1978) notes:

> The eco-map [sic] portrays an overview of the family in their situation; it pictures the important nurturant or conflict-laden connections between the family and the world. It demonstrates the flow of resources, or the lack of and deprivations. This mapping procedure highlights the nature of the interfaces and points to conflicts to be mediated, bridges to be built, and resources to be sought and mobilized. (p. 467)

Ecomaps shift the emphasis away from the historical genogram to the current functioning of the family and its environmental context. This focus on the present is an important message in our outcome-based health-care climate. The ecomap depicts reciprocal relationships between family members and broader community institutions such as schools, courts, health-care facilities, and so forth.

How to Use an Ecomap

As with the genogram, family members can actively participate in working on the ecomap during the assessment process.

The family genogram is placed in the center circle, labeled "Family or household." The outer circles represent significant people, agencies, or institutions in the family's context. The size of the circles is not important. Lines are drawn between the family and the outer circles to indicate the nature of the connections that exist. Straight lines indicate strong connections, dotted lines indicate tenuous connections, and slashed lines indicate stressful relations. The wider the line, the stronger the tie. Arrows can be drawn alongside the lines to indicate the flow of energy and resources. Additional circles may be drawn as necessary, depending on the number of significant contacts the family has.

An ecomap for the Lamensa family is illustrated in Figure 3-10:

- Raffaele, Silvana, Gemma, and Antonio are placed in the center circle.
- Raffaele has strong connections with his workplace, where he is a foreman and a union representative. He has moderately strong bonds with his "drinking buddies." These relationships, however, are stressful for him.

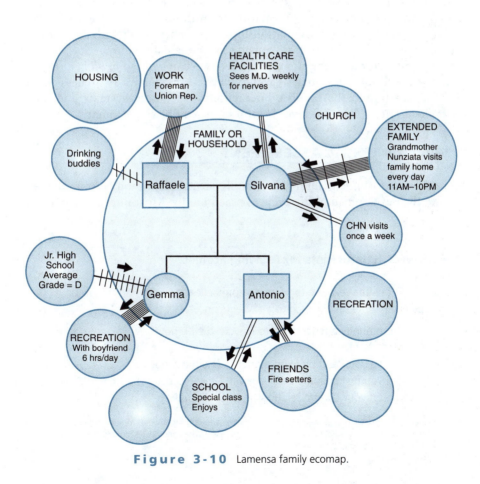

Figure 3-10 Lamensa family ecomap.

- Silvana's connections are mainly with her mother and the health-care system. She sees her family physician every week "for nerves" and sees a community health nurse (CHN) once a week. Silvana's mother, Nunziata, visits Silvana every day from 11 a.m. to 10 p.m. There is a strong connection between Silvana and her mother, but Silvana says she really "doesn't like Mom coming over so often."
- Antonio has a few friends, most of whom set fires. He is in a special class for his learning disability and enjoys both the teacher and the school.
- Gemma is in junior high school, where she maintains an average grade of D. She frequently does not attend school, and when she does attend, she participates little. She spends about 6 hours a day with her boyfriend.

When the CHN completed the ecomap with the Lamensa family, Mrs. Lamensa (Silvana) commented, "I seem to spend all my time with medical or health people." Mr. Lamensa (Raffaele) then said, "You're also so busy with your mother that you don't have time for anybody else." The nurse was able to use this information from the ecomap to discuss further with the family the types of relationships they wanted both with those inside their household and with those outside the immediate family.

In summary, the genogram and the ecomap can be used in *all* health-care settings, especially in primary care, to increase the nurse's awareness of the whole family and the family's interactions with larger systems and their extended family. Box 3-2 gives helpful hints for drawing ecomaps.

DEVELOPMENTAL ASSESSMENT

In addition to understanding the family structure, the nurse must understand the developmental life cycle for each family. Most nurses are familiar

---

Box 3-2 Helpful Hints for Drawing Ecomaps

Pose questions that explore the family's connections to other individuals or groups outside the family, such as:

- "What community agencies are you involved with now? Which are most and least helpful?"
- "How would you describe your relationship with school staff?"
- "How did you first become involved with Child Protective Services? What is the nature of your current relationship with them?"

Levac, A.M., Wright, L.M., & Leahey, M. (2002). Children and families: Models for assessment and intervention. In J. Fox (Ed.), Primary healthcare of infants, children and adolescents (p. 14). St. Louis, MO: Mosby. Copyright 2002. Adapted with permission.

with the stages of child development and the literature in the area of adult development. Many are becoming interested in the burgeoning literature about development in the senior years, an interest that has been fostered by the aging of the baby boomer generation. But what of family development? It is more than the concurrent development at different phases of children, adults, and seniors who happen to call themselves "family." We believe families are people who have a shared history and a shared future.

KEY CONCEPT DEFINED

Developmental Assessment

One of the categories of the Calgary Family Assessment Model (CFAM) that nurses use to identify the developmental life cycle for each family.

Family development is an over-arching concept, but each family has its own developmental path, influenced by its past and present context and its future aspirations. McGoldrick, Garcio Preto, and Carter (2016) believe that "individuals and families transform, and need to transform, their relationships as they evolve, to adapt to changing circumstances over the life course" (p. 7). There is no single family developmental life cycle or model. This is especially evident as our population ages. The natural sequential phases of generational boundaries are not as clear as in the past with, for example, children maturing at earlier ages but living at home longer, the trend toward later marriages, and seniors continuing to work well into their 60s. This blurring of boundaries can sometimes lead to tension and confusion within families.

KEY CONCEPT DEFINED

Family Development

The unique path constructed by a family that is shaped by predictable and unpredictable events and societal trends.

In keeping with postmodernist ideas, we believe that there are limits to describing family development in precise, absolute, universal ways. Postmodernists differ from modernists in that exceptions interest them more than rules; specific, contextualized details more than grand generalizations; difference rather than similarity. We are not concerned with authoritative truth, facts, and rules but rather with the meaning a family gives to its particular story of development over time.

We have found it useful to distinguish between *family development* and *family life cycle*. Family development emphasizes the *unique* path constructed by a family. It is shaped by predictable and unpredictable events, such as illness, catastrophes (e.g., terrorist attacks, fires, earthquakes, hurricanes, floods), and societal trends (e.g., Internet and cell-phone usage, stock market fluctuations, company mergers, changes in crime and birth rates).

Family life cycle refers to the *typical* path most families go through. The typical life-cycle events are connected to the comings and goings of family members. For example, most families experience certain events in their life cycle, such as birth, child-rearing, departure of children from the household, retirement, and death. These events generate changes requiring a formal reorganization of roles and rules within the family. The life-cycle course of families evolves through a generally predictable sequence of stages, despite cultural and ethnic variations. Although individual variations, timing, and coping strategies exist, biological time clocks and societal expectations for events such as entrance into elementary school and retirement from work are relatively typical in North America.

KEY CONCEPT DEFINED

Family Life Cycle

The typical path most families follow; generally predictable sequence of stages connected to the comings and goings of family members, such as birth, child-rearing, departure of children from the household, retirement, and death.

Given our keen interest in a particular family's specific development over time, it might be questioned why we include a family developmental section in the CFAM at all. We take the position that an informed "not-knowing" stance is useful when working with families. That is, we seek to be informed by the literature, research, and other families' stories of development. Yet, we are "not knowing" but curious about this particular family's developmental story in terms of how the family members progressed through time.

A rich history about family development still pervades clinicians' thinking. It is useful for nurses to have some understanding of this history. The early proponents of the family life cycle (Duvall, 1977) developed a four-stage model that was subsequently expanded into an eight-stage model featuring successive stages in the progression of primary marriages. With the increase in various family forms, more complex designs were created. Most recently, the Multicontextual Life Cycle Framework for Clinical Assessment developed by McGoldrick et al (2016) has become a helpful framework for conceptualizing the complexities of the life cycle. It provides a visual of the individual within the context of the multigenerational family system, which is embedded in the larger social context, all moving through time simultaneously.

In the field of family therapy, there were "pioneers" in applying the family development framework. Much was written about the interface among family development, functioning, and therapy. Carter and McGoldrick (1988) believed that the family life-cycle perspective viewed symptoms in relation to normal functioning over time and that "therapy" helped to reestablish the family's developmental momentum. Family therapists such as Haley (1977), Minuchin (1974), and Selvini, Boscolo, Cecchin, and Prata (1980) noted the frequency of symptom appearance with the addition or loss of a family member. These therapists worked with families that did not move smoothly or automatically from one stage in the family life cycle to another, and they focused on the stressful transition points between stages. In doing an assessment and in planning interventions, these therapists paid considerable attention to life-cycle events as markers of change. Although their approaches differed, they similarly sought to understand the relationship between psychopathology and the family's developmental life-cycle stage.

Family development is now seen as an interactive process in which the historian influences which stories of development are told and emphasized. All of these changes have required a critical rethinking of our assumptions about "normality" and the idea of "family" development. The relationship between demographic changes and alterations in the prevalence, timing, and sequencing of some key family transitions must also be noted.

In our clinical work with families presenting in various forms and at all stages of development, we have found it useful to adopt Falicov's (2012) ideas about family development. She emphasizes culture and gender relativity rather than universality, transitions rather than stages, dimensions and processes rather than markers, and a resource rather than a deficit orientation. We concur with her idea that a systems approach to family development calls for a dialectical integration of two tendencies: stability and change. The emphasis is on both tendencies rather than one or the other. Change and stability must be addressed simultaneously. We do not find it clinically useful to think of families as "stuck" and unable to bring about change. Rather, we find it clinically useful to look for patterns of continuity, identity, and stability that can be maintained while new behavioral patterns are changing.

There is much evidence to support the position that nurses will find heuristic value in the family development category of the CFAM. They should be aware, however, of some of the problems in its indiscriminate adoption and application. We find it indefensible for some nurses to make sweeping generalizations such as, "The family life cycle is genetically determined," or, "The family life cycle is culturally universal." We urge nurses to carefully consider the implications of a family's ethnicity, race, and social class in applying the family development category.

We also caution nurses against *indiscriminately* applying the family development category and overemphasizing *smooth progression*. Contradictions and difficulties inherent in progressing through the life cycle are normal. Families are complex systems that need to deal with many different progressions at once—that is, there are biological, psychological, sociological, and cultural progressions. Tensions and continuing change brought about by contradictions between these progressions are normal. Family life is seldom smooth or bland; rather, it is zestful and active. We therefore encourage nurses, when using the family development category, to have families discuss their joys and satisfactions as well as their tensions and stresses. The family developmental story told by one family member is from that member's "observer perspective" (Maturana & Varela, 1992).

In addition to delineating stages and tasks implicit in the family life cycle, we have found it useful to notice the attachments between family members. *Attachment* refers to a relatively enduring, unique emotional tie between two specific persons. Each person has the need for emotional connection while also remaining secure in his or her own individuality.

Bowlby (1977) notes:

Affectional bonds and subjective states of a strong emotion tend to go together.... Thus many of the most intensive of all emotions arise during the formation, the maintenance, the disruption and renewal of affectional bonds which for that reason are sometimes called emotional bonds. In terms of subjective experience the formation of a bond is described as falling in love, maintaining a bond as loving someone, and losing a partner as grieving over someone. Similarly the threat of loss arouses anxiety and actual loss causes sorrow, while both situations are likely to arouse anger. Finally the unchallenged maintenance of a bond is experienced as a source of security and renewal of a bond as a source of joy. (p. 203)

Although the terms *bonding* and *attachment* are sometimes used to describe different relationships, we have chosen in this book and in our clinical work to make no distinction between these terms. We recognize the complexity of relationships that arise from international connections between family members and the relationship stresses and the hard choices economic and social immigrants face with separations and reunions of parents, young children, and elderly family members. When working with a family, we tend to pay the most attention to the reciprocal nature of an attachment and the quality of the affectional tie.

We illustrate these bonds between family members by drawing attachment diagrams. The symbols used in these diagrams (Figure 3-11) are similar to those used in the structural assessment diagrams. It is important for us to emphasize that there is no one right level of attachment or best attachment configuration.

We are partial to the idea of the network paradigm as a useful base to integrate attachment and family systems theories. Such a paradigm integrates dyadic and family systems as simultaneously distinct and yet interconnected. The clinician holds multiple perspectives in mind, considers each system level as both a part and a whole, and shifts the focus between levels

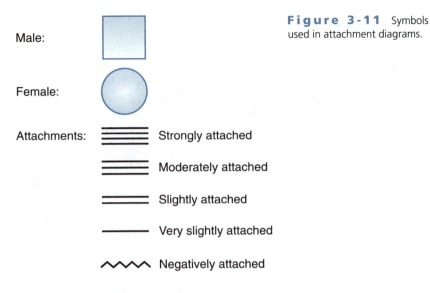

Figure 3-11 Symbols used in attachment diagrams.

as required. We like this concept because it expands attachment to include multiple system levels and networks, which is especially important as the baby boomer cohort increases in age. Attachment theory is relevant to more than just parent-infant bonding; it is important for all ages. The key elements of attachment processes (affect regulation, interpersonal understanding, information processing, and the provision of comfort within intimate relationships) are as applicable to family systems as they are to individual development.

In the CFAM developmental category, we discuss family life-cycle stages, the emotional process of transition (namely, key principles), and second-order changes—the issues dealt with and tasks often accomplished during each stage. In an effort to emphasize the variability of family development, we discuss six sample types of family life cycles:

1. Middle-class North American family life cycle
2. Divorce and post-divorce family life cycle
3. Remarried family life cycle
4. Professional and low-income family life cycles
5. Adoptive family life cycle
6. Lesbian, gay, bisexual, queer, intersex, transgender and twin-spirited family life cycles

Middle-Class North American Family Life Cycle

We are grateful to McGoldrick et al (2016) for delineating six phases in the North American middle-class family life cycle (summarized in Table 3-1). We highlight the expansion, contraction, and realignment of relationships as

TABLE 3-1	Phases of the Family Life Cycle	
FAMILY LIFE CYCLE PHASE	**EMOTIONAL PROCESS OF TRANSITION: KEY PREREQUISITE ATTITUDES**	**SECOND-ORDER TASKS/ CHANGES OF THE SYSTEM TO PROCEED DEVELOPMENTALLY**
Emerging young adults	Accepting emotional and financial responsibility for self	a. Differentiation of self in relation to family of origin b. Development of intimate peer relationships c. Establishment of self in respect to work and financial independence d. Establishment of self in community and larger society e. Establishment of one's worldview, spirituality, religion, and relationship to nature f. Parents shifting to consultative role in young adult's relationships
Couple formation: the joining of families	Commitment to new expanded system	a. Formation of couple system b. Expansion of family boundaries to include new partner and extended family c. Realignment of relationships among couple, parents and siblings, extended family, friends, and larger community
Families with young children	Accepting new members into the system	a. Adjustment of couple system to make space for children b. Collaboration in child-rearing and financial and housekeeping tasks c. Realignment of relationships with extended family to include parenting and grandparenting roles d. Realignment of relationships with community and larger social system to include new family structure and relationships
Families with adolescents	Increasing flexibility of family boundaries to permit children's independence and grandparents' frailties	a. Shift of parent–child relationships to permit adolescent to have more independent activities and relationships and to move more flexibly into and out of system b. Families helping emerging adolescents negotiate relationships with community c. Refocus on midlife couple and career issues d. Begin shift toward caring for older generation

TABLE 3-1	Phases of the Family Life Cycle—cont'd	
FAMILY LIFE CYCLE PHASE	**EMOTIONAL PROCESS OF TRANSITION: KEY PREREQUISITE ATTITUDES**	**SECOND-ORDER TASKS/ CHANGES OF THE SYSTEM TO PROCEED DEVELOPMENTALLY**
Launching children and moving on at midlife	Accepting a multitude of exits from and entries into the system	a. Renegotiation of couple system as a dyad b. Development of adult-to-adult relationships between parents and grown children c. Realignment of relationships to include in-laws and grandchildren d. Realignment of relationships with community to include new constellation of family relationships e. Exploration of new interests/ career, given the freedom from childcare responsibilities f. Dealing with care needs, disabilities, and death of parents (grandparents)
Families in late middle age	Accepting shifting generational roles	a. Maintaining or modifying own and/or couple and social functioning and interests in the face of physiological decline: exploration of new familial and social role options b. Supporting more central role of middle generations c. Making room in the system for the wisdom and experience of the elders d. Supporting older generation without overfunctioning them
Families nearing the end of life	Accepting the realities of family members' limitations and death and the completion of one cycle of life	a. Dealing with loss of spouse, siblings, and other peers b. Making preparations for death and legacy c. Managing reversed roles in caretaking between middle and older generations d. Realignment of relationships with larger community and social system to acknowledge changing life cycle relationships

McGoldrick, Monica; Carter, Betty; Garcia-Preto, Nydia. (Eds.). (2016). The Expanded Family Life Cycle: Individual, Family and Social Perspectives, 5th edition, copyright 2016, pp 24 - 25. Reprinted by permission of Pearson Education, Inc. Upper Saddle River, NJ.

entries, exits, and development of family members occur. Although the relationship patterns and family themes may sound familiar, we wish to emphasize that the structure and form of the North American family are changing radically. It is important for nurses to have a positive conceptual framework for what *is*: dual-career families, permanent single-parent households, unmarried couples, homosexual couples, remarried couples, and sole-parent adoptions. Transitional crises should not be thought of as permanent traumas. It is imperative that the use of language that links us to previous stereotypes be dropped. For example, we try to eliminate such phrases as "children of divorce," "working mother," "out-of-wedlock child," "fatherless home," and so forth, from the language we use about families. Also, we urge nurses to critically reflect on how culture, ethnicity, gender, race, and sexual orientation influence a family's developmental stages and tasks as well as attachments.

Phase One: Emerging Young Adults

In outlining the phases of the middle-class North American family life cycle, we have chosen to start with the stage of young adults. The primary task of young adults is to come to terms with their family of origin by remaining connected and yet separate, without cutting off or fleeing reactively to a substitute emotional source. The family of origin has a profound influence on who, when, how, and whether the young adult will marry. There have been sharp increases in the proportion of never married, primarily among men and women in their late 20s and early 30s who continue to live in the family home.

This phase may last for several years in a family's development. It is an opportunity for young adults to sort out emotionally what they will take along from the family of origin, what they will leave behind, and what they will establish for themselves as they progress through succeeding stages of the family life cycle. For both men and women, this is a particularly critical phase. During this stage, men sometimes have difficulty committing themselves to relationships and form a pseudoindependent identity centered on work. Women may choose to define themselves in relation to a man and postpone or forgo establishing an independent identity. We find it helpful to be curious in our clinical work and try to understand the client's views and legacies regarding marital status and the flexibility of the young person's expectations about pathways to adulthood.

Tasks

1. **Differentiation of self in relation to family of origin.** The young adult's shift toward adult status involves the development of a mutually respectful form of relating with his or her parents in which the young adult's parents can be appreciated for who they are. The young adult adjusts the view of the parents by neither making them into what they are not nor blaming them for what they could not be. The complexity of this task is not to be underestimated. Each ethnic and racial group has norms and

expectations regarding acceptable ways to be attached and connected to family and about issues of dependence versus independence.

2. **Development of intimate peer relationships.** The emphasis is on the young adult's passing from an individual orientation to an interdependent orientation of self. There is no single template of social experience for young adults to follow as they develop intimate relationships. During this task, young adults strive to bridge the gap between autonomy and attachment as they share themselves with others rather than using others as the source of self. With the increased use of Internet dating sites, social media, and chat rooms, the young adult will be exposed to a wide variety of personal styles and personalities.

3. **Establishment of self in respect to work and financial independence.** In a young adult's 20s and 30s, the "trying on" of various identities to test or refine career skills and interest is typical. The young adult who is committed to a career path or occupational choice by his or her late 20s or early 30s is less vulnerable to self-doubt or decreased self-esteem than the young adult without direction. Issues of competitiveness, expectations, and differences regarding work and financial goals require sorting through by the young adult and his or her family of origin.

4. **Establishment of self in community and larger society.** The future of how young adults relate to others as a responsible citizen depends on the development of self management.

5. **Establishment of one's worldview, spirituality, religion and relationship to nature.** The social responsibility gets determined in this phase where young adult's development of self management shifts.

6. **Parents shifting to consultative role in young adult's relationships.** The relationship between parents and the young adult changes. Parents role shifts as the young adult develops new ways to relate.

Attachments

There are no right or wrong attachments for young adults in stage one. Rather, it is important for the nurse to draw forth from family members their beliefs about attachment to one other and how they regard these attachments. These beliefs are influenced by culture, gender, race, sexual orientation, and social class as well as by whether the young adult lives at home. Some sample attachments for phase one are given in Figure 3-12. The first diagram illustrates a young adult who is bonded equally with her father and mother. The second diagram illustrates a young adult who is more closely attached to each parent than the parents are to each other; the parents are negatively bonded. Of significance in the second diagram is that there was a death of a sibling during the childhood of the young adult. It could be hypothesized that his difficulties in establishing his own identity are related to the family's hesitancy to come to grips with his deceased sister and the parents' living alone without children.

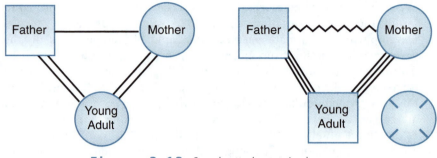

Figure 3-12   Sample attachments in phase one.

Questions to Ask the Family.

- "Which of your parents is most accepting of your career plans? How does he or she show this?"
- "What does your sister, Maria, think of your parents' reaction to your career plans?"
- "If your father were more accepting of your desire to move into an independent living situation with people not of the Jewish faith, how do you think your mother would react?"
- "If you continue to wear hijab because it is integral to your religious beliefs, would this reassure your parents?"

Phase Two: Couple Formation: The Joining of Families

Many couples believe that when they marry, it is just two individuals who are joining together. However, both spouses have grown up in families that have now become interconnected through marriage. Both spouses, although in some ways differentiated from their families of origin in an emotional, financial, and functional way, carry their whole family into the relationship. This is particularly relevant if the marriage is an arranged one. Marriage is a two-generational relationship with a minimum of three families coming together: one spouse's family of origin, the other spouse's family of origin, and the new couple. Given the current prevalence of stepfamilies, the likelihood of several families coming together is increased exponentially. Also, the certainty that the couple will be heterosexual is not evident because, in both the United States and in Canada, same-sex marriages and civil unions have increasingly been formally recognized.

Tasks

1. **Formation of couple system.** The new couple must establish itself as an identifiable unit. This requires negotiation of many issues that were previously defined on an individual level. These issues include routine matters such as eating and sleeping patterns, sexual contact, and use of space and time. The couple must decide which traditions and rules to retain from

each family and which ones they will develop for themselves. They must develop acceptable closeness-distance styles and recognize individual differences in adult attachment styles. Although the majority of studies on the quality and stability of marriage focus on couple communication, we believe that love is the decisive factor for quality and stability. For some cultures, however, the concept of a "love marriage" as compared to an arranged marriage is quite different.

2. **Expansion of family boundaries to include new partner and extended family.**

3. **Realignment of relationships among couple, parents and siblings, extended family, friends, and larger community.** A renegotiation of relationships with each spouse's family of origin has to take place to accommodate the new spouse. This places no small stress on both the couple and each family of origin to open itself to new ways of being. Some couples deal with their parents by cutting off the relationship in a bid for independence. Other couples choose to handle this task of realignment by absorbing the new spouse into the family of origin. The third common pattern involves a balance between some contact and some distance.

Attachments

Figure 3-13 illustrates a sample attachment for a couple in phase two: the development of close emotional ties between the spouses. The first diagram illustrates how they do not have to break ties with their families of origin but rather maintain and adjust ties with them. The second diagram illustrates a different type of attachment that can occur if both members of a couple do not align themselves together. The wife is more heavily bonded to her family of origin than she is to her husband. The husband is more tied to outside interests (such as work and friends) than to his wife. We have found that negative attachment-related events occurring early in the marriage are especially distressing for the couple. These and other attachment injuries can be characterized by a betrayal of trust during a critical moment of need.

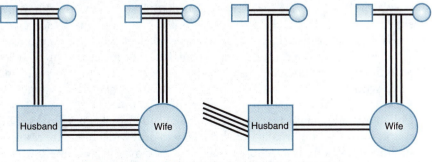

Figure 3-13 Sample attachments in phase two.

Questions to Ask the Family.

- "Which family members were most in favor of your marriage?"
- "How did you incorporate Greek and American traditions in your marriage?"
- "How did your siblings show that they supported your marriage?"
- "What does your spouse think of your parents' marital relationship?"
- "If you two as a couple were to model your marriage on your parents' marriage, what would you incorporate into your marriage?"
- "How did the diagnosis of multiple sclerosis influence your bonding as a couple?"

Phase Three: Families With Young Children

During this stage, the adults now become caregivers to a younger generation. The birth and rearing of a baby present varying challenges. Moreover, taking responsibility for and dealing with the demands of dependent children are challenging for most families when financial resources are stretched and the parents are heavily involved in career development. The disposition of child-care responsibilities and household chores in dual-career households is a particular struggle. We have found that men and women often differ in the coping strategies they use to deal with this issue. Women with young children tend to use cognitive restructuring, delegation, limiting of avocational activities, and social support significantly more often than do men. The work-family issue of juggling child care and other household accountabilities is a social problem to be dealt with by the couple, not a "woman's problem" for her to struggle with alone.

Tasks

1. **Adjustment of couple system to make space for children.** The couple must continue to meet each other's personal needs as well as their parental responsibilities. With the introduction of the first child, challenges for personal space, sexual and emotional intimacy, and socializing exist. Both mothers and fathers are increasingly aware of the need for emotional integration of the child into the family. Children can be brought into three types of environments: (1) there is no space for them, (2) there is space for them, or (3) there is a vacuum that they are expected to fill. If the child has a disability, the couple may face more stress as they adjust their expectations and deal with their emotional reactions. We have found that normal family processes in couples becoming parents include shifts in the sense of self, shifts in relationships with families of origin, shifts in relation to the child, changes in stress and social support, and changes in the couple.

2. **Collaboration in child-rearing and financial and housekeeping tasks.** The couple must find a mutually satisfying way to deal with child-care responsibilities and household chores that does not overburden one partner. Balancing the budget and juggling family and other responsibilities is a

major task. The emotional and financial cost of solutions to deal with child-care responsibilities must be addressed. Parents contribute to the child's development and can do so in different or similar ways. Physical and playful stimulation of the child complements verbal interaction. Parents can either support or hinder their children's success in developing peer relationships and doing well academically at school. Some families, responding to intense pressure from the school system, tend to stress the values of academic achievement and productivity, whereas other families may respond to this pressure with feelings of alienation. Recent immigration experiences and whether the children are documented or undocumented can also influence peer and school interaction.

3. **Realignment of relationships with extended family to include parenting and grandparenting roles.** The parents must design and develop their new parenting roles in addition to the marital role rather than replacing it. Members of each family of origin also take on new roles, for example, grandfather or aunt. In some cases, grandparents who perhaps were opposed to the marriage in the beginning become very interested in the young children. For many older adults, this is an especially gratifying time because it allows them to have intimacy with their grandchildren without the responsibilities of parenting. It also permits them to develop a new type of adult-adult relationship with their children. Opportunities for intergenerational support or conflict abound as expectations about child-rearing and health-care practices are expressed.

4. **Realignment of relationships with community and larger social system to include new family structure and relationships.**

Attachments

Parents need to maintain a marital bond and continue personal, adult-centered conversations in addition to child-centered conversations. Space for privacy and time spent together are important needs.

Children require security and warm attachments to adults, as well as opportunities to develop positive sibling relationships. We believe teaching interdependence is a central goal of parenting, helping children see themselves as part of a community and living cooperatively with others.

In Figure 3-14, sample attachment diagrams are given for this phase. A competitive, negative relationship (illustrated by the wavy line) exists between the children and spouses in the second diagram. The mother is overbonded to the daughter, and the father is underinvolved with the daughter. The father is overattached to the son, and the mother is underinvolved with the son. This is an example of same-sex coalitions existing cross-generationally.

Questions to Ask the Family.

- "What percentage of your time do you spend taking care of your children?"
- "What percentage do you spend taking care of your marriage? Is this a comfortable balance for the two of you?"

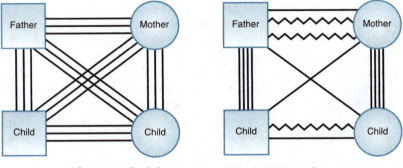

Figure 3-14 Sample attachments in phase three.

- "What effect does this pattern have on your children?"
- "If your children thought that you should be closer, how might they tell you this?"
- "What impact did the miscarriages have on your marriage?"

Phase Four: Families With Adolescents

This period has often been characterized as one of intense upheaval and transition, in which biological, emotional, and sociocultural changes occur with great and ever-increasing rapidity. Peers; Internet technology, such as instant messaging, social media, pornography, and sports; and other activities all compete for the adolescent's attention. This stage is highly influenced by socioeconomic level. Adolescence can begin early within poor, inner-city, or rural communities where, at a very young age, children are often faced with pressures related to sexuality, household responsibility, drugs, and alcohol use. In many middle-class families, adolescence can last well into the young adult's 20s and 30s, with the young person being financially dependent on the parents and continuing to live in the family home.

Tasks

1. **Shift in parent-child relationships to permit adolescent to have more independent activities and relationships and to move more flexibility into and out of system.** The family must move from the dependency relationship previously established with a young child to an increasingly independent relationship with the adolescent. Growing psychological independence is frequently not recognized because of continuing physical dependence. Conflict often surfaces when a teenager's independence threatens the family. For example, teenagers may precipitate marital conflict when they question who makes the family rules about the car: Mom or Dad? Families frequently respond to an adolescent's request for increasing autonomy in two ways: (1) they abruptly define rigid rules and recreate an earlier stage of dependency, or (2) they establish

premature independence. In the second scenario, the family supports only independence and ignores dependent needs. This may result in premature separation when the teenager is not really ready to be fully autonomous. The teenager may thus return home defeated. Parents need to shift from the parental role of "protector" to that of "preparer" for the challenges of adulthood. The challenge for parents to shift responsibility to their teens in a balanced way is often complicated if there are health problems.

2. **Families helping emerging adolescents negotiate relationship with community.**
3. **Refocus on midlife couple and career issues.** During this stage, parents are often struggling with what Erickson (1963) calls *generativity,* the need to be useful as a human being, partner, and mentor to another generation. The socially and sexually maturing teenager's frequent questioning and conflict about values, lifestyles, career plans, and so forth can thrust the parents into an examination of their own marital and career issues. Depending on many factors, including cultural and gender expectations, this may be a period of positive growth or painful struggle for men and women.
4. **Begin shift toward caring for older generation.** As parents are aging, so too are the grandparents. Parents (especially women) sometimes feel that they are besieged on both sides: teenagers are asking for more freedom, and grandparents are asking for more support. With the trend of women having children later in life and seniors living longer, this double demand for attention and resources most likely will intensify. Celebrating the wisdom of seniors and intergenerational reciprocity are key tasks.

Attachments

All family members continue to have their relationships within the family, although teenagers become increasingly more involved with their friends than with family members. These transitions through the family life cycle can be stressful because they challenge attachment bonds among family members. We advocate open communication and the addressing of primary emotions. A decrease in parental attachment is normative and developmentally appropriate for adolescents. The young person's widening social network, however, does not preclude strong family relationships, although family relationships are altered. The husband and wife need to reinvest in the marital relationship while this is taking place.

An example of an attachment pattern is illustrated in Figure 3-15. In the second diagram, the mother is overinvolved with the eldest son and has a negative relationship with the husband. The father tends to be minimally involved with all family members. There is conflict between the two sons.

Questions to Ask the Family.

- "What privileges do your teenagers have now that they did not have when they were younger?"

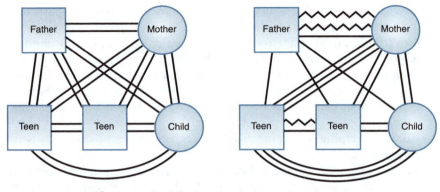

Figure 3-15   Sample attachments in phase four.

Ask the adolescents:

• "How do you think your parents will handle it when your younger sister, Nena, wants to date? Will it be different from when you wanted to date?"
• "On a scale of 1 to 10, with 10 being the highest, how much confidence do your parents have in your ability to say no to marijuana?"

Phase Five: Launching Children and Moving On at Midlife

Many middle-class North Americans whose children are grown up used to assume they would have an empty nest. However, this expectation is in the process of change. Adult children may return to the family home after graduating from college; they may return, along with their children, after their marriages end; or they may never have moved out. Rising housing costs and beginning pay rates that have not risen as fast as those of more experienced workers have been singled out as some of the causes of this trend. A different explanation is that young North Americans are having difficulty growing up and are unwilling to go out on their own and settle for less affluence than their parents afford them.

Tasks

1. **Renegotiation of couple system as a dyad.** In many cases, a thrust to alter some of the basic tenets of the marital relationship occurs. This is especially true if both partners are working and the children have left home. The couple bond can take on a more prominent position. The balance between dependency, independency, and interdependency must be re-examined.
2. **Development of adult-to-adult relationships between parents and grown children.** The family of origin must relinquish the primary roles of parent and child. They must adapt to the new roles of parent and adult child. This involves renegotiation of emotional and financial commitments. The key emotional process during this stage is for family members to deal with a multitude of exits from and entries into the family system.

3. **Realignment of relationships to include in-laws and grown children.** The parents adjust family ties and expectations to include their child's spouse or partner. This can sometimes be particularly challenging if the parents' expectation is for a heterosexual son-in-law or daughter-in-law of the family's race, religion, and ethnicity and the child chooses someone different. The once-prevalent idea that the time after a grown child marries is a lonely, sad time, especially for women, has been replaced. Increases in marital satisfaction have frequently been noted.

4. **Realignment of relationships with community to include new constellation of family relationships.**

5. **Exploration of new interests/career, given the freedom from child care responsibilities.**

6. **Dealing with health needs, disabilities, and death of parents (grandparents).** Many families regard the disability or death of an elderly parent as a natural occurrence. It can be a time of relishing and finding comfort in the happy memories, wisdom, and contributions of the elder. If, however, the couple and the elderly parents have unfinished business between them, there may be serious repercussions, not only for the children but also for the new third generation. The type of disability afflicting the seniors determines the effects on the immediate family. For example, caregivers who do not understand Alzheimer dementia and its effects on cognitive function and behavior often attempt to deal with inappropriate or disruptive behavior in ineffective and counterproductive ways. Thus, they inadvertently intensify their own stress.

We recommend that health professionals, in addition to attending to the family's multigenerational legacies of illness, loss, and crisis, also note intergenerational strengths and wisdom. Tracking key events, transitions, and coping strategies helps elicit resiliencies.

Attachments

Each family member continues to have outside interests and establish new roles appropriate to this phase. Sample attachment patterns are illustrated in Figure 3-16. A problem may arise when both husband and wife hold on

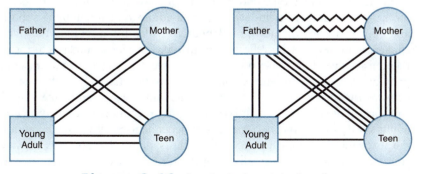

Figure 3-16 Sample attachments in phase five.

to their last child. They may avoid conflict by allowing the eldest child to leave home and then focusing on the next child.

Questions to Ask the Family.

- "How did your parents help you to leave home?"
- "What is the difference between how you left home and how your son, Zubin, is leaving home?"
- "Will your parents get along better, worse, or the same with each other once you have left home?"
- "Who, between Mom and Dad, will miss the children the most?"
- "As you see your child moving on with a new relationship, what would you like your child to do differently than you did?"
- "If your parents are still alive, are there any issues you would like to discuss with them?"

Phase Six: Families in Later Life

This stage can begin with retirement and last until the death of both spouses. It is hard to say, however, when the stage actually begins for each family because it is dependent on social, economic, and personal factors relative to each family. Potentially, this stage can last 20 to 30 years for many couples. Key emotional processes in this stage are to flexibly adjust to the shift of generational roles and to foster an appreciation of the wisdom of the elders.

Tasks

1. **Maintaining or modifying own and/or couple and social functioning and interests in the face of physiological decline: exploration of new familial and social role options.** Marital relationships continue to be important, and marital satisfaction contributes to both the morale and ongoing activity of both spouses. We have noted that the husband's morale is often strongly associated with health, socioeconomic status, income, and to a lesser extent, family functioning. The wife's morale is most strongly associated with family functioning and, to a lesser extent, with health and socioeconomic status.

   As the couple in later life find themselves in new roles as grandparents and mother-in-law and father-in-law, they must adjust to their children's spouses and open space for the new grandchildren. Difficulty in making the status changes required can be reflected in an older family member refusing to relinquish some of his or her power, for example, refusing to turn over a company or make plans for succession in a family business. The shift in status between the senior family members and the middle-aged family members is a reciprocal one. Difficulties and confusion may occur in several ways. Older adults may give up and become totally dependent on the next generation, the next generation may not accept the seniors' diminishing powers and may continue to treat them as totally competent, or the next generation may see only the seniors' frailties and may treat them as totally incompetent.

2. **Supporting more central role of middle generations.**
3. **Making room in the system for the wisdom and experience of the elders.** The task of supporting the older generation without overfunctioning for them is particularly salient because, in general, people are living longer. It is not uncommon for a 90-year-old woman to be cared for by her 70-year-old daughter, with both of them living in close proximity to a 50-year-old son and grandson. The "young-old" age group, those between 55 and 75 years of age, are often highly motivated to participate in self-help groups and are generally interested in improving their quality of life through counseling, traditional and alternative health activities, and education. Many have found "new" family connections through the use of e-mail, social media, and cell phones. They do not live by the aging myths of the past. Rather, as consumers, they expect and demand a good quality of life. Many grandparents continue to be involved in child-rearing.
4. **Supporting older generations without overfunctioning for them.**

Attachments

The couple reinvests and modifies the marital relationship based on the level of functioning of both partners. This phase is characterized by an appropriate interdependence with the next generation. The concept of interdependence is particularly important for nurses to understand when working with families with adult daughters and their parents. Middle-class older men and women seem equally likely to aid and support their children, especially daughters. Frequency of contact, however, tends to be higher with daughters than with sons. Thus, the possibility of strong intergenerational attachments between a daughter and her parents exists. In the attachment patterns illustrated in Figure 3-17 and shown previously in Figure 3-16, the couple project their conflicts onto the extended family. This causes difficulty for the succeeding generations.

Questions to Ask the Family.

* "When you look back over your life, what aspects have you enjoyed the most?"

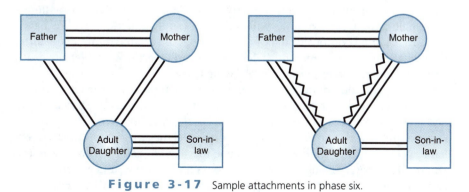

Figure 3-17 Sample attachments in phase six.

- "What has given you the most happiness?"
- "About what aspects do you feel the most regret?"
- "What would you hope that your children would do differently than you did? Similarly to what you did?"
- "As your health is declining, what plans have you and your daughter, Aminah, made for her because of her schizophrenia?"

Phase Seven: Families Nearing the End of Life

During this phase, one has to deal with the realities of family member's limitations and death and completion of one cycle of life.

1. **Dealing with loss of spouse, siblings, and other peers.** This is a time for life review and taking care of unfinished business with family as well as with business and social contacts. Many people find it helpful to discuss their lives, review life events, and enjoy the opportunity of passing this information along to succeeding generations.
2. **Making preparation for death and legacy.**
3. **Managing reversed roles in caretaking between middle and older generation.**
4. **Realignment of relationships with larger community and social system to acknowledge changing life cycle relationships.**

Divorce and Post-Divorce Family Life Cycle

Many changes in marital status and living arrangements are prevalent in North America today, such as increased divorce rates and single-parent families. Whether divorce rates or the number of single-parent families will level off, climb, or decline is a matter of speculation that can be backed up by various theories. Families experiencing divorce are often under enormous pressure. Single-parent families, whether a result of divorce or unmarried parents separating, must accomplish most of the same developmental tasks as two-parent families but without all the resources. This places extra burdens on the remaining family members, who must compensate with increased efforts to accomplish family tasks such as physical maintenance, social control, and tension management. We caution nurses, however, not to assume that single-parent status alone will influence family functioning. We have found that family composition alone is too broad a variable to predict health outcomes, and we recommend a focus on more specific variables such as parental cooperation in parenting following divorce.

Single-parent households generally experience challenges in managing shortages of time, money, and energy. Some parents voice serious concerns about the failure to meet perceived family and societal expectations for living "in a normal family" with two parents. Some women feel they must display behaviors that are contradictory to those they assume they should exhibit if they were to remarry. They perceive ongoing pressure from family, friends, and possibly their faith community to marry again to give their children a "normal" family. These women report being caught in a double-bind, trying to demonstrate behaviors such as compliance that might attract a new husband while trying to use seemingly opposing behaviors such as assertiveness to successfully manage their lives. We encourage nurses working with single-parent families to explore the parent's feelings about opposing expectations. This is a way of helping these parents plan their responses to various paradoxical situations.

It is also important for nurses engaged in relational family nursing practice to focus on the positive changes experienced by many separated spouses. Separated women often use growth-oriented coping, such as becoming more autonomous and furthering their education, and experience positive changes, such as increased confidence and feelings of control, in the post-separation phase.

Resilience in the post-divorce period is another focus for nurses. Resilience commonly depends on the ability of parents and children to build close, constructive, mutually supportive relationships that play a significant role in buffering families from the effects of related adversity. Factors that promote resiliency and positive adjustment to divorce include those associated with children's living arrangements. Whether family relationships post-divorce improve, remain stable, or get worse is dependent on a complex interweaving of many factors.

In our clinical supervision with nurses, we encourage focusing on the siblings, a subsystem that generally remains undisrupted during the process of family reorganization. Siblings are often the unit of continuity. We also try to notice and support cooperative post-divorce parenting environments such as mutual parental support; teamwork; clear, flexible boundaries; high information exchange; constructive problem solving; and knowledgeable, experienced, involved, and authoritative parenting. Because many fathers are not used to taking care of their children without their wives orchestrating things, fathers often fade out of their children's lives. They want to avoid ex-wives and conflict and may feel uncomfortable if they have an unclear role of authority in their children's lives. Nurses can be extremely helpful in intervening in these situations and fostering mutually agreeable post-divorce arrangements for the benefit of the children. For families locked in intractable disputes, we encourage them to develop a good-enough climate in which parents maintain distance from one another and conflict and triangulation are minimized.

Divorce may occur at any stage of the family life cycle and with any family, irrespective of socioeconomic status, ethnicity, or race. However, it has a different impact on family functioning depending on its timing and the diversity of individuals involved in the process. The marital breakdown may be sudden, or it may be long and drawn out. In either case, emotional work is required so that the family may deal with the shifts, gains, and losses in family membership. Some additional phases involved in divorce and post-divorce are depicted in Table 3-2. Column 1 lists the phase. Column 2 gives the prerequisite attitudes that will assist family members to make the transition and come through the developmental issues listed in column 3 en route to the next phase. We believe that clinical work directed at column 3 will not succeed if the family is having difficulty dealing with the issues in column 2.

TABLE 3-2	The Developmental Tasks for Divorcing and Remarrying Families		
PHASE	**TASK**	**PREREQUISITE ATTITUDE TRANSITION**	**DEVELOPMENTAL ISSUES**
Divorce	Decision to divorce	Acceptance of inability to resolve marital problems sufficiently to continue relationship	Acceptance of one's own part in the failure of the marriage
	Planning breakup of the system	Supporting viable arrangements for all parts of the system	a. Working cooperatively on problems of custody, visitation, and finances b. Dealing with extended family about the divorce
	Separation	a. Willingness to continue cooperative co-parental relationship and joint financial support of children b. Working on resolution of attachment to spouse	a. Mourning loss of original family; b. Restructuring marital and parent–child relationships and finances; adaptation to living apart c. Realignment of relationships with extended family; staying connected with spouse's extended family
	Divorce	Working on emotional divorce: overcoming hurt, anger, guilt, etc.	a. Mourning loss of original family; giving up fantasies of reunion b. Retrieving hopes, dreams, expectations from the marriage c. Staying connected with extended families
Post-divorce family	Single parent (custodial household or primary residence)	Willingness to maintain financial responsibilities, continue parental contact with ex-spouse, and support contact of children with ex-spouse and his or her family	a. Making flexible visitation arrangements with ex-spouse and family b. Rebuilding own financial resources c. Rebuilding own social network

TABLE 3-2	The Developmental Tasks for Divorcing and Remarrying Families—cont'd		
PHASE	**TASK**	**PREREQUISITE ATTITUDE TRANSITION**	**DEVELOPMENTAL ISSUES**
	Single parent (non-custodial)	Willingness to maintain financial responsibilities and parental contact with ex-spouse and to support custodial parent's relationship with children	a. Finding ways to continue effective parenting b. Maintaining financial responsibilities to ex-spouse and children c. Rebuilding own social network
Remarriage	Entering new relationship	Recovery from loss of first marriage (adequate emotional divorce)	Recommitment to marriage and to forming a family with readiness to deal with the complexity and ambiguity
	Conceptualizing and planning new marriage and family	Accepting one's own fears and those of new spouse and children about forming new family Accepting need for time and patience for adjustment to complexity and ambiguity of: 1. Multiple new roles 2. Boundaries: space, time, membership, and authority 3. Affective issues: guilt, loyalty conflicts, desire for mutuality, unresolvable past hurts	a. Working on openness in the new relationships to avoid pseudo-mutuality b. Planning for maintenance of cooperative financial and coparental relationships with ex-spouses c. Planning to help children deal with fears, loyalty conflicts, and membership in two systems d. Realignment of relationships with extended family to include new spouse and children e. Planning maintenance of connections for children with extended family of ex-spouses

Continued

TABLE 3-2	The Developmental Tasks for Divorcing and Remarrying Families—cont'd		
PHASE	**TASK**	**PREREQUISITE ATTITUDE TRANSITION**	**DEVELOPMENTAL ISSUES**
	Remarriage and recon-struction of family	Resolution of attachment to previous spouse and ideal of original family; Acceptance of different model of family with permeable boundaries	a. Restructuring family boundaries to allow for inclusion of new spouse-stepparent b. Realignment of rela-tionships and financial arrangements to permit interweaving of several systems c. Making room for relationships of all children with all parents, grand-parents, and other extended family d. Sharing memories and histories to enhance stepfamily integration.
	Renego-tiation of remarried family at all future life cycle transitions	Accepting evolv-ing relationships of transformed remarried family	a. Changes as each child graduates, marries, dies, or becomes ill b. Changes as each spouse forms new couple relationship, remarries, moves, becomes ill, or dies

McGoldrick, Monica; Carter, Betty; Garcia-Preto, Nydia. (Eds.). (2016). *The Expanded Family Life Cycle: Individual, Family and Social Perspectives*, 5th edition, copyright 2016, pp 413 - 414. Reprinted by permission of Pearson Education, Inc. Upper Saddle River, NJ.

Questions to Ask the Family.

- "How do you explain to yourself the reasons for your divorce?"
- "Who initiated the idea of divorce? Who left whom?"
- "Who was most supportive of developing viable arrangements for every-one in the family? How did your ex-husband, Luis, show his willingness to continue a cooperative co-parental relationship with you? How did you respond to this?"
- "As you changed your attachment to Luis, what changes did you notice in your children? What would your in-laws say about how you have fostered your children's relationship with them? What would your children say?"

- "What methods have you found most successful in resolving conflicting issues with Luis? What advice would you give to other divorced parents on how to resolve conflictual issues with their ex-partners?"
- "How have your children helped you and your ex-spouse to maintain a supportive environment for them?"

Remarried Family Life Cycle

The family emotional process at the transition to remarriage consists of struggling with fears about investment in new relationships: one's own fears, the new spouse's fears, and the fears of the children (of either or both spouses). It also consists of dealing with hostile or upset reactions of the children, extended families, and ex-spouse. Unlike biological families, in which family membership is defined by bloodlines, legal contracts, and spatial arrangements and is characterized by explicit boundaries, the structure of a stepfamily is less clear. Nurses must address the ambiguity of the new family organization, including roles and relationships.

We have found it helpful to use attachment theory as a framework for conceptualizing the impact of structural change and loss on stepfamily adjustment. We believe nurses can assist stepfamilies in increasing emotional connectivity and stability.

Ahrons and Rodgers (1987) have advocated for models of healthy, well-functioning binuclear families. Having been angered by a predominant emphasis on pathology in the divorce literature, Ahrons began to study what she calls "binuclear families." This term not only refers to joint-custody families or to families in which the relationship between ex-spouses is friendly but indicates a different familial structure, without inferring anything about the nature or quality of the ex-spouses' relationship. Ahrons (1999) advocates a normative process model of divorce rather than focusing on evidence of pathology or dysfunction.

We encourage nurses working with divorced and remarried families to bring to their patients research knowledge of what works and does not work to foster continuing family relationships. Nurses should be cautious, however, because complex problems seldom have simple answers. For example, predictors such as a child's age and gender, the frequency and regularity of father/mother-child visitation, father/mother-child closeness, and the effect of parental legal conflict on the child's self-esteem have different implications for different groups of 6- to 12-year-old children and for children in different situations.

We also encourage nurses working with stepfamilies to increase their knowledge about stepfamily issues and respect the uniqueness of complex stepfamily life. We encourage nurses to educate themselves about the beliefs of a particular stepfamily because uninformed clinicians may unwittingly increase rather than decrease family tensions if they communicate to stepfamilies that they should be like biological families.

Questions to Ask the Family.

- "Reeves, what were the differences between you and your wife, Lily, in how you each successfully recovered from your first marriage?"
- "What most helped each of you deal with your own fears about remarriage? About forming a stepfamily?"
- "How did Lily invite your children to adjust to her?"
- "What do your children think was the most useful thing you did in helping them deal with loyalty conflicts?"
- "What advice do you have for other stepfamilies on how to create a new family?"
- "What are you most proud of in how you have helped your stepfamily successfully make the transition from what they were before to what they are now?"

Professional and Low-Income Family Life-Cycle Stages

We align with Madsen (2013), who uses the term "families living in poverty" and who states that progression throughout the family life-cycle phases is often more accelerated for those families living in poverty than for those in working-class and middle-class families. As such, the family life cycle of families living in poverty can be organized into three stages (McGoldrick et al, 2016):

Stage 1: Adolescence and emerging adulthood
Stage 2: Coupling and raising young children
Stage 3: Families in later life

We encourage nurses to consider the effects of ethnicity and religion, socioeconomic status, race, and environment on when and how a family makes transitions in its life cycle. This is especially important in relational family nursing practice in primary care.

Adoptive Family Life Cycle

In adoption, the family boundaries of all those involved are expanded. Reitz and Watson (1992) define adoption as

a means of providing some children with security and meeting their developmental needs by legally transferring ongoing parental responsibilities from their birth parents to their adoptive parents; recognizing that in so doing we have created a new kinship network that forever links those two families together through the child, who is shared by both. (p. 11)

We agree with this definition. As with marriage, the new legal status of the adoptive family does not automatically sever the psychological ties to the earlier family. Rather, family boundaries are expanded and realigned. We believe that nurses should be aware of the trends and special circumstances in forming adoptive families. For example, most agencies offer adoption services along a continuum of openness. Some potential benefits of open adoption for birth parents include increased empathy for adoptive parents, reassurance that the child is safe and loved, and a reduction of shame and guilt. For adoptive parents, benefits include increased empathy for the birth parents, reduced stress imposed by secrecy and the unknown, and an embracing from the start of an affirmative acceptance of the child's cultural heritage. For the child, benefits include increased empathy for the adoptive parents, enriched connections with them, and reduced stress of disconnection. Simultaneously, the child experiences increased empathy for the birth parents, a reduction in fantasies about them, and—with clear, consistent information—increased control in dealing with adoptive issues. We believe that these potential benefits are very significant, especially for families adopting babies from different cultures and races. Adoptive families can include divorced, single-parent, married, or remarried families as well as extended families and families with various forms of open dual parentage.

The adoption process, including the decision, application, and final adoption, can be a stressful as well as joyful experience for many couples. During the preschool developmental phase, the family must acknowledge the adoption as a fact of family life. The question of the permanency of the relationship sometimes arises from both the child and the parents. In our clinical work with adoptive families, we have found it useful to consider many aspects of the adoption, including the following:

1. Genetic, hereditary factors in the child
2. Deficiencies in the child's prenatal and perinatal care
3. Adverse circumstances of adoption, including the child's having had multiple disruptions in early life
4. Conditions in the adoptive home, including pre-existing and current family resiliencies, problems, and strengths
5. Temperamental similarities and differences between the adoptee and the adoptive parents or family
6. Fantasy system and communication regarding adoption, including parental attitudes about adoption
7. Difficulties establishing a firm sense of identity during adolescence
8. Greater age difference than usual between parents and adoptees

We believe that it is important in relational family nursing practice to recognize adoptive families' strengths and resources as they deal with challenging issues. During the adolescent stage of family development, a major task is to increase the flexibility of family boundaries. In adoptive families, altercations may give rise to threats of desertion or rejection. During the young adult or launching phase, the young adult may "adopt" the parents in a recontracting phase.

As the adopted child proceeds to develop his or her own family of procreation, the integration of the adoptee's biological progeny can be a developmental challenge for everyone. Adoptive parents may be delighted with the psychological and social continuity. Simultaneously, they may mourn the loss of biological grandchildren and the pain of genealogical discontinuity. For the adoptee, reproduction includes the thrill of a biological relationship and possibly some fears of the unknowns in their own genetic history.

We believe that nurses can play an important role in helping families navigate the complexities of the adoption process and life cycle. When complexity is accepted, when the losses are acknowledged and resolved, when parents and their children feel satisfied with adoption as a legitimate route to becoming a family, and when the community of family, friends, and professionals who surround them is affirming, then the outcomes for adoptive families are very positive.

Lesbian, Gay, Bisexual, Queer, Intersex, Transgender, Twin-Spirited Family Life Cycles

Until recently, popular culture has ignored LGBQITT people in couple or family relationships or has portrayed them as part of an invisible subculture. Much of what we see, read, and hear in the media and society at large expresses a patriarchal, Anglo-Saxon, white, Christian, male, middle-class, ableist, and heterosexual view of the world. More recently, with open discussion about same-sex marriage or union, more attention is being focused on these relationships and their structures, developmental life cycles, challenges, strengths, and issues. We believe that the popular family life-cycle model may not apply to lesbians and gays because it is based on the notions that child-rearing is fundamental to family and that blood and legal ties constitute criteria for definition as a family.

Furthermore, the transmission of norms, rituals, folk wisdom, and values from generation to generation is not typically associated with lesbian and gay life. In many cases, the family of origin may not know what name to call their daughter's partner or spouse.

We believe, however, that more differences exist *within* traditionally defined families than *between* LGBQITT families and those families designated as traditional. There are also many differing beliefs *within* diverse couples. For many clinicians, sexual nonexclusivity challenges fundamental beliefs. Our view of family life is socially constructed, as is the view held by each nurse. Managing multiple views of relationships is an important task for nurses working with families.

The stages of the traditional family life cycle can be applied to lesbians and gays, with some unique differences. During adolescence, which can be a tumultuous time for most families, gays and lesbians face similar identity and individuation tasks as heterosexuals but often without the support of such rituals as proms or "going steady." Parents frequently struggle more with parenting to "protect" than to "prepare" the young person to live in a homophobic social environment.

The stages of leaving home, single young adulthood, and coupling present challenges for the young person who needs to learn from the gay/lesbian world about dating and cannot rely on the family of origin for modeling in this area. Couch-surfing and seeking hospitality from friends' parents, LGBQITT-friendly shelters, and transitional living programs are examples of the living-arrangement options for what some have called "throwaway" youth (i.e., LGBQITT youth in crisis). These are young people who have "come out" to their families and were then pushed out of the family home.

In discussing their same-sex relationship with their parents, many lesbian and gay couples have found it useful to focus on the strengths of their relationship. When parents see that the relationship has such strengths and can be beneficial for their son or daughter, they often adjust more easily. Dealing with the core issues of coupling—money, work, and sex—involves addressing gender scripts. During midlife and later life, the LGBQITT family continues to adapt and renegotiate with their families of origin. These relationships may be influenced by illness within either the aging family or the midlife chosen family. Intergenerational responsibility for caregiving and legacy issues may need to be addressed. We believe nurses engaged in relational practice can be helpful in providing a context for these conversations between family members.

We recommend an oppression-sensitive approach to working with LGBQITT families. This approach invites a stance of respectful curiosity for exploring domains of convergence and difference.

Questions to Ask the Family.

- "In what area do you feel privileged? Oppressed?"
- "How do you as a couple deal with these similarities and differences?"
- "How does the more privileged one respond to the other's sense of oppression?"
- "How does each member of the couple deal with heterosexism? With your families of origin? With the dominant gay culture?"
- "What are your strengths as a couple?"
- "How does spirituality influence your relationship?"

We encourage nurses to avoid the alpha bias of exaggerating differences between groups of people and the beta bias of ignoring differences that do exist. In their privileged role in working with families who are dealing with health issues, nurses can play a significant part in modeling inclusivity and respect for diversity.

In this CFAM developmental category, we have presented six sample types of family life cycles. Nursing is beginning to recognize the special characteristics of diverse family forms, such as lesbian and gay couples. We encourage nurses to broaden their perspectives when interacting with various family forms. What we do know is that great variety exists: the poor and homeless family, the lesbian or gay couple, the single parent, the adopted child with parent, the stepfamily, the divorced family, the separated family, the foster family, the nuclear family, the extended family, the household of children raising children without a parent present, and so forth.

FUNCTIONAL ASSESSMENT

The family functional assessment deals with how individuals *actually* behave in relation to one another. It is the here-and-now aspect of a family's life that is observed and that the family presents. There are two basic aspects of family functioning:

- Instrumental
- Expressive

KEY CONCEPT DEFINED

Functional Assessment

One of the categories of the Calgary Family Assessment Model (CFAM) that nurses use to identify how individuals actually behave in relation to one another; the here-and-now aspect of a family's life that is observed and that the family presents.

Instrumental Functioning

The instrumental aspect of family functioning refers to routine activities of daily living, such as eating, sleeping, preparing meals, giving injections, changing dressings, and so forth. For families with health problems, this area is particularly important. The instrumental activities of daily life are generally more numerous and more frequent and take on a greater significance because of a family member's illness.

Examples:

- A quadriplegic requires assistance with almost every instrumental task.
- If a baby is attached to an apnea monitor, the parents almost always alter the manner in which they take care of instrumental tasks. (For instance, one parent will leave the apartment to do a load of wash only if the other parent is sufficiently awake to attend to the infant.)
- If a senior family member is unable to distinguish what medication to take at a specific time, other family members often alter their daily routines to telephone or drop in on the senior.

The interaction between instrumental and psychosocial processes in clients' lives is an important consideration for nurses. For example, nurses can pay attention to a family's routines around eating and bedtime rituals and incorporate new health-care practices into the family's routine rather than "adding on" to the family's already busy schedule.

We recommend that health professionals understand that caregiving, whether given to a spouse who has cancer by an elderly spouse or to a parent by his or her partner, constitutes a major challenge in adaptation. Elderly spouses often rate the overall burden of caregiving and personal strain (the subjective component) as heavier than do their children and the cancer patients themselves. The importance of family nursing care is thus highlighted.

As the nurse hypothesizes about the family's possible stage of health and illness and inquires into their ordinary routines of living alongside illness, the nurse and family will discover resiliencies and areas for possible assistance. Effective assistance consists of a series of events rather than single interactions. The trajectory of cardiac illness, for instance, suggests that interventions may be most effective when provided during all stages of illness and may best be tailored to meet the specific needs of individuals and families in each stage.

Expressive Functioning

The expressive aspect of functioning refers to nine categories:

1. Emotional communication
2. Verbal communication
3. Nonverbal communication
4. Circular communication
5. Problem solving
6. Roles
7. Influence and power
8. Beliefs
9. Alliances and coalitions

These nine subcategories are derived in part from the Family Categories Schema developed by Epstein, Sigal, and Rakoff (1968) and later published by Epstein, Bishop, and Levin (1978). These categories were expanded by Tomm (1977) and later published by Tomm and Sanders (1983). Early work (Westley & Epstein, 1969) suggested that several of these categories distinguished emotionally healthy families from those that were experiencing more than the usual emotional distress.

We have expanded on these works in our earlier editions of *Nurses and Families* to include nonverbal and circular communication, beliefs, and power. However, we do not use any of these categories as determinants of whether a family is emotionally healthy. Rather, it is the family's judgment of whether they are functioning well that is most salient. With the exception, of course, of issues such as violence and abuse, we encourage nurses to find ways to support the family's definition of health versus imposing their own definition on the family.

Before discussing each subcategory, we would like to point out that most families must deal with a combination of instrumental and expressive issues.

Example: A 79-year-old woman has a burn. The instrumental issues revolve around dressing changes and an exercise program. The expressive or affective issues might center on roles or problem solving. The family might be considering the following questions:

- "Whose role is it to change Gram's dressing?"
- "Are women better 'nurses' than men?"
- "Whose turn is it to call the physical therapist?"
- "Why is it that Jas never gets involved in Gram's care?"
- "How can we get Jas to drive Gram to her doctor's visit?"

If a family is not coping well with instrumental issues, expressive issues almost always exist. However, a family can deal well with instrumental issues and still have expressive or emotional difficulties. Therefore, it is useful for the nurse and the family together to delineate the instrumental from the expressive issues. Both need to be explored when the nurse and the family have a conversation about family functioning.

Although both past behaviors and future goals are taken into consideration in the functional assessment, the primary focus is on the here and now. It is helpful for both the nurse and family to identify a family's strengths and limitations in each of the aforementioned subcategories. We find it helpful to remember that the very conversation the nurse and family have about the family system shapes that system. People continually and actively reauthor their lives and stories. Our commitment to families is to show curiosity, delight, interest, and appreciation for their resiliency. Naturally, this does not mean that we condone family violence or abuse. Rather, it means that we recognize that families are trying to make sense of their lives and stories. Our job is to witness this.

Patterns of interaction are the main thrust of the expressive part of the functional assessment category. Families are obviously composed of individuals, but the focus of a family assessment is less on the individual and more on the interaction *among* all of the individuals within the family. Thus, the family is viewed as a system of interacting members. In conducting this part of the family assessment, the nurse operates under the assumption that individuals are best understood within their immediate social context. The nurse conceives of the individual as defining and being defined by that context. Each individual's relationships with family members and other meaningful members of the larger social environment are thus very important. If we do not attend to ideas and practices at play in the larger social context, we run the risk of focusing too narrowly on small, rather tight, recursive feedback loops. We have found this to be especially important considering current social, political, environmental, and economic trends because families may struggle to adapt to constant changes.

By interviewing family members together, the nurse can observe how they spontaneously interact with and influence each other. Furthermore, the nurse can ask questions about the impact family members have on one another and on the health problem. Reciprocally, the nurse can inquire about the impact of the health problem on the family. If the nurse thinks "interactionally" rather than "individually," each individual family member's behavior will not be considered in isolation but rather will be understood in context.

It is important for nurses to remember that if they embrace a postmodernist worldview, they will not be able to conduct an objective family evaluation. Rather, the nurse and the family, in talking about the family's patterns of interacting, will bring forth a new story, rich in contextualized details. Particular attention is paid to the ways that even the small and the ordinary—single words, single gestures, minor asides, trivial actions—can provide opportunities for generating new meanings. Unlike modernist nurses who define themselves as separate from the family with whom they are working, nurses with postmodernist views assume that each participant in the family interview—wife, husband, partner, nurse—makes an equal and often different contribution to the process. It is the nurse's task to help family members engage in conversations to make sense of their lives rather than to explain their behavior.

Emotional Communication

This subcategory refers to the range and types of emotions or feelings that families express or the practitioner observes. Families generally express a wide spectrum of feelings, from happiness to sadness to anger, whereas families with difficulties commonly have quite rigid patterns within a narrow range of emotional expression. For example, some families experiencing difficulties almost always argue and rarely show affection. In other families, parents may express anger but children may not, or the family may have no difficulty with women expressing tenderness but feel that men are not permitted to express it.

Questions to Ask the Family.

- "Who in the family tends to start conversations about feelings?"
- "How can you tell when your dad is feeling happy? Angry? Sad? How about your mom? What effect does your anger have on your son Noah?"
- "What does your mom do when your dad is angry?"
- "If your grandmother were to express sadness about her upcoming chemotherapy to your parents, how do you think your parents would react?"
- "When your brother Henry was killed in the accident, what most helped your family to cope with the grief?"

Verbal Communication

This subcategory focuses on the meaning of an oral (or written) message between those involved in the interaction. That is, the focus is on the meaning of the words in terms of the relationship.

Direct communication implies that the message is sent to the intended recipient. An elderly woman may be upset by what her husband is saying but corrects her grandson's inconsequential fidgeting with the comment, "Stop doing that to me." This could represent a displaced message, whereas the same statement directed at her husband would be considered direct.

Another way of looking at verbal communication is to distinguish between clear versus masked messages. In a clear message, there is a lack of distortion in the message. A father's statement to his child, "Children who cry when they get needles are babies" may be masked criticism if the child is fighting back tears at the time of his injection. The old child management strategy of "say what you mean, and mean what you say" is a good guideline for clear, direct communication.

Questions to Ask the Family.

- "Who among your family members is the most clear and direct when communicating verbally?"
- "When you state clearly to your young adult son that he has to pay rent to you, what effect does that have on him?"
- "When your teenagers talk directly to each other about the use of condoms, what do you notice?"
- "If your adolescents were to talk more with you and your husband about safer sex, what do you think your husband's reaction might be?"
- "What ways have you found for you and Manuel to have good, direct conversations? In person? On the cell phone? By e-mail? Through text messaging?"

Nonverbal Communication

This subcategory focuses on the various nonverbal and paraverbal messages that family members communicate. Nonverbal messages include body posture (slumped, fidgeting, open, closed), eye contact (intense, minimal), touch (soft, rough), gestures, facial movements (grimaces, stares, yawns), and so forth. Personal space, the proximity or distance between family members, is also an important part of nonverbal communication. Paraverbal communication includes tonality, guttural sounds, crying, stammering, and so forth. Nurses must remember that nonverbal communication is highly influenced by culture. Nurses should note the sequence of nonverbal messages as well as their timing.

> *Example:* When an older man starts to talk about his terminal illness and his adult daughter turns her head and casts her tear-filled eyes toward the floor, the nurse can infer that the daughter is sad about her father's impending death. The daughter's sequence of nonverbal behavior is congruent with sadness and the topic of conversation. Note, however, that this behavior sequence may not necessarily be the most supportive for her father.

Nonverbal communication is closely linked to emotional communication. We encourage nurses to inquire about the meaning of nonverbal communication when it is inconsistent with verbal communication.

Questions to Ask the Family.

- "Who in your family shows the most distress when your foster father is drinking?"
- "How does Sheldon show it?"
- "What does your foster mother do when your foster father is drinking?"
- "When your sister Seema turns her head and stares out the window as your stepfather is talking, what effect does it have on you?"
- "If your dad were to stop talking at the same time as your stepmother, would you think she might move closer to him?"

Circular Communication

Circular communication refers to reciprocal communication between people (Watzlawick, Beavin, & Jackson, 1967). A pattern exists in most relationship issues. For example, a common circular pattern occurs when a wife feels angry and criticizes her husband; in return, the husband feels angry and avoids both the issues and her. The more he avoids, the angrier she becomes. The wife tends to see the problem only as her husband's, whereas the husband identifies the wife's criticism as the only problem. This type of pattern is often called the demand/withdraw pattern. The circularity of this pattern is the most important aspect in understanding interaction in dyads. Each person influences the behavior of the other. More information about this topic is available in Chapter 2.

KEY CONCEPT DEFINED

Circular Communication

Reciprocal communication between people; a subcategory of expressive functioning in the functional assessment category of the Calgary Family Assessment Model (CFAM).

Circular communication patterns can also be adaptive. For example, an older parent feels competent and negotiates well with the landlord; the adult son feels proud and praises his parent. The more reinforcement the adult son gives, the more confident and self-assured the senior feels. This pattern is diagrammed in Figure 3-18.

Circular pattern diagrams (CPDs) concretize and simplify the repetitive sequences noted in a relationship. This method of diagramming interaction patterns, first developed by Tomm in 1980, may be applied to relationships between family members or between the nurse and the family. Because the nurse and the family also mutually influence each other, the nurse is encouraged to think interactionally about situations and offer the family an opportunity to think interactionally.

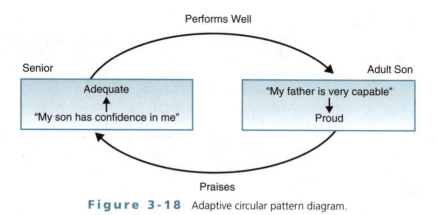

Figure 3-18 Adaptive circular pattern diagram.

KEY CONCEPT DEFINED

Circular Pattern Diagrams (CPDs)

A method of diagramming interaction patterns developed by Tomm (1980); may be applied to relationships between family members or between the nurse and the family.

The simplest CPD includes two behaviors and two inferences of meaning. The inferences can be cognitive, affective, or both. Inferences about cognition refer to ideas, concepts, or beliefs, whereas inferences about affect refer to emotional states. Affect and/or cognition propels the behavior. Figure 3-19 illustrates the relationship between these elements. As noted by Tomm (1980), "The inference is entered inside the enclosure and represents some internal process (what is going on inside each interactant). The connecting arrows represent information conveyed from each person to the other through behavior. The circular linkage implies an interaction pattern that is repetitive, stable, and self-regulatory" (p. 8). CPDs encourage a position of curiosity rather than a passion for particular values and a stand against others.

Although CPDs can be used to foster circular thinking, one must be mindful of their limitations. CPDs can tempt us to look within families for collaborative causation of problems. This may distract from personal responsibility for unacceptable behavior such as violence. Small, tight feedback loops may be highlighted, and the "big picture" of the negative influence of particular values, institutions, and cultural practices may be forgotten. Another limitation of CPDs is that they may encourage nurses to believe that they are outside the family system. As a participant observer in the larger system, the nurse is shown and hears about circular

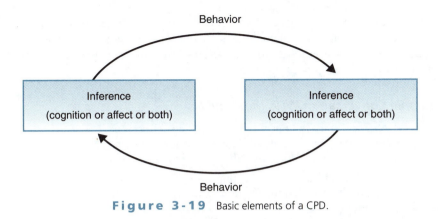

Figure 3-19 Basic elements of a CPD.

patterns reflecting family functioning. The interdependence of the nurse interviewer and family must be recognized. Both the nurse and family members cannot be decontextualized from their social and historical surroundings.

In what has come to be called the "feminist critique" of systems, some have taken exception to the simplistic causation ideas advanced by a circular perspective. CPDs, by virtue of their neutral context, ignore power differentials and imply a discourse or relationship between equals. These writers criticize circularity for not being transparent about responsibility and minimizing power differentials in relationships. Of particular concern are such issues as incest, abuse, violence, intimidation, and battering.

Despite these valid criticisms, we believe that it is still useful in clinical work with families to subscribe to the notion of circularity but simultaneously hold to the idea of personal responsibility. An example of a circular argument is illustrated in Figure 3-20. Each party blames and threatens the

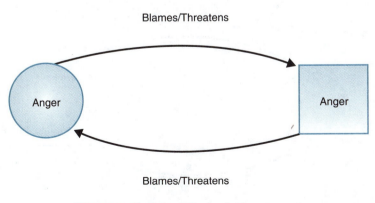

Figure 3-20 CPD of a circular argument.

other. An example of a supportive relationship is illustrated in Figure 3-21. The husband trusts his wife and reveals his needs and fears. She is concerned and, in turn, sustains and supports him. This leads him to trust her more, and the relationship progresses.

Sample Conversation With the Family

Nurse: You say your wife "always" criticizes you. *(Nurse conceptualizes Figure 3-22). What do you do then? (Nurse tries to fill in the husband's behavior in Figure 3-23.)*

Niz: I don't like to discuss things. I avoid conflict. I leave. I go in the other room. What else can I do? She is always telling me what I did wrong. I go to the computer.

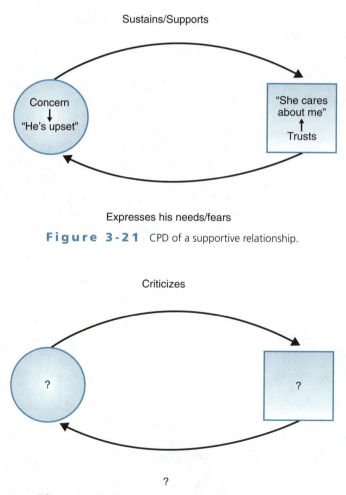

Sustains/Supports

Concern
↓
"He's upset"

"She cares about me"
↑
Trusts

Expresses his needs/fears

Figure 3-21   CPD of a supportive relationship.

Criticizes

?

?

?

Figure 3-22   Beginning conceptualization of CPD.

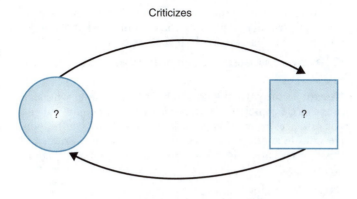

Figure 3-23 CPD illustrating husband's and wife's behaviors.

Nurse: So she expresses her needs, and you leave. How do you think that makes her feel? *(Nurse tries to fill in the inferred emotion in the wife's circle in Figure 3-24.)*

Zara: I'll tell you. I get annoyed. I feel ignored, rejected.

Nurse: So you're annoyed when he leaves and ignores you. And then you become more critical. Is that right?

Zara: Well I don't really criticize, I just…

Niz: Yeah, you got it, Nurse.

Nurse: So, when you try to express your concerns, how do you think it makes him feel? *(Nurse tries to fill in the inference in the square in Figure 3-24.)*

Zara: I don't know.

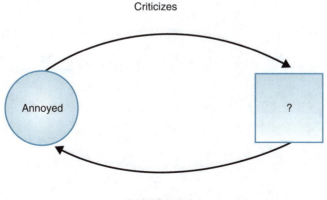

Figure 3-24 CPD illustrating wife's emotion.

Nurse: If he thinks you're lecturing and avoids the issues by leaving the room and going to the computer, what effect do you think your talking might be having on him?

Zara: Well, I suppose he could be feeling frustrated. He sulks.

Nurse: So the pattern seems to be that, no matter who starts it, the circle completes itself. Sometimes you're annoyed and you criticize. Your husband feels frustrated and ignores you. He sulks in another room. Other times he avoids issues, and this arouses your frustration and criticism. *(Nurse explains Figure 3-25.)*

Zara: It's a vicious circle.

Niz: I don't want it to go on this way anymore. We both get too upset.

   Once the nurse has elicited a CPD, the nurse should ask the family members to contextualize their discussion. One context might be that Zara is exhausted by her factory job and all the housework and child care. Niz does not see why he should change his life because his wife has a stressful job and works long hours. They may engage in this particular negative circular interaction pattern every night while caring for their 3-year-old child with asthma.

Problem Solving

This subcategory refers to the family's ability to solve its own problems effectively. Family problem solving is strongly influenced by the family's beliefs about its abilities and past successes. How much influence the family

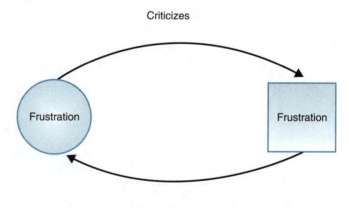

Figure 3-25 Nurse's conceptualization of this couple's communication pattern.

believes it has on the problem or illness is useful to know. Who identifies the problems is important. Is it characteristically someone from outside the family or from inside the family?

Once the problems are identified, are they mainly instrumental (routine, day-to-day logistics) or emotional problems? Families sometimes encounter difficulties when they identify an emotional problem as an instrumental one. *Examples:*

- A mother who states that she cannot get her child who has food allergies to maintain the diet is really discussing an emotional issue rather than an instrumental one; she has difficulty influencing her child. As more families cope with issues such as childhood obesity, this is a particularly important distinction for nurses to notice. *Is the obesity an instrumental or emotional problem? An individual, family, or societal problem?*
- A couple dealing with the wife's myeloma might decide to harvest stem cells as a proactive measure. *What are the family's solution patterns? Are they proactive in planning for issues that might arise?*
- Older parents move to a retirement community. The wife breaks her hip. The husband is used to being self-reliant or, in a pinch, depending on his middle-aged daughter. The older couple know few people in their new community. The husband is reluctant to accept help from the visiting nurse. He states that he can manage all of his wife's care despite the fact that he is losing weight and getting insufficient rest. The husband's solution pattern conflicts with that of the nurse. Many close-knit extended families rely on relatives for assistance in time of need. Others tend to seek help from professionals. Knowing a family's usual solution style can give the nurse insight into why this family may seem to be "stuck" at this particular time with this particular issue.
- A 68-year-old grandmother tells Katherine, the nurse, "I can't afford to let myself cry about the death of my son's newborn baby. I have to go on for the sake of my other children." Knowledge of whether a family evaluates the cost of its solutions can be helpful to the nurse. Katherine was able to evaluate with the grandmother the cost of her solution pattern. Neither the grandmother nor the son discussed the baby's death with each other. The grandchildren's questions about why the baby did not come home from the hospital were left unanswered. There was considerable tension between the son and the grandmother, and the son was particularly overprotective of his 4-year-old boy (the only surviving male child). By gently exploring the cost of the solution (tension and overprotection), the nurse was able to suggest other solution patterns (e.g., shared grieving).

Questions to Ask the Family.
- "Who first noticed the problem?"
- "Are you the one who usually notices such things?"

- "What most helped you to take the first step toward eliminating the addiction and violence pattern?"
- "What effect did it have when Toya also took steps to stop the cycle of violence in your family?"
- "How did the relationship between your son, Jeremiah, and your husband change when the violence stopped? When the addiction stopped?"
- "If a violent episode were to occur again, how do you think you and your daughter would deal with it?"
- "If his cocaine addiction were to flare up again, what steps would you take to protect your family?"

Roles

This subcategory refers to the established patterns of behavior for family members. A role is consistent behavior in a particular situation. Roles, however, are not static but are developed through an individual's interactions with others. Roles are thus influenced by culture, race, and others' sanctions and norms. In Hispanic families, for example, *machismo* can be very significant for the hierarchical male role, and *simpatía,* or the avoidance of conflict and the ability to get along well, is often highly valued in the female role.

The psychological cost of providing care for a parent with Alzheimer disease is often anxiety, depression, guilt, and resentment in the caregiver. The fact that women dominate as adult caregivers reflects a North American pattern. The gender differences clearly profile women's more frequent, intensive, affective involvement with the caregiver role.

Women's roles have changed in recent years and are now less defined by the men in their lives. The birth rate has fallen below replacement levels, and many more women are concentrating on jobs and education. In many cases, a husband's income is negatively related to role sharing, and a wife's education is positively related to role sharing.

Although role change is increasingly prevalent for both men and women in today's society, what is important for nurses to assess is how family members cope with their roles. Nurses should consider the following:

- Does role conflict or cooperation exist?
- Are roles determined solely by age, rank order, or gender?
- Do additional criteria, such as social class and culture, influence roles?
- Are the women in the family more involved with a wider network of people for whom they feel responsible?
- Do the men hear less than the women in the family about stress in their family network?

Formal roles are those for which the community has broadly agreed on a norm. Examples include the roles of mother, husband, and friend. Informal roles refer to the established patterns of behavior that are idiosyncratic to particular individuals in certain settings. Examples include the roles of "bad kid," "angel," and "class clown." These serve a specific function in a particular family. If Dad is the "softie," most likely Mom is the "heavy." If Giffy is the "good daughter," Kweisi is probably the "black sheep." The roles of "parentified child," "good child," and "symptomatic child" have been identified in many families. Auxiliary roles of "child advocate," "analyst," "peacemaker," and "therapist" have also been described.

It is helpful for the nurse to learn how family roles evolved, their impact on family functioning, and whether the family believes they need to be altered. It is important for nurses to conceptualize the functional assessment category of roles in a family-oriented rather than an individual-oriented way. According to Hoffman (1981):

> The individual-oriented approach badly misrepresents the subject. For instance, to speak of the "role of the scapegoat" is to present the deviant as a person with fixed characteristics rather than a person involved in a process. "Scapegoating" technically applies to only one stage of a shifting scenario—the stage where the person is metaphorically cast out of the village. After all, the term originates from an ancient Hebrew ritual in which a goat was turned loose in the desert after the sins of the people had been symbolically laid on its head. The deviant can begin like a hero and go out like a villain, or vice versa. There is a positive-negative continuum on which he can be rated depending on which stage of the deviation process we are looking at, which sequence the process follows, and the degree to which the social system is stressed.
>
> At the time, the character of the deviant may vary in another direction, depending on the way his particular group does its typecasting. Which symptoms crop up in members of a group is itself a kind of typecasting. Thus the deviant may appear in many guises: the mascot, the clown, the sad sack, the erratic genius, the black sheep, the wise guy, the saint, the idiot, the fool, the imposter, the malingerer, the boaster, the villain, and so on. Literature and folklore abound with such figures. (p. 58)

Questions to Ask the Family.

- "To whom do most of you go when you need someone to talk to?"
- "What effect does it have on Maxine when Ken helps with the baby's care?"
- "When Maxine and Ken collaborate instead of competing, who would be the first to notice? If Ken were to be more responsible for initiating contact with the relatives around Cherie's day-care arrangements and babysitting, how do you think Maxine would feel?"

Influence and Power

This subcategory refers to behavior used by one person to *influence* or affect another's behavior. *Power* is the ability of a person to regulate the criteria by which differing views of "reality" are judged and resources apportioned. Power addresses hierarchical and egalitarian positions in relationships. In a hierarchical relationship, a person can be in a one-up or a one-down position in the relationship and can be dominant in one context and subordinate in another. In an egalitarian relationship, there is equality in the relationship. In an egalitarian relationship, a give-and-take negotiation of individual needs, goals, and desires with an expectation of reciprocal attunement to the needs of the relationship or each other occurs.

Gender, race, and cultural issues are frequently intermingled with power issues. For example, in many relationships, women tend to raise issues and draw men out in the early phase of a discussion, whereas men tend to control the content and emotional depth of the later discussion phases and largely dominate the outcome. Shifts in power are preceded by changes in "reality," an expansion from a single perspective to a multiverse. We encourage nurses to adopt a postmodernist worldview because it offers useful ideas about how power and "truth" are socially constructed, constituted through language, organized, and maintained in families and larger cultural contexts.

A nurse who is unaware of power differences among family members, in terms of roles, gender, economics, or social class, can inadvertently encourage family members in positions of less power to accept goals that decrease their power and constrain their choices.

Whether all family members contribute equally to problems and share responsibility for resolution is something that the nurse can pose for consideration. We believe that the most clinically useful stance to take with regard to the idea of power is to say, "Power is...." It can be used positively or negatively, overtly or covertly, to enhance or constrain options. Power relations exist among family members, their health-care providers, and institutions. McGoldrick et al. (2008, p. 78) have depicted a negative power and control pyramid that includes eight levels and combines racism, heterosexism, and sexism:

1. "Isolation, controlling whom she can see and when and where
2. Sexual abuse, abusive touching, sexual acts against her will, having affairs, exposing her to HIV
3. Using children, being abusive, controlling, guilt-inducing or under-responsible regarding visitation, etc.
4. Physical abuse, hitting, shoving, choking, kicking, grabbing, etc.
5. Economic abuse, controlling her financially, not sharing financial information or resources, challenging her every purchase
6. Threats and intimidation, threatening to hurt her physically, to commit suicide, have an affair, divorce, report her to welfare, take away children or cut off her emotional support system, putting her in fear by looks, actions, destroying property, stalking, driving car too fast
7. Using immigration status, using her undocumented status to threaten deportation, loss of children, job, healthcare, etc.

8. Emotional abuse and use of male privilege, putting her down, name calling, making her think she's crazy, playing mind games, stonewalling, treating her like a servant, assuming right to make all major decisions or to neglect '2nd shift' home responsibilities such as housework and childcare."

Instrumental influence, power, or control refers to the use of objects or privileges (e.g., money; television watching; computer, car, or cell-phone use; candy; vacations; and so forth) as reinforcers. Psychological influence or power refers to the use of communication and feelings to influence behavior. Examples include directives, praise, criticism, threats, and guilt induction. Corporal control refers to actual body contact, such as hugging, spanking, and so forth. It is important to note the positive and negative influences used in the family, especially with infants and seniors. Abuse of seniors by informal and sometimes formal caregivers is not infrequent, and abuse by family members may occur as well.

We have found that the most important positive predictors of compliance for children are consistency of enforcement of rules, encouragement of mature action, use of psychological rewards such as praise and approval, and play with the child. The most important negative one is the amount of physical punishment. The use of praise is positively related to success, whereas physical punishment and verbal, psychological punishment are constraining influences.

Questions to Ask the Family.

- "Which of your parents is best at getting Nirvana to take her medication?"
- "When Devin dominates the conversation, what effect does that have on Jamie?"
- "What does your mother feel about how your stepfather disciplines your sister?"
- "If your stepfather were to be more positive with your sister Tiffany, how might his relationship with your mother change?"
- "Whose interests are most reflected in major decisions in the Veliz family?"
- "Who is more likely to accommodate to the other person, Gustavo or Fines?"

Beliefs

This subcategory refers to fundamental attitudes, premises, values, and assumptions held by individuals and families. Beliefs are the blueprint from which people construct their lives and intermingle them with the lives of others. Families co-evolve an ecology of beliefs that arise from interactional, social, and cultural contexts (Wright & Bell, 2009). When illness arises, our beliefs about health are challenged, threatened, or affirmed. During times of illness, nurses may assess the beliefs of patients, family members, or even their own beliefs to be constraining or facilitating. Constraining beliefs can enhance suffering and decrease solution options, whereas facilitating beliefs can soften illness suffering and increase solution options for managing an illness (Wright & Bell, 2009). Which illness beliefs are determined to be constraining or facilitating is determined by the clinical judgment of the nurse in collaboration with the family.

Beliefs and behaviors are intricately connected. Every action and every choice that families and individuals make evolves from their beliefs. Consequently, beliefs shape the way in which families adapt to chronic and life-threatening illness. For example, if a family believes that the best treatment for colon cancer is a nontraditional approach, it makes good sense for the family to pursue acupuncture. Because North American culture tends to use a paradigm of control about symptoms (it is good to be in control and bad to be out of control), nurses might find it useful to explore family members' beliefs about control and mastery over their symptoms.

Beliefs are intricately intertwined with familial and socioeconomic contexts.

Examples:

- The meaning of pregnancy loss is intricately intertwined with the woman's emotional needs at the time of the loss. If a mother was very happy about being pregnant and felt devastated by her miscarriage, then her emotional needs would differ dramatically from those of another mother who did not want to be pregnant and felt relieved by her miscarriage. Feelings about pregnancy loss can range from feelings of devastation to relief.

- A 51-year-old father of two teenage girls wrote to a nurse about his beliefs about his chronic pain:

  I think each person has a different threshold of pain. Every day I try to disassociate the pain…. I try to "get into" my work and life. I am not always successful … but I try as hard as I can. The why, is because of my family, friends, and faith (gushy, eh?, but it's true). I think you have to find out what is important in your life and let it motivate you, as terrible as this will be to say, there are always thoughts of "ending it all" … but then you think about the sadness you would leave with the ones you love … it keeps you going. I really think the key is to find one important thing as a start, and let that be the fuel that keeps you motivated to do the things you would like to do. I wish there were more I could say…. It's a day to day struggle.

Wright and Bell (2009) have suggested that the most relevant beliefs to explore with patients and their families are beliefs about etiology, diagnosis, prognosis, healing, and treatment; spirituality and religion; mastery and control; role of family members; and role of health-care providers.

Box 3-3 provides a list of areas for nurses to explore when assessing family beliefs about the health problem.

Questions to Ask the Family.

- "What do you believe is the cause of your sexual addiction?
- "How much control do you believe your family has over chronic pain?
- "How much control does chronic pain have over your family?
- "What do you believe the effect, if any, would be on chronic pain if you and your wife agreed on treatment?
- "Who do you believe is suffering the most in your family because of the changes in your family life due to your multiple sclerosis?
- "What do you believe has been the most useful thing health professionals have offered to help you cope with your suffering from fibromyalgia? What has been the least helpful?"
- "Have any of your Buddhist beliefs helped you to cope with the tragic loss of your son?"

Box 3-3 Beliefs About the Health Problem

A. Beliefs about:
 1. Diagnosis
 2. Etiology
 3. Prognosis
 4. Healing and treatment
 5. Mastery, control, and influence
 6. Religion and spirituality
 7. Place of illness in lives and relationships
 8. Role of family members
 9. Role of health-care professionals
B. Influence of the family on the health problem
 1. Resource utilization
  a. Internal (to family)
  b. External
 2. Medication and treatment
C. Influence of the health problem on the family
 1. Client response to the illness
 2. Family members' responses to illness
 3. Perceived difficulties and changes related to the health problem
D. Strengths related to the health problem at present
E. Concerns related to the health problem at present

Adapted from Family Nursing Unit records, Faculty of Nursing, University of Calgary, Calgary, Alberta.

Alliances and Coalitions

This subcategory focuses on the directionality, balance, and intensity of relationships between family members or between families and nurses. *Complementary* and *symmetrical* are terms used to describe a two-person relationship (see Chapter 2). A term commonly used to distinguish a three-person relationship is *triangle*, a term first coined by Bowen (1978). Bowen, a psychiatrist and family therapist, explains:

> The two-person relationship is unstable in that it has a low tolerance for anxiety and it is easily disturbed by emotional forces within the twosome and by relationship forces from outside the twosome. When anxiety increases, the emotional flow in a twosome intensifies and the relationship becomes uncomfortable. When the intensity reaches a certain level the twosome predictably and automatically involves a vulnerable third person in the emotional issue. The twosome might "reach out" and pull in the other person, the emotions might "overflow" to the third person, or the third person might be emotionally programmed to initiate the involvement. With involvement of the third person, the anxiety level decreases. It is as if the anxiety is diluted as it shifts from one to another of the three relationships in a triangle. The triangle is more stable and flexible than the twosome. It has a much higher tolerance of anxiety and is capable of handling a fair percentage of life stresses. (p. 400)

Most family relationships are organized around threesomes or triangles. Triangular alliances can be helpful or unhelpful. We have learned that in families of combat veterans experiencing post-traumatic stress disorder, the veteran can sometimes become triangulated with a dead buddy without the spouse's knowledge. With soldiers returning from the Iraq or Afghanistan War, the ongoing impact of their military alliances may be a useful area for the nurse to explore if the family is having difficulty realigning as a unit. Restless days, fractured relationships, and vials of pills that help with some types of pain, but not all types, have commonly been reported by these families. Relationships are not unidirectional, even if one member of the triangle is an infant, an older person, or a person who has a handicap. The intensity of each relationship and the total amount of interaction are often fairly balanced. If one relationship becomes more intense, another one or two become less intense. Also, if one member of a threesome withdraws, the other two become closer.

We believe that it is important for the nurse to note the degree of flexibility and fluidity within the family as they adjust to new arrivals, death, or illness. Experienced community health nurses have often noticed triangulation in infancy support. For example, if the father acts intrusively while playing with his baby, the infant often averts and turns to the mother. The regulation of this intrusion-avoidance pattern at the family level sheds some light on the couple alliance. When co-parenting is supportive, the mother validates the infant's bid for help without interfering with the father. Thus, the problematic pattern is contained within the dyad of father-baby. If co-parenting is hostile/competitive, the mother ignores the infant's bid or engages with her in a way that interferes with her play with her father. In this case, triangulation occurs and tension is lessened, but at a cost. The nurse can identify these patterns with the couple and then collaborate with them to design effective interventions.

As nurses address this functional subcategory of alliances and coalitions, they will be aware of its interconnection with structural and developmental categories. The structural subcategory of boundaries is an important part of the alliance or coalition subcategory. The boundary defines who is part of the triangle and who is not. Of course, there are many triangles and many shifting alliances and coalitions within families. What is important for the nurse and family to note, therefore, is whether these are problematic or enriching.

An example of what can inadvertently occur in a family is if a patient's illness is seen as "his problem" versus "our challenge." If the condition becomes defined as the affected patient's problem, a fundamental split occurs between the patient, the well partner, and other family members. By introducing the concept of "our challenge" early on, the nurse can provide an opportunity for all family members to examine cultural and multigenerational beliefs about the rights and privileges of ill and well family members. An alternate example of a positive coalition is when family members join together to help another family member stop smoking or stop drinking alcohol. They collectively voice their concerns to the individual and their intent to provide support and help.

We have observed that cross-generational coalitions sometimes coincide with symptomatic behavior. In addition to noting the connection between the structural subcategory of boundaries and the functional subcategory of alliances and coalitions, nurses should be aware of the interconnection with the developmental subcategory of attachments. Family attachments, or underlying emotional bonds that have an enduring or stable quality, are similar to alliances in that they are both unions. Attachments tend to differ from coalitions, however, in that the latter implies an alignment between two members, with a third member being split off or opposed.

Questions to Ask the Family.

- "When Deanna and Logan argue, who is most likely to get in the middle of the fight?"
- "If the children are playing very well together, who would most likely come along and *start* them fighting? Who would *stop* them from fighting?"
- "What impact has Don's brain tumor had on family members coming together or becoming further distanced?"

CASE SCENARIO: JOHN AND VALERIE

John and his wife, Valerie, were very excited about having their first baby. Valerie's pregnancy was uneventful, and the labor and delivery were normal. They happily welcomed Hannah, a beautiful baby girl. Valerie was doing well at the hospital with feeding Hannah and, with the exception of a couple of unexplained crying spells that the nurses explained to her as "the baby blues," she was coping well.

Two weeks after they got home with the baby, John started feeling down. He was tired and feeling useless in helping Valerie and in caring for her and their new daughter. John was feeling as though he couldn't be the father and husband he dreamed of when Valerie was pregnant. John was trying to balance long hours at work, helping Valerie around the house, and spending time cuddling his new baby. Valerie's mother lives a distance away and planned to come for a couple of weeks, but unfortunately, Valerie's father fell ill, and her mother had to stay and take care of him. As the weeks went by, John was feeling overwhelmed, useless, and anxious about not fulfilling his role. One night, John told Valerie that he thought they had made a mistake in having the baby. "I am just not a good dad," he said, "and I'm afraid that you and Hannah are going to hate me."

Valerie and John have brought Hannah to the well-child clinic for her 2-month appointment. During the infant assessment, John shares his thoughts about being a failure as a father with the public health nurse. Valerie tells the public health nurse that she is concerned about John. She did not expect this to happen. John has always been such a competent, strong husband who wanted nothing more than to have a family. She was sure he would be happy and would be a wonderful dad. She did not know what to do to help him.

Reflective Questions

1. How would constructing a genogram and ecomap with John and Valerie be helpful for the nurse?
2. What questions could the nurse ask John and Valerie in order to assess the structural components of their family, such as roles, subsystems, and boundaries?
   a. How can the nurse use this information when working with John and Valerie?

CRITICAL THINKING QUESTIONS

1. Identify a family in your clinical practice and complete the three major categories of the CFAM:
   a. Structural (including a genogram and ecomap)
   b. Developmental
   c. Functional
2. What are three questions you would ask the family from each of the categories in order to obtain information?

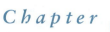
The Calgary Family Intervention Model

Learning Objectives

- Explain the Calgary Family Intervention Model (CFIM).
- Identify the domains of family functioning.
- Describe examples of interventions directed at each domain of family functioning.
- Compare the difference between linear and circular questions.

Key Concepts

Affective domain of family functioning

Behavioral domain of family functioning

Behavioral-effect questions

Calgary Family Intervention Model (CFIM)

Circular questions

Cognitive domain of family functioning

Commendations

Difference questions

Hypothetical or future-oriented questions

Illness narrative

Linear questions

The Calgary Family Intervention Model (CFIM) is a companion to the Calgary Family Assessment Model (CFAM) (see Chapter 3). To our knowledge, the CFIM is the first family intervention model to emerge within nursing. There is increasing evidence of the importance of nursing interventions with families in the literature; more detail can be found

139

in Chapter 1. In addition, the focus of health-care providers has shifted from deficit- or dysfunction-based family assessments to strengths- and resiliency-based family interventions. For example, the McGill Model of Nursing developed by faculty and students from McGill University under the guidance of Dr. Moyra Allen states that one of its goals is to "help families use the strengths of the individual family members and of the family as a unit, as well as resources external to the family system" (Feeley & Gottlieb, 2000, p. 11). Gottlieb and Gottlieb (2017) identify strengths-based nursing as family nursing, and it is a growing movement across disciplines.

KEY CONCEPT DEFINED

Calgary Family Intervention Model (CFIM)

An organizing framework conceptualizing the intersection between a particular domain—cognitive, affective, or behavioral—of family functioning and a specific intervention offered by health-care professionals; a companion to the Calgary Family Assessment Model (CFAM).

The CFIM is a strengths- and resiliency-based model. We believe that this type of shift in emphasis from deficits and dysfunction to strengths and resiliency in family nursing practice greatly influences the types of interventions offered to and chosen by families within our model. It is important to note that Gottlieb (2012) has devoted an entire book to the importance of focusing on strengths in nursing care and continues to advocate for its importance (Gottlieb & Gottlieb, 2017).

This chapter presents our definition and description of the CFIM, examples of interventions in three domains of family functioning, and actual clinical examples using the CFIM. This chapter concludes with intervention ideas for family situations that nurses commonly encounter.

DEFINITION AND DESCRIPTION

If a comprehensive family assessment has been completed and family intervention is indicated, a nurse must then consider how to intervene to facilitate change. The CFIM is an organizing framework for conceptualizing the intersection between a particular domain of family functioning and the specific intervention offered by the nurse (Figure 4-1). The elements of the CFIM are as follows:

- Interventions
- Domains of family functioning
- "Fit" or meshing (i.e., effectiveness)

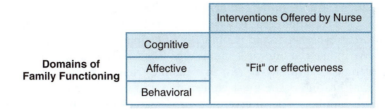

Figure 4-1   CFIM: Intersection of domains of family functioning and interventions.

The CFIM visually portrays the fit or meshing between a domain of family functioning and a nursing intervention; it answers these questions:

- In what domain of family functioning does this intervention intend a change?
- Is it a fit for this family?

The CFIM focuses on promoting, improving, and sustaining effective family functioning in three domains or areas:

- Cognitive
- Affective
- Behavioral

Interventions can be designed to promote, improve, or sustain family functioning in any or all of the three domains, but a change in one area can affect the other domains. We believe that the most profound and sustaining changes are the ones that occur within the family's beliefs (cognition) (Bell & Wright, 2011; Wright, 2015; Wright & Bell, 2009). In other words, as a family thinks, so it *is*. In many cases, one intervention can actually simultaneously influence all three domains of family functioning.

We believe that nurses can only offer interventions to the family within a relational stance; they cannot instruct, direct, demand, or insist on a particular kind of change or way of family functioning. Such directive practices by nurses do not result in satisfying family-nurse relationships for either the nurse or the family, nor do they result in beneficial outcomes. Families are more open to the ideas offered by nurses when the relationships are in the context of collaborative interaction (e.g., inviting, asking, encouraging, supporting) rather than instructive interaction (e.g., instructing, directing, lecturing, demanding).

Whether the family is open to an intervention also depends on its genetic makeup and the family's history of interactions among family members and between family members and health professionals (Maturana & Varela, 1992). Openness to certain interventions is also profoundly influenced by the relationship between the nurse and the family (Bell, 2016; Moules & Johnstone, 2010; Sigurdardottir, Svavarsdottir, Rayens, & Adkins, 2013; Svavarsdottir & Sigurdardottir, 2013; Sveinbjarnardottir, Svavarsdottir, & Saveman, 2011;

Wright, 2015) and the nurse's ability to help the family reflect on their health problems (Bell & Wright, 2011; Wright & Bell, 2009; Wright & Levac, 1992). Second-order cybernetics and the biology of cognition (Maturana & Varela, 1992) have influenced our ideas in this area (see Chapter 2).

Intervening in a family system in a manner that promotes or facilitates change and healing is the most challenging and exciting aspect of clinical work with families. The intervention process represents the core of clinical practice with families. It provides an appropriate context in which the family can make necessary changes that enhance the possibilities of healing. Myriad interventions are possible, but nurses need to tailor their interventions to each family and to the chosen domain of family functioning.

An awareness of ethical considerations is necessary for the nurse. Specific interventions usually vary for each family, although in some instances the same intervention may be used for several families and for different problems. We wish to emphasize, however, that each family is unique and that although labeling particular interventions is an important part of putting our practice into language, it does not represent a "cookbook" approach. We also wish to emphasize that the interventions we list are examples of interventions that can be used; they are not intended to be all-inclusive. The interventions that we cite are based on several important theoretical foundations: postmodernism, systems theory, cybernetics, communication theory, change theory, and the biology of cognition (see Chapter 2).

In summary, the CFIM is not a list of family functions or a list of nursing interventions. Rather, it provides a means to conceptualize a fit or meshing between domains or areas of family functioning and selected interventions offered by the nurse. The CFIM assists in determining the domain of family functioning that predominantly needs changing, usually where there is the greatest suffering, and the most useful interventions to effect change in that domain.

We use the qualitative terms *fit* or *meshing* to emphasize whether or not the interventions effect change and/or ease suffering in the presenting problem. *Fit* involves recognizing reciprocity between the nurse's ideas and opinions and the family's illness experience. Therefore, determining fit or meshing may involve some experimentation or trial and error. It also entails a belief by nurses that each family is unique and has particular strengths. In Chapter 7, we outline techniques for enhancing the likelihood that interventions will stimulate change in the desired domain of family functioning.

INTERVENTIVE QUESTIONS

One of the simplest but most powerful nursing interventions for families experiencing health problems is the use of interventive questions. These questions are intended to actively effect change in any or all of the three domains. However, nurses conducting family interviews should remember that knowing when, how, and why to pose questions is more important than simply choosing one type of question over another (Wright & Bell, 2009).

KEY CONCEPT DEFINED

Linear Questions

Questions asked by the nurse during family interviews that are meant to inform the nurse about the family's descriptions or perceptions of a problem.

Linear Versus Circular Questions

Interventive questions are usually of two types (Tomm, 1987, 1988):

- Linear (investigative)
- Circular (reveal explanations)

KEY CONCEPT DEFINED

Circular Questions

Questions asked by the nurse during family interviews that are meant to reveal the family's understanding of its problems.

The important difference between these kinds of questions is their intent. Linear questions are meant to inform the nurse, whereas circular questions are meant to effect change (Tomm, 1985, 1987, 1988).

Linear Questions

These types of questions explore and investigate a family member's descriptions or perceptions of a problem.

> *Example:* When exploring parents' perceptions of their daughter Cheyenne's anorexia nervosa, the nurse could begin with linear questions, such as: *"When did you notice that your daughter had changed her eating habits?"* and *"What do you think caused your daughter to stop eating as she normally would?"*

These linear questions inform the nurse of the history of the young woman's eating patterns and help illuminate family perceptions or beliefs about eating patterns. Linear questions are frequently used to begin gathering information about a family's problems, whereas circular questions reveal a family's understanding of problems.

Circular Questions

These types of questions aim to reveal explanations of problems.

> *Example:* With the same family, the nurse could ask: *"Who in the family is most worried about Cheyenne's anorexia?"* and *"How does Mother show that she is the one who worries the most?"*

Circular questions help the nurse to discover valuable information because they seek out information about relationships between individuals, events, ideas, and/or beliefs.

The effect of these different question types on families is quite distinct. Linear questions tend to limit any further understanding, whereas circular questions are generative and open possibilities for new understandings. Circular questions introduce new cognitive connections or a change in the illness beliefs of families, paving the way for new or different family behaviors. Linear questioning implies that the nurse knows what is best for the family and is therefore operating under the "sin of certainty" or objectivity without parentheses (Maturana & Varela, 1992). It also implies that the nurse has become purposive and invested in a particular outcome. Linear questions are intended to correct behavior; circular questions are intended to facilitate behavioral change.

The primary distinction between circular and linear questions lies in the notion that information reveals differences in relationships (Bateson, 1979). With circular questions, a relationship or connection between individuals, events, ideas, or beliefs is always sought and in a context of compassion and curiosity. With linear questions, the focus is on cause and effect. The idea of circular questions evolved from the concept of circularity and the method of circular interviewing developed by the originators of Milan Systemic Family Therapy (Selvini-Palazzoli, Boscolo, Cecchin, & Prata, 1980; Tomm, 1984, 1985, 1987).

Circularity involves the cycle of questions and answers between families and nurses that occurs during the interview process. The nurse's skillful questions are based on thoughtful assessment, conceptualization, and hypotheses that can foster understanding and that can obtain information the family gives in response to the questions the nurse asks, and thus the cycle continues. The family's responses to questions provide information for the nurse and the family. The nurse is not an outside interpreter or narrator in this process but rather a participant in the relationship and interaction. Questions in and of themselves can also provide new information and answers for the family, and so they become interventions. Interventive questions may encourage family members to perceive their problems in a new way, which eases their suffering and allows them to see new solutions. Thus, as the family's answers provide information for the nurse, the nurse's questions may provide information for the family.

Circular questions have various applications in family nursing and family therapy. Østergaard et al (2018) conducted a randomized multicenter trial to explore the effect of family nursing therapeutic conversations on health-related quality of life, self-care, and depression among outpatients with heart failure. Circular questions were used as an intervention, with a focus on commendations, strengths, and resources within the family, which was beneficial to building family relationships. Wright and Bell (2009) demonstrated the therapeutic aspect of circular questions with families experiencing chronic illness, life-threatening illness, and psychosocial problems. In family therapy, Spain et al (2017) conducted a literature review to evaluate the effectiveness of enhanced communication and coping for individuals with autism spectrum disorder (ASD) and their family members and found that family therapists utilized various interventions, such as circular and reflective questions. Utilizing the CFIM, Duhamel and Talbot (2004) found that nurses considered interventive questioning useful because it stimulated discussion on specific topics: "One of the questions was formulated as 'What were the most significant changes that occurred in the family since the onset of the illness?' This question led to the identification of efforts made by the couples to comply with medical recommendations, and of their progress in the rehabilitation process" (p. 23).

KEY CONCEPT DEFINED

Commendations

Comments by the nurse during family interviews and counseling that emphasize observed positive patterns of behavior, such as family and individual strengths, competencies, and resources.

Tomm (1987) embellished the types of circular questions used by the Milan Systemic Family Therapy team and identified, defined, and classified various circular questions. The ones we have found most useful in relational clinical practice with families are as follows:

- **Difference questions**
- **Behavioral-effect questions**
- **Hypothetical or future-oriented questions**

KEY CONCEPT DEFINED

Difference Questions

Questions asked by the nurse during family interviews that explore differences between people, relationships, time, ideas, and/or beliefs.

> **KEY CONCEPT DEFINED**
>
> ## Hypothetical or Future-Oriented Questions
>
> Questions asked by the nurse during a family interview that explore family options and alternative actions or meanings in the future.

We have expanded the use of circular questions by providing examples of questions that can be asked to intervene in the cognitive, affective, and behavioral domains of family functioning (Table 4-1).

> **KEY CONCEPT DEFINED**
>
> ## Behavioral-Effect Questions
>
> Questions asked by the nurse during family interviews that explore the effect of one family member's behavior on another.

TABLE 4-1   **Circular Questions to Invite Change in the Cognitive, Affective, and Behavioral Domains of Family Functioning**

1. Type: Difference Question

Definition: Explores differences between people, relationships, time, ideas, and/or beliefs.

COGNITIVE	AFFECTIVE	BEHAVIORAL
■ What is the best advice that you have received about managing your son's HIV?	■ Who in the family is most worried about how HIV is transmitted?	■ Who in the family is best at getting your son to take his medication on time?
■ What is the worst advice you have received?	■ Who finds your disclosure of sexual abuse most difficult?	■ When you first disclosed your sexual abuse, what actions by professionals were most helpful?
■ What information would be most helpful to you about managing the effects of sexual abuse?		
■ Who in the family would benefit most from the information?		

TABLE 4-1	Circular Questions to Invite Change in the Cognitive, Affective, and Behavioral Domains of Family Functioning—cont'd

2. Type: Behavioral-Effect Question

Definition: Explores the effect of one family member's behavior on another.

COGNITIVE	AFFECTIVE	BEHAVIORAL
▪ How do you make sense of your husband not visiting your son in the hospital?	▪ What do you feel when you see your son crying after his treatments?	▪ What do you do when your husband does not visit your son in the hospital?
▪ What do you know about the effect of life-threatening illness on children?	▪ How does your mother show that she is afraid of dying?	▪ What could your father do to indicate to your mother that he understands her fears?

3. Type: Hypothetical/Future-Oriented Question

Definition: Explores family options and alternative actions or meanings in the future.

COGNITIVE	AFFECTIVE	BEHAVIORAL
▪ What do you think will happen if these skin grafts continue to be so painful for your son?	▪ If your son's skin grafts are not successful, what do you think his mood will be? Sad? Angry? Resigned?	▪ How much longer do you think it will be before your son engages in treatment for his contractures?
▪ If the worst occurs, how do you think your family will cope?	▪ If your grandmother's treatment does not go well, who will be most affected?	▪ How long do you think your grandmother will have to remain in the hospital?
▪ If you decide to have your grandmother institutionalized, with whom would you discuss the decision?		▪ If your grandmother stays longer in the hospital, what new self-care behaviors will she be doing?

In summary, difference questions, behavioral-effect questions, and hypothetical questions can be used to facilitate change in any or all of the domains of family functioning. Figure 4-2 illustrates the intersection of various types of circular questions and the domains of family functioning. We strongly emphasize that the effectiveness, usefulness, and fit of the question, rather than the specific question itself, are most critical in effecting change.

	Interventions Offered by Nurse: Circular Questions			
	Difference	Behavioral Effect	Hypothetical	Triadic
Cognitive				
Affective				
Behavioral				

*(Left label: **Domains of Family Functioning**)*

Figure 4-2   Intersection of circular questions and domains of family functioning.

Other Examples of Interventions

To illustrate the intersection of the three domains or areas of family functioning (cognitive, affective, and behavioral) and various interventions, we have chosen a few examples of interventions that can be used in addition to circular questions. This list is not exhaustive; rather, it is a selection of interventions that we have found useful and effective in our clinical practice and research. Examples include the following:

- Commending family and individual strengths
- Offering information and opinions
- Validating, acknowledging, or normalizing emotional responses
- Encouraging the telling of illness narratives
- Drawing forth family support
- Encouraging family members to be caregivers and offering caregiver support
- Encouraging respite
- Devising rituals

These interventions can influence change in any or all of the domains of family functioning. For example, the nurse can offer information to promote change in cognitive, affective, or behavioral family functioning (Figure 4-3).

The following section describes each intervention and offers a case example illustrating its application. We have grouped the sample interventions around a particular domain of family functioning. However, we do not wish to imply that one intervention can be used to facilitate change in only one domain of family functioning or that one intervention is a "cognitive intervention" and another an "affective intervention." Rather, these are examples of the fit between a specific problem or illness, a particular intervention, and a domain of family functioning.

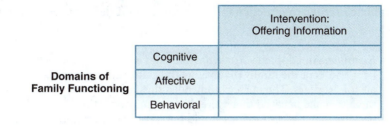

Figure 4-3 Intersection of intervention (offering information) and domains of family functioning.

INTERVENTIONS TO CHANGE THE COGNITIVE DOMAIN OF FAMILY FUNCTIONING

Interventions directed at the cognitive domain of family functioning usually offer new ideas, opinions, beliefs, information, or education on a particular health problem or risk. The treatment goal or desired outcome is to change the way in which a family perceives its health problems so that members can discover new solutions to these problems. The following interventions are examples of ways to change the cognitive domain of family functioning.

> **KEY CONCEPT DEFINED**
>
> **Cognitive Domain of Family Functioning**
>
> Interventions used in the Calgary Family Intervention Model (CFIM) that offer new ideas, opinions, beliefs, information, or education on a particular health problem or risk.

Commending Family and Individual Strengths

We routinely commend family and individual strengths, competencies, and resources observed during interviews. Commendations differ from compliments and are instead an observation of *patterns* of behavior that occur across time. Example of a commendation: *"Your family members are very loyal to one another."* A compliment is usually an observation of a one-time event. Example of a compliment: *"You were very praising of your son today."*

Families coping with chronic, life-threatening, or psychosocial problems commonly feel defeated, hopeless, or unsuccessful in their efforts to overcome or live with these problems. We choose to emphasize strengths and resilience rather than deficits, dysfunctions, and deficiencies in family members.

> *Example:* An adopted son's behavioral and emotional problems had kept the family involved with health-care professionals for 10 years. The nurse commended this family by telling them that she believed they were the best family for this boy because many other families would not have been as sensitive to his needs and probably would have given up years ago. Both parents became tearful and said that this was the first positive statement made to them as parents in many years.

By commending a family's competence, resilience, and strengths and offering them a new opinion or view of themselves, a context for change is created that allows families to then discover their own solutions to problems and enhance healing. Box 4-1 suggests helpful hints for offering commendations. Further discussion about commendations can found in Chapter 9.

Offering Information and Opinions

The offering of information and opinions from health-care professionals is one of the most significant needs for families experiencing illness, especially if the illness is complex.

Adams, Mannix, and Harrington (2017) conducted a literature review on nurses' perceptions of their role when communicating with families in adult intensive care units (ICUs). This review found that intensive care nurses wanted to help families to understand a broader picture of their patients'

Box 4-1 Helpful Hints for Offering Commendations

- Be a "family strengths" detective and look for opportunities to commend families when strengths are discovered and uncovered.
- Ensure that sufficient evidence for the commendation is present; otherwise it may sound insincere and overly ingratiating.
- Use the family's language and integrate important family beliefs to strengthen the validity of the commendation.
- Offer commendations within the first 10 minutes of meeting with a family to enhance the practitioner-family relationship and to increase family receptivity to later ideas.
- Routinely include commendations to families at the end of an interaction or meeting and before offering an opinion.

From Levac, A. M. C., Wright, L. M., & Leahey, M. (2002). Children and families: Models for assessment and intervention. In J. Fox (Ed.), Primary health care of infants, children, and adolescents (2nd ed.). St. Louis, MO: Mosby, p. 13. Reprinted by permission.

situations and prioritized their role as interpreters of information and plans while also having an active role in providing information to families.

> **Example:** *Families with young children*
> Nurses working with families with young children often provide important information to parents about the following:
>
> - Child's current health situation
> - Treatment plans, medications, diagnostic screening
> - Health education and promotion
> - Physiological, emotional, and cognitive development
> - Developmental milestones

In this example, the information provided by the nurse can influence the way in which the parents may think about or understand a situation and in turn impact decisions.

> **Example:** *Families with a chronic or acute illness*
> Families with a chronic or acute illness often identify that obtaining information is a high priority. Many families have expressed to us their frustration at their inability to readily obtain information or opinions from health-care professionals. Nurses can offer information about the impact of chronic or life-shortening illnesses on families.

> **Example:** *Families with complex health issues*
> A family of two aging parents who are the caregivers of their 34-year-old son, who has severe multiple sclerosis, has not had any respite for several months. The nurse asked the son if he would be willing to challenge his beliefs about his "helplessness." The nurse asked him to take the leadership role in exploring possible resources for caregivers so that his parents could have a vacation. Because of his search, the son discovered that he was eligible for many financial benefits of which he had previously been unaware, including benefits to hire professional caregivers. Shortly afterward, the son arranged for 24-hour in-home nursing care when his parents took a vacation. His parents reported that they felt much less stressed and that their son was much happier. He began making efforts to walk using parallel bars, which he had not done in several months.

In this example, the nurse was able to empower the son to change his thinking about his current situation. The intervention fit the cognitive domain, and results took place in the affective and behavioral domains of family functioning.

In all of these examples, nurses are able to empower families to obtain information and resources that impact health outcomes. Box 4-2 suggests helpful hints for offering information and opinions.

Box 4-2 Helpful Hints for Offering Information and Opinions

- Use language that is relevant, clear, and specific.
- Provide easy-to-read literature; write out key points on a small card.
- Inform families of community support groups and resources. Determine if these resources have been helpful to families who have used them and how they were helpful.
- Build on family abilities by encouraging family members to independently seek resources. Inquire about the family's reaction after seeking resources.
- Offer ideas, information, and reflections in a spirit of learning and wondering (e.g., "I wonder what would happen if you tried a slightly different approach to talking with Manisha about sex and birth control. Perhaps you might…").
- Do not be invested in the outcome. If the family does not apply the teaching materials, be curious about what did not fit for them rather than becoming judgmental and angry with them.

From Levac, A. M. C., Wright, L. M., & Leahey, M. (2002). Children and families: Models for assessment and intervention. In J. Fox (Ed.), Primary health care of infants, children, and adolescents (2nd ed.). St. Louis, MO: Mosby, p. 13. Reprinted by permission.

INTERVENTIONS TO CHANGE THE AFFECTIVE DOMAIN OF FAMILY FUNCTIONING

Interventions aimed at the affective domain of family functioning are designed to reduce or increase intense emotions that may be blocking families' problem-solving efforts. The following interventions are examples of ways to change the affective domain of family functioning.

KEY CONCEPT DEFINED

Affective Domain of Family Functioning

Interventions used in the Calgary Family Intervention Model (CFIM) that reduce or increase intense emotions that may be blocking families' problem-solving efforts.

Validating, Acknowledging, or Normalizing Emotional Responses

Validation or acknowledgment of intense affect can reduce or cushion feelings of isolation and loneliness, ease suffering, and help family members to make the connection between a family member's illness and their emotional response (Wright, 2008).

Example: *Diagnosis of a life-shortening illness*

Families frequently feel out of control or frightened for a period of time after learning of this kind of diagnosis. It is important for nurses to acknowledge these strong emotions and to reassure and offer hope to families that, in time, they can adjust and learn new ways to cope. A nurse may say: *"Feeling overwhelmed and frightened is common because there can be a lot of emotions and feelings of uncertainty at this time. Let's talk about some of the changes that are occurring and strategies that might help you cope."*

Encouraging the Telling of Illness Narratives

Too often, family members are encouraged to tell only the medical story or narrative of their illness rather than the story of their own unique experience of their illness, or illness narrative. However, when nurses encourage family members to tell their illness narratives, not only are stories of sickness and suffering told but also stories of strength and tenacity (Wright & Bell, 2009). Through therapeutic conversations, nurses can create a trusting environment for open expression of family members' fears, anger, and sadness about their illness experience (Sigurdardottir et al, 2013; Svavarsdottir & Sigurdardottir, 2013; Wright & Bell, 2009).

KEY CONCEPT DEFINED

Illness Narrative

An individual's story of his or her own unique experience of illness.

These conversations are particularly important for complex family types involving multiple parents and siblings. Having an opportunity to express the illness's impact on the family and the influence of the family on the illness from each family member's perspective validates their experiences.

Listening to, witnessing, and documenting illness stories can also have a profound impact on the nurse. This approach is very different from limiting or constraining family stories to symptoms, medication use, and physical treatments. By providing a context for family members to share the illness experience, nurses allow intense emotions to be legitimized.

Drawing Forth Family Support

Nurses can enhance family functioning in the affective domain by encouraging and helping family members to listen to each other's concerns and feelings. This technique can be particularly useful because talking can be healing. By fostering opportunities for family members to express feelings about a painful or positive experience, the nurse can enable them to draw forth their own strengths and resources to support one another. The nurse can be the catalyst that facilitates communication between family members or between the family and other health-care professionals. This type of family support can prevent families from becoming unduly burdened or defeated by an illness. Intervening in this manner is especially important in primary health-care settings.

INTERVENTIONS TO CHANGE THE BEHAVIORAL DOMAIN OF FAMILY FUNCTIONING

Interventions directed at the behavioral domain help family members to interact with and behave differently in relation to one another. This change is most often accomplished by inviting some or all the family members to engage in specific behavioral tasks. Some tasks are given during a family meeting so that the nurse can observe the interaction; other tasks or homework assignments are given for family members to complete between interactions. In some cases, the nurse must review with the family the details of the particular task or experiment in order to verify that the family understands what has been suggested. The following interventions are examples of ways to change the behavioral domain of family functioning.

KEY CONCEPT DEFINED

Behavioral Domain of Family Functioning

Interventions used in the Calgary Family Intervention Model (CFIM) that help family members interact with and behave differently in relation to one another and are most often accomplished by inviting some or all of the family members to engage in specific behavioral tasks.

Encouraging Family Members to Be Caregivers and Offering Caregiver Support

Family members are often timid or afraid to become involved in the care of their ill family member unless a nurse supports them. However, in our experience, we have found that family members greatly appreciate opportunities to help their hospitalized family member. They report that it makes them feel less helpless, anxious, and out of control. Of course, family caregivers are also susceptible to the well-known phenomenon of caregiver burden. Health professionals must be alert to the risks involved in family caregiving and be willing to intervene when necessary by offering caregiver support, which means providing the necessary information, advocacy, and support to facilitate patient care by people other than health-care professionals (Barbabella et al, 2016; Blanton, Dunbar & Clark, 2018; Ducharme, 2011). In a study about grandparents' experience of childhood cancer in their grandchildren, grandparents revealed their often unattended and unacknowledged role of both providing and needing support (Moules et al, 2012). Therefore, these authors recommended that an inquiry regarding the resources and support needs of grandparents is essential for optimal family care. We encourage nurses to weigh with family members the ethical, emotional, and physical balance between too much caregiving and not enough caregiving.

Encouraging Respite

Family caregivers commonly do not allow themselves adequate respite. Too frequently, family members feel guilty if they need or want to withdraw themselves from the caregiving role. This is especially true of female caregivers. Even the ill member must occasionally disengage himself or herself from the usual caregiving and reject another person's assistance. Each family's need for respite varies. Factors affecting respite include the severity of the chronic illness, availability of family members to care for the ill person, and financial resources. All of these issues must be considered before a nurse can recommend a respite schedule. Caregiving, coping, and caring for one's own health need to be balanced.

> *Examples:* The following examples of "time-outs" or "times away" can be essential for families facing excessive caregiving demands:
>
> • A family could buy a less expensive prosthesis and use the extra money for a family vacation.
> • A couple with a child with leukemia have the grandparents babysit for a day while the couple spends time together.
> • A postpartum mother is extremely exhausted and has her partner take their newborn to a close friend's house to allow her to rest.

Devising Rituals

Families engage in many types of rituals: daily (e.g., bedtime reading), yearly (e.g., vacation), and cultural (e.g., festivals, celebrations). Roberts (2003) defines rituals as

> co-evolved symbolic acts that include not only the ceremonial aspects of the actual presentation of the ritual, but the process of preparing for it as well. It may or may not include words, but does have both open and closed parts which are "held" together by a guiding metaphor. Repetition can be a part of rituals through the content, the form, or the occasion.

There should be enough space in therapeutic rituals for the incorporation of multiple meanings by various family members and clinicians, as well as a variety of levels of participation. (p. 9)

The findings of Smith et al (2017) suggest that structure provided through family routines and family rituals creates meaning within the family and can support family health. Santos, Crespo, Canavarro, Alderfer, and Kazak (2016) explored family rituals in relation to financial burden and mothers' adjustment in pediatric cancer cases. They concluded that the relationship between financial burden and anxiety symptoms was buffered for mothers who reported high levels of family ritual meaning during their children's cancer treatments and within 5 years after the end of treatment. In our clinical practice, we have observed that chronic illness and psychosocial problems frequently interrupt the usual rituals and routines a family may have. Nurses may want to suggest therapeutic rituals that are not or have not been observed by the family as an intervention to influence the behaviors.

> *Example:* Parents in a new blended family who cannot agree on parenting practices commonly give conflicting messages to their families. This can result in chaos and confusion for their children. The introduction of an odd-day/even-day ritual (Selvini-Palazzoli et al, 1978) can typically assist the family. The mother could experiment with being responsible for the children on Mondays, Wednesdays, and Fridays and the father on Tuesdays, Thursdays, and Saturdays. On Sundays, they could behave spontaneously. On their "days off," parents could be asked to observe, without comment, their partner's parenting.

CLINICAL EXAMPLES

The following clinical examples illustrate the use of the CFIM. These examples of interventions were chosen to facilitate change in all three domains (cognitive, affective, and behavioral) of family functioning. Remember, it is not always necessary or efficient to try to "fit" interventions to all three domains of family functioning simultaneously. Whether this can be done successfully depends on how well the family is engaged and on prior assessment of the nature of the illness, problems, or concerns.

Clinical Example 1: Difficulty Putting 3-Year-Old Child to Bed

To illustrate a specific family intervention aimed at all three domains of family functioning, consider a parenting problem commonly presented to community health nurses (CHNs): parents having difficulty putting their young children to bed each night. The parents' efforts are generally met with annoyance from the child, then anger, and then tears. In their efforts, the parents also become frustrated and commonly end up angry with each other and with their child. The family intervention offered was in the form of information and opinions. In describing this case example, we will also discuss executive skills the nurse can use to operationalize the intervention. These skills are also outlined in Chapter 5.

Parent-Child System Problem

Parents' chronic inability to get their 3-year-old to go to bed and stay there at required time. See Table 4-2 for parent-child interventions.

Clinical Example 2: Elderly Father Complains His Children Do Not Visit Often Enough

This example demonstrates the intervention of encouraging family members to be caregivers and offering caregiver support. This intervention entails inviting family members to be involved in the emotional and physical care of the patient and offering support. Again, the accompanying executive skills to operationalize the interventions are given.

TABLE 4-2	Interventions
DOMAINS OF FAMILY FUNCTIONING	**INTERVENTIONS: OFFERING INFORMATION AND OPINIONS**
Cognitive	■ Offer information, such as a parenting book that explains what bedtime means to children with suggestions on how to put children to bed.
Affective	■ Discuss with the parents the importance of admitting their frustrations to each other, especially if one spouse made an effort to put the child to bed but was not successful. ■ The other parent may give emotional support (e.g., "You tried really hard; he was being very difficult").
Behavioral	■ Teach the parents that, when they put their son to bed, they should not respond to his efforts to gain attention (e.g., asking for a glass of water). Rather, parents should be sure that these needs have been attended to as part of his bedtime rituals. ■ Discuss with parents that, before they can change their child's behavior of leaving his bed or continually calling them to his bedroom, his behavior will worsen for a few nights while he makes greater efforts to get his parents to respond. If the parents continue in a matter-of-fact way to put him back in his room and respond "no" to any further requests, his behavior should improve dramatically in a few nights.

Parent-Child System Problem

Elderly father wants his adult children to visit him more often. The adult children do not enjoy visiting their father at the long-term care center because he always complains that they do not visit often enough. See Table 4-3 for parent-child interventions.

It is important to note that in the examples provided, many other interventions and executive skills could have been offered. There is no one "right" intervention, only "useful" or "effective" interventions. How useful or effective an intervention is can be evaluated only after it has been implemented. The element of time must be taken into account. With some interventions, the change or outcome may be noted immediately. However, in many cases, changes (outcomes) are not noticed for a long time. Most problems do not occur overnight; therefore, their resolutions also require reasonable lengths of time.

Clinical Example 3: Enuresis and Discipline Problems With a Child

To illustrate that change is observed over time, we now offer two more actual case examples, from beginning to end, with the emphasis on the interventions that were used.

TABLE 4-3	Interventions
DOMAINS OF FAMILY FUNCTIONING	**INTERVENTIONS: ENCOURAGING FAMILY MEMBERS TO BE CAREGIVERS AND OFFERING CAREGIVER SUPPORT**
Cognitive	■ Discuss with the adult children that their father may have difficulty remembering their visits (short-term memory deficits), a normal change associated with aging.
Affective	■ Empathize with the father by saying that you understand that it must be lonely at times being a resident in a long-term care center. The adult children might appreciate knowing that their parent is lonely so that they can respond appropriately. ■ Encourage the father to let his children know how lonely he feels at times and that he is happy that they come to visit rather than complaining to the children that they do not visit often enough.
Behavioral	■ Encourage the adult children to stop giving excuses for why they cannot visit more often. Instead, obtain a guest book or calendar and write down each visit. Write down who visited, on what day, and perhaps any interesting news so that the aging parent may read this between visits.

A family was referred to one of our graduate nursing students with the complex presenting problems of enuresis and disciplinary problems at school in the elder child, an 8-year-old boy. The family was composed of the father, age 28, self-employed; the stepmother, age 21, homemaker; and two sons, ages 8 and 6. The couple had been married for approximately 1 year. The family was seen (both as a whole family and in various subsystems) for six sessions over 13 weeks from initial contact to termination. A thorough family assessment (using the CFAM model) revealed problems in the whole family system, in the parent-child subsystem, and at the individual level.

Whole-Family System Problem

Adjustment to Being a Stepfamily

When the couple married, a new family was formed, and all family members had to adjust to a new family structure.

After being married for only a short time, the stepmother found herself thrust into a parenting role when she and her husband became responsible for his two children. The birth mother had deserted the children after living with them for 2 years in her home. The children had to adjust to a new set of parents, new surroundings, and no contact with their biological mother. See Table 4-4 for family interventions.

Providing information about the adjustment process seemed to relieve the parents a great deal. Initially, the parents were hesitant about the children having contact with the biological mother, but they later stated that they understood this contact was important for the children. The eldest child's enuresis was conceptualized as a response to the adjustment to a stepfamily and the loss of his mother. This new opinion, also directed at the cognitive domain of family functioning, had a very positive effect on the family. The enuresis improved dramatically over the course of treatment.

TABLE 4-4	Interventions
DOMAINS OF FAMILY FUNCTIONING	**INTERVENTIONS: OFFERING INFORMATION AND OPINIONS**
Cognitive	■ Acknowledge that the problems the family members are experiencing are a usual part of the adjustment process of stepfamilies and provide them information about the adjustment process.
Behavioral	■ Encourage the parents to allow the children to have contact with their biological mother when she again seeks them out.

Parent-Child Subsystem Problem

Maladaptive Interactional Pattern Between Stepmother and Eldest Son (see Figure 4-4) Because of the initial experience of the loss of their father (as a result of the biological parents' divorce) and then the abandonment by their biological mother, the children, particularly the elder child, feared being abandoned again. Thus, the elder child, hoping to be reassured that he would not be abandoned again, frequently reminded his young stepmother that she was not his real mother.

Initially, the stepmother made efforts to reassure him, but she eventually withdrew in frustration and felt rejected. This encouraged the child to maintain the maladaptive interactional pattern because he perceived this withdrawal as further evidence that he would again be abandoned. The vicious cycle was evident.

In deciding which interventions to offer the family, the graduate nursing student was at first overwhelmed by the complexity of their situation. Then she considered which area had the most leverage for change. See Table 4-5 for parental interventions.

The stepmother reported that when she offered more reassurance to the boy, he stopped rejecting her. With decreased rejection, the stepmother was able to offer even more reassurance. Thus, a virtuous cycle began.

Individual Problem

Elder Child's Behavioral Problems at School

To further assess this behavioral problem, the graduate nursing student met with the child's teacher at school and also discussed the problem twice with the teacher by telephone. The stepmother was also present during the session at school.

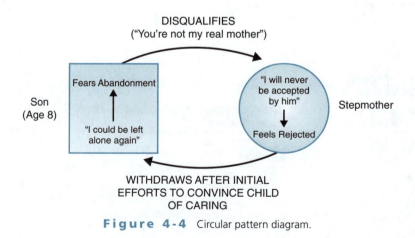

Figure 4-4 Circular pattern diagram.

TABLE 4-5	Interventions
DOMAINS OF FAMILY FUNCTIONING	**INTERVENTIONS: PROVIDING PARENT SUPPORT AND EDUCATION**
Cognitive	■ Encourage the stepmother to stop withdrawing and to offer the child continual and sustained reassurance by stating: *"I know I am not your mother, but your father and I love and care for you and want to look after you. We will not leave you."* ■ Provide commendations of family strengths to the stepmother for her efforts to fulfill her role.
Affective	■ Encourage the stepmother to stop withdrawing and to offer the child continual and sustained reassurance by stating: *"I know I am not your mother, but your father and I love and care for you and want to look after you. We will not leave you."*
Behavioral	■ Encourage the stepmother to stop withdrawing and to offer the child continual and sustained reassurance by stating: *"I know I am not your mother, but your father and I love and care for you and want to look after you. We will not leave you."*

The main objective of the interventions was to enhance the elder child's self-esteem by focusing on his positive behavior. See Table 4-6 for interventions.

On termination with this family, the graduate student recommended to the parents some readings on stepfamilies and informed them of a self-help group for stepfamilies. These two interventions of offering ideas and opinions in books and providing information on community resources were targeted at all three domains of family functioning: cognitive, affective, and behavioral.

It might seem that the interventions the graduate student chose in this example were "simple." However, in many cases, nurses either try to use

TABLE 4-6	Interventions
DOMAINS OF FAMILY FUNCTIONING	**INTERVENTION: ENHANCE ELDEST CHILD'S SELF-ESTEEM**
Behavioral	■ Encourage the teacher to acknowledge the child's positive behavior in front of his classmates to give him a different status than *"class clown."* ■ Recommend that the stepmother minimize her contact with the school and allow the teacher to assume more responsibility for the boy's behavior in class.

overly complex interventions to address issues or they have difficulty collaborating with the family to determine areas with leverage for change. In both cases, nurses commonly become frustrated and immobilized by the complexity of the family situation. A thorough exploration of the presenting issue and then an offering of interventions designed to ameliorate that problem generally works best to foster change.

Clinical Example 4: Social Isolation and Physical Complaints of Elderly Woman

During one of our undergraduate nursing students' field placement in a community-health facility, she encountered a family whose presenting problems were social isolation and frequent physical complaints from the 78-year-old widowed mother. The widow lived in a government-subsidized, one-bedroom apartment. She had six adult children (sons ages 51, 48, 41, 37, and 35 years and a daughter, age 44 years) and 12 grandchildren. Five of the children were married, and all six lived in the same city as their mother. The family was seen as a whole and in various subsystems for eight home visits over a period of 2 months. After a thorough family assessment (using the CFAM model) and individual assessments, the following core problem was identified.

Whole-Family System Problem

The Mother's Lack of Social Contact Beyond Her Immediate Family.

It became apparent that this older woman was overly dependent on her adult children and, therefore, did not make an effort to be involved with her peers or in social activities appropriate to her age group. This resulted in frequent disagreements between the mother and the children over the frequency of visits with the mother.

The problem was further exacerbated by the fact that the mother had no friends. After the death of her husband, approximately 10 years earlier, she had lived intermittently with some of her children but had been living alone for the past 4 years. At the time of intervention, the youngest son visited most often and did the mother's grocery shopping.

The nursing student's first significant intervention was to broaden the context in order to expand her view and understanding of this family's concerns. Thus, the student initially interviewed the mother alone and then interviewed her with her youngest son (the adult child who visited most frequently). Then the student took on the ambitious task of arranging an interview with the mother and her six children. This was a significant effort on the student's part to create a context for change by obtaining each family member's view of the problem. In the interview with the mother and her youngest son, the mother agreed to contact the children. However, when the student followed up with the mother, the mother said that she had not called any of her children because she expected her youngest son to do it. This was further evidence of the mother's overdependence on her children. Because the youngest son was anxious to have the meeting take place, he had taken on the task of inviting all of his siblings to an interview with his mother and the nursing student.

At the family interview, all of the siblings were present, and two of their spouses attended as well. Interestingly, the daughters-in-law were more vocal than their husbands and stated that they were very involved with their mother-in-law. In this large family interview, the mother's social isolation (apart from her family) was discussed. Through the process of circular questioning, the expectations for family contact of both the mother and children were assessed. Initially, the student encouraged the family to explore solutions to their mother's lack of social activities and peer interactions (an intervention aimed at the behavioral domain of family functioning). To this intervention, the family responded that they had no ideas beyond what they had already tried. Therefore, the student suggested more specific interventions in an attempt to uncover solutions to the mother's social isolation.

This interview revealed that the woman had always relied on her children for her main social interaction. She had never been a "joiner." In the past few years, she had even discontinued her attendance at church. Throughout her life, she had few close friends. The assessment also revealed that, collectively, the children had generally been supportive of their mother. Each week, she had lunch with one or more of them. They included her in all special family occasions. However, the children always had to initiate contact. They were genuinely concerned about their mother's loneliness and lack of additional social contact but had exhausted their ideas for changing her situation.

One of the first interventions the nursing student attempted was directed at both the cognitive and behavioral domains of family functioning: offering information regarding community resources that are available to older people. Specifically, the student made the family aware of the Community Services Visitor Program. The mother agreed to contact this program, and the children agreed to provide support. The mother also expressed interest in becoming involved in a choir again. The student offered to accompany her to a senior citizens' choir practice and introduce her to other participants.

The final major intervention discussed in that family session was directed at the behavioral domain. The student nurse asked the mother if she would initiate contact with one of her children during the next week. After the contact, the child would ask the mother to come for a visit as soon as possible. This intervention was important because the interest of family members in an older parent's activities typically increases the parent's motivation. It is important to emphasize that the mother was involved in and receptive to these interventions.

The effects and outcomes of these interventions were as follows:

- The mother followed through on contacting the Community Services Visitor Program. The coordinator of the program then contacted the mother and arranged for a regular visitor.
- The student nurse accompanied the mother to the senior citizens' choir. The older woman enjoyed the experience and telephoned two of the other women in the choir afterward!
- The mother took the initiative to contact a couple of her children, and they, in turn, invited her for a family visit, which she accepted. The children reported that they enjoyed having their mother call them, and this new dynamic appeared to increase their own desire to have more frequent contact with her.

In subsequent interviews, the student nurse encouraged the mother to reconnect with her church. The student also solicited the support of the children in this endeavor by requesting that they take an interest in and inquire about their mother's church and choir activities when they called her.

Because this mother was accustomed to a good deal of family support, it was not appropriate to remove that support totally. However, physical instrumental support (i.e., doing things for the mother) was reduced without the mother feeling abandoned. Verbal (emotional) support for the mother's attempts at independence was most appropriate. When the mother began to increase her social contacts and activities, her nonspecific physical complaints decreased.

The student concluded treatment with this woman in a face-to-face interview. To involve the children in the termination process, the student sent a therapeutic letter to each of them. The letter highlights the major interventions and solicits further assistance from the children and includes some of the family strengths.

> *Dear...:*
> *I wish to thank you for your help and cooperation in my family assignment. I enjoyed meeting each of you and appreciated your individual input and assessment of your family. Your willingness to work together is certainly an excellent family strength.*
> *I visited your mother on several occasions during my time with the Outreach Program. She continued to express her desire to be more socially independent. She has been able to make some increased community contact. She attended the choir and several of the choir ladies have called her to encourage her in continued participation. She met with the gentleman from the church and spoke with his wife. The coordinator of the visitor program visited; she is arranging for*

a friend who will visit with your mother. Hopefully, they will develop some outside interests together. She has also been out to shop on her own on a few occasions.

I did contact Kerby Centre, as well as other seniors from Carter Place who go there, but was unable to find anyone going to the Wednesday lunch or any other suitable transportation. I have discussed this with your mother and she felt it might be something she could pursue on her own in the future.

Your mother expressed positive feelings about her attempts to be more socially active. However, she still looks to her children for her main support. At times, I found she needed more encouragement not to overly worry about her health to the point that she thinks she is unable to participate in any activities. I believe that each of you may help your mother by encouraging her in this area. I might suggest that if she says that she is unwell that she see her doctor. If there is no serious problem, gentle support for her independent activities might be helpful. This may be somewhat difficult at first, but if you are able to present a united front to your mother and support each other in a mutual approach to her being more socially active, she may be more able to accomplish this.

I am very impressed with the cohesiveness of your family and the continued concern and support you show toward your mother. Thank you very much again for letting me work with you.

Yours truly,
Leslie Henderson
Undergraduate Nursing Student
Faculty of Nursing, University of Calgary

This therapeutic letter sent by the student is an intervention in and of itself (Bell, Moules, & Wright, 2009; Moules, 2009; Wright & Bell, 2009). Several interventions were outlined in the letter, and these interventions were aimed at all three areas of family functioning. Specifically, the student offered commendations and opinions directed at the cognitive domain of functioning. She invited the adult children to encourage their mother, which aimed at changes in the behavioral domain. By summarizing the clinical work with the family in the form of a therapeutic letter, the student intended to effect changes in both the affective and cognitive domains of family functioning. This clinical example demonstrates how to effectively involve families in health care by the use of family assessment and intervention models with clear treatment goals.

CASE SCENARIO: HARVEY JOHNSON

Harvey Johnson is an 85-year-old male who lives alone in his own home. His wife of 65 years, Patricia, recently was moved into a long-term care facility after she was diagnosed with Alzheimer disease, and Harvey was no longer able to care for her at home. Patricia's memory has declined rapidly, and she no longer remembers who Harvey is or where she is. Harvey and Patricia's four children live 30 minutes away and have families of their own. They visit Harvey regularly but have recently been concerned about how their father is coping at home alone. Their oldest son has requested that a home-care nurse visit Harvey at home. During an initial phone conversation with the son, the home-care nurse was able to find out that Harvey and Patricia had never spent a night apart until Patricia moved to the long-term care facility. They were devoted to each other and mostly kept to themselves. They were like "teenagers in love" even after 65 years of marriage. Their son stated that Harvey has become increasingly irritable, appears very tired, and has lost weight since Patricia was moved to long-term care.

When the home-care nurse arrives at Harvey's home, there are dishes piled in the kitchen sink and newspapers piled on the kitchen table, and the temperature is very cold in the home. The home-care nurse asks Harvey about how he is coping, and he states: "It doesn't matter anymore how I am. Patricia doesn't remember who I am, and the kids are so busy with their own families. What is the point?"

Reflective Questions

1. What are three linear questions and three circular questions the nurse could ask Harvey to gain further understanding of the family's concerns?
2. Identify a potential intervention and expected outcome aimed at each domain of family functioning.
3. How can the nurse involve Harvey's children in the development and implementation of the interventions?

CRITICAL THINKING QUESTIONS

1. Reflect on an interaction you had with a family:
   a. How did you use intervention questions?
   b. What linear questions did you ask?
   c. What circular questions did you ask?
2. Consider your own clinical practice to answer the following question:
   a. What interventions do you implement to direct change at the cognitive, affective, and behavioral domains of family functioning?

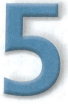

Chapter **5**

Family Nursing Interviews: Stages and Skills

Learning Objectives

- Explain the four evolving stages of a family nursing interview.
- Describe perceptual, conceptual, and executive skills used in each stage of a family nursing interview.
- Describe educational approaches for nurses to develop family interview skills.

Key Concepts

Assessment stage	Executive skills	Termination stage
Conceptual skills	Intervention stage	
Engagement stage	Perceptual skills	

Once nurses have a clear conceptual framework for assessing and intervening with families, they can then begin to consider the various new competencies and skills needed for family interviews. The clinical skills deemed necessary by various authors on family work reflect each author's theoretical orientation and preference regarding how to approach and resolve relational, family, and individual problems. Therefore, the skills delineated in this chapter are based on our postmodernist worldview. This includes, but is not limited to, the theoretical foundations of systems theory, cybernetics, communication theory, the biology of cognition, and change theory that inform the Calgary Family Assessment Model (CFAM) and the Calgary Family Intervention Model (CFIM).

We favor an approach that is strengths and resiliency based, problem *and* solution focused, and time effective. Families possess the ability to solve their own problems and/or diminish their suffering but often lack the confidence or belief in their strengths due to the oppression felt by families that often follows when illness arises. Our task as nurses is to help families find and facilitate their own solutions to their emotional, physical, or spiritual suffering through compassionate and competent therapeutic conversations. We do not propose that we know what is "best" for families. Rather, we embrace the notion that the world has multiple realities—in other words, that each family member and nurse sees a world that he or she brings forth by interacting with others through language. We encourage openness in ourselves, our students, and our families to the diversity of difference among us. However, to be involved in helping families change requires that nurses possess certain essential competencies and skills.

In the previous chapters, we discussed the theoretical knowledge base that is necessary to begin to competently assess and intervene with families. Two practice models (the CFAM and CFIM) were offered as frameworks to conceptualize family dynamics and offer specific family interventions. This chapter focuses on the specific beginning-level skills necessary for relational family nursing interviews. In Chapter 10 we discuss how to move beyond basic skills and offer ideas for tailoring advanced skills to the unique client and clinical practice setting.

The International Council of Nurses (ICN) published a document entitled *The Family Nurse: Frameworks for Practice* developed by Madrean Schober and Fadwa Affara (2001). These ideas were further expanded in 2002 when the ICN selected the theme for International Nurses Day to be "Nurses Always There for You: Caring for Families" and produced a document with the same title (ICN, 2002). In this document, the roles of the "nine-star family nurse" were identified, as shown in Box 5-1.

In 2015, The International Family Nursing Association (IFNA) released a document entitled *Position Statement on Generalist Competencies for Family Nursing Practice*. This statement identified five family nursing competencies for undergraduate-level and generalist-level family nursing practice (p. 3):

1. Enhance and promote family health.
2. Focus nursing practice on family strengths, the support of family and individual growth, the improvement of family self-management abilities, the facilitation of successful life transitions, the improvement and management of health, and the mobilization of family resources.
3. Demonstrate leadership and systems-thinking skills to ensure the quality of nursing care with families in everyday practice and across every context.
4. Commit to self-reflective practice based on examination of nurse actions with families and family responses.
5. Practice using an evidence-based approach.

When nurses use conceptual practice models such as the CFAM/CFIM in combination with competencies and skills, they are able to enhance and

> **Box 5-1 Nine-Star Family Nurse**
>
> - Educator
> - Care provider and supervisor
> - Family advocate
> - Case finder and epidemiologist
> - Researcher
> - Manager and coordinator
> - Counselor
> - Consultant
> - Environmental modifier

promote family health more effectively and efficiently. The skills described in this chapter emerge from our theoretical orientation and application of the CFAM and CFIM practice models. These skills become the nurse behaviors that are unique to working with families. Of course, each nurse also has a unique genetic and personality makeup and history of interactions, and these personalize the application of these skills.

> **KEY CONCEPT DEFINED**
> **Engagement Stage**
> The stage during the family interview in which the family is greeted and made comfortable and the relationship continues; based on compassion, collaboration, and consultation.

> **KEY CONCEPT DEFINED**
> **Assessment Stage**
> A stage during the family interview when problem identification and exploration occurs, including delineation of strengths; an ongoing process.

EVOLVING STAGES OF FAMILY NURSING INTERVIEWS

Four major stages of family nursing interviews can be identified:

- Engagement
- Assessment
- Intervention
- Termination

> **KEY CONCEPT DEFINED**
>
> ## Intervention Stage
>
> The stage during a family interview in which the nurse and the family collaborate on areas for desired change.

These stages evolve throughout the interview. They tend to follow a logical sequence during both the course of a given interview and the overall course of contact. For example, a nurse engages family members and terminates with them at the end of each interview and at the beginning and end of the entire contact. Of course, there are times when a nurse may have to return to a previous stage. For example, interventions may be offered too quickly before a thorough assessment has been completed. Other times, the nurse might want to revisit the engagement stage if a new family member attends a meeting. Table 5-1 further explains the stages of family nursing interviews.

> **KEY CONCEPT DEFINED**
>
> ## Termination Stage
>
> The stage during the family interview when the therapeutic relationship between the nurse and the family is ended.

TYPES OF SKILLS

Each stage of family interviewing requires three types of skills:

1. Perceptual
2. Conceptual
3. Executive

> **KEY CONCEPT DEFINED**
>
> ## Executive Skills
>
> Observable therapeutic interventions that a nurse carries out in a family interview that elicit responses from family members and are the basis for the nurse's further observations and conceptualizations.

Cleghorn and Levin's (1973) identification and categorization of these three skill types are considered a seminal contribution. Tomm and Wright (1979) used the perceptual, conceptual, and executive skills framework as a guide for their comprehensive outline, which offered examples of therapist

TABLE 5-1	Stages of Family Nursing Interviews

ENGAGEMENT

- The nurse and the family begin to establish a therapeutic relationship using compassion, collaboration, and consultation (Leahey & Harper-Jaques, 1996).
- The nurse demonstrates curiosity and interest in the family through questioning.
- The nurse must consider equality and respect for the family's resiliency and resourcefulness.
- The nurse brings to the relationship expertise about promoting health and managing illness.
- Family members bring their own unique expertise about their understanding of health and their illness experiences.

ASSESSMENT

- Problem identification and exploration occur, including delineation of strengths.
- The nurse enables the family to tell the story about their particular situation. The story is different for each family.
- The conversation between the nurse and the family is in and of itself part of the therapeutic discourse (Wright & Bell, 2009) and moves beyond focusing only on signs and symptoms of a disease.
- Beginning nurse interviewers generally lack a clear, stepwise rationale to guide the collecting and processing of data during an interview and may spend an inordinate amount of time collecting vast amounts of information or rush into inappropriate treatment because they do not have a clear formulation of the presenting problem.
- Assessment is an ongoing process; the strengths and problems list may change over time.

INTERVENTION

- Provides a context in which the family may make small or significant changes.
- Treatment plans should be co-constructed and tailored by the nurse and family to match each family situation.
- Different styles of questioning can be used as interventions in family interviewing.

TERMINATION

- Termination is the process of ending the therapeutic relationship between the nurse and the family.
- The family continues to maintain constructive changes, new understandings, and facilitating beliefs.
- Therapeutic termination encourages the family's ability to solve problems in the future.

functions, competencies, and skills in each category over the evolution of a family interview. The skills that we have identified fit within the context of our particular practice models—namely, the CFAM and CFIM. Perceptual and conceptual skills are paired because what we perceive is so intimately interrelated with what we think; in many cases, separating the perceptual from the conceptual component is difficult. Perceptual and conceptual skills are then matched with executive skills. Table 5-2 further explains the skills required for family interviewing.

TABLE 5-2	Skills Required for Family Interviewing

PERCEPTUAL SKILLS

- Perceptual skills include nurse's ability to make relevant observations.
- Factors that may influence a nurse's perceptions include the following:
  - Age, ethnicity, gender, sexual orientation, race, class, culture, religion, education
- The perceptual skills required in individual interviewing are different from those required in family interviewing.
  - Family interviewing: The nurse is involved in observing multiple interactions and relationships simultaneously; the interaction among family members and the interaction between the nurse and the family are simultaneous.

CONCEPTUAL SKILLS

- Conceptual skills involve the ability to give meaning to the nurse's observations.
- Conceptual skills involve the ability to formulate one's observations of the family as a whole, as a system. (Meanings derived from observations are not "the truth" about the family; instead, they represent efforts to make sense of observations.)
- Students entering the nursing profession may have intuitive perceptual and conceptual skills from previous life experiences that they may not be aware of.
- Nurses need to develop an overt awareness of the perceptual process, which takes time and is the basis of the executive skills.

EXECUTIVE SKILLS

- Executive skills involve the observable therapeutic interventions that a nurse carries out in an interview (implementation).
- Skills and interventions elicit responses from family members and are the basis for the nurse's further observations and conceptualizations.
- The interview process embedded within the therapeutic conversation is a circular phenomenon between the nurse and family.
- Executive skills develop over time with practice and experience.

KEY CONCEPT DEFINED

Conceptual Skills

Nurses' ability to formulate observations of a family as a whole and as a system and to give meaning to their observations during a family interview.

KEY CONCEPT DEFINED

Perceptual Skills

The nurse's ability to make relevant observations when working with families.

Specific skills for interviewing families are summarized in a logical sequence in Table 5-3. However, during the course of an actual interview, the

(Text continued on page 179)

TABLE 5-3	**Family Interviewing Skills for Nurses**

STAGE 1: ENGAGEMENT

Perceptual/Conceptual Skills	*Executive Skills*
1. Recognize that an individual family member is best understood in the context of the family. ■ No individual exists in isolation.	**1.** Invite all family members who are concerned or involved with the problem, suffering, or illness to attend the first interview. ■ Grandparents or other relatives or friends living inside or outside of the home should also be invited to attend if they are involved with the problem or illness.
2. Appreciate that initial efforts to involve *both* spouses/parents enable (from the onset) a more holistic view of the family and increase engagement. ■ All family members should be involved for effective family work.	**2.** Employ all efforts to initially involve *both* spouses/parents in early sessions. ■ The spouses/parents have the greatest influence on the identification, understanding, and resolution of the problem; easing suffering; and/or managing illness.
3. Recognize that providing a clear structure to the interview reduces anxiety and increases engagement. ■ The uncertainty of being in a new setting and of not knowing how to behave in the situation can result in anxiety. ■ Structure is particularly important if the family is experiencing a crisis.	**3.** Explain to family members the purpose, length, and structure of the interview and ask if they have any questions relating to the interview. ■ Say: *"I thought we could spend about 10 minutes together discussing the issues that you are concerned about."*
4. Recognize that initially, members are most comfortable talking about the structural aspects of the family. ■ Note nonverbal cues indicating level of comfort, such as taking coat off, adequate versus minimal time spent talking, and participating in versus ignoring conversation.	**4.** Ask each family member to briefly relate information with regard to name, age, work, or school; years married; and so forth. ■ Introduce yourself directly by giving your name and shaking hands. ■ Ask questions about information that is familiar to all family members because this type of conversation is least threatening.

Continued

TABLE 5-3	Family Interviewing Skills for Nurses—cont'd

STAGE 2: ASSESSMENT

Perceptual/Conceptual Skills	*Executive Skills*

1. Realize the importance of having a conceptual assessment map to understand family dynamics.
 	
   ■ A conceptual assessment map provides the nurse with several possible courses for focused exploration.
	1. Explore the components of the structural, developmental, and functional aspects of the CFAM to assess strengths and problem areas.
	   ■ Not all components of the CFAM need to be explored if they are not relevant to the present issues, problems, or illness.

2. Begin a family assessment by obtaining a detailed description and history of the presenting problem, concern, or illness.
   ■ The presenting problem usually serves as an entry point for the family to seek help. Focusing on addressing the problem is time-effective.
	2. Ask each family member, including the children, to share his or her knowledge and understanding of the presenting concern.
	   ■ Ask each family member: *"How do you see the problem?"*
	   ■ Ask the whole family: *"What is the main problem or issue that each of you would like to see changed?"*

3. Realize that the presenting problem is commonly related to other concerns in the family.
   ■ A child's temper outbursts may be related to family conflict (e.g., the child may be triangulated into a family conflict over caring for the grandmother).
	3. Explore with the family if there are other problems or concerns connected to the presenting problem.
	   ■ Say: *"We have been talking for some time about the problem of Theo's refusal to take his meds in the mornings. I am wondering if there are any other problems the family is presently concerned about or that relate to Theo's issue?"*

4. Realize that eliciting differences generates more specific information for family assessment.
   (a) Clarification of differences between individuals is a source of information about family functioning.
 	
   (b) Clarification of differences between relationships is a source of information about family structure and alliances.
	4. Inquire about differences between individuals, between relationships, and between various points in time.
	   (a) To explore differences between individuals, ask the child: *"What is expected of you before you go to bed at night?"* and then ask, *"Who is the best, mother or father, at getting you to do those things in the evening?"*
	   (b) To explore differences between relationships, ask: *"Do your father and Ingo argue more or less than your father and Hannah about how to care for your younger sister?"*

TABLE 5-3	**Family Interviewing Skills for Nurses—cont'd**

STAGE 2: ASSESSMENT

Perceptual/Conceptual Skills	*Executive Skills*
(c) Clarification of differences in family members or in relationships at various points in time is a source of information about family development.	(c) To explore differences before or after important points in time, ask: "*Do you worry more, less, or the same about your husband's health since his heart attack?*"
5. Use the information obtained from the family assessment to begin formulating hypotheses in the form of a strengths and problems list. ■ Offering conclusions or a summary of the nurse's assessment ideas enhances engagement and collaboration and allows for self-correction—structural, developmental, and functional strengths and problems may be present at various systems levels. For example, whole-family-system issues include the following: (a) Structural: Adjusting to new family form of single-parent household (b) Developmental: Family in life-cycle stage of children leaving home (c) Functional: Family belief that "Father would be displeased with us for still crying about his death"	5. Obtain verification of the nurse's understanding of strengths and problems by listing them to the family for their agreement and eventually recording them. ■ For example, say: "*We have identified that being a new single parent and also having to cope with your child (who has a developmental delay) leaving home are your two major concerns. We have also discussed that your family is very well respected in the Latino community. Have I understood things correctly?*"
6. Assess whether any of the identified problems are beyond the scope of the nurse's competence. ■ Consider referral when medical symptoms have not been fully assessed or long-standing emotional or behavioral problems exist.	6. Tell the family whether you will continue to work with them on problems. (If a decision is made to refer them to another professional, proceed to Stage 4: Termination.) ■ Say to the family: "*Now that I have a more complete understanding of your concerns, I think it is necessary to have your son's headaches checked out medically. I would like to refer you to a pediatrician.*"

Continued

TABLE 5-3	Family Interviewing Skills for Nurses—cont'd

STAGE 2: ASSESSMENT

Perceptual/Conceptual Skills	*Executive Skills*
7. Recognize that a more extensive inquiry into the most pressing problems is necessary before intervention plans can be implemented. ■ Initially, families are usually most concerned with the presenting problem or the area of greatest suffering.	7. Seek the family's opinion of which issue they perceive as most important and/or where there is the greatest suffering, and explore it in depth. If the family cannot agree, then discuss the lack of consensus. ■ Ask: *"About which of the problems we have discussed today are you most concerned?"*
8. Recognize that the assessment is complete when sufficient information has been obtained to formulate a treatment plan. ■ Nurses may rush into inappropriate treatment because they are without a clear understanding of the presenting problem or other significant related problems.	8. State your integrated understanding of problems to the family, and obtain their commitment to work on a specific problem. ■ Say: *"Because everyone agrees that Soon's bulimia is connected to the other addictions in the family, I would like to suggest that we focus on this problem for three interviews. Would you be willing?"*

STAGE 3: INTERVENTION

Perceptual/Conceptual Skills	*Executive Skills*
1. Recognize that families possess problem-solving abilities. ■ Families possess the capability to change and can identify and implement solutions for how to change; this helps the nurse avoid becoming overcontrolling or over-responsible.	1. Encourage family members to explore possible solutions to problems and to ease suffering. ■ Say: *"Shaheena, you have mentioned that your mother is too blaming of herself. Do you have any ideas of what she could do to blame herself less about experiencing a chronic illness?"*
2. Recognize that interventions are focused on the cognitive, affective, and behavioral domains or areas of functioning in families, as described in the CFIM. ■ It is not always necessary or efficient to design interventions for all three domains of functioning simultaneously.	2. Plan interventions to influence any one or all three of the domains of functioning described in the CFIM. ■ For example: (a) Cognitive: Invite the family to think differently. (b) Affective: Encourage different affective expression.

TABLE 5-3	Family Interviewing Skills for Nurses—cont'd

STAGE 3: INTERVENTION

Perceptual/Conceptual Skills	*Executive Skills*
	(c) Behavioral: Ask the family to perform new tasks either within or outside of the interview.
3. Recognize that lack of information of an educational nature can inhibit the family's problem-solving abilities. ■ Many families can provide their own creative and unique solutions to problems when given additional information.	3. Provide information to family members that will enhance their knowledge and facilitate further problem solving. ■ Ask family members if they would like to hear about some typical reactions of a 3-year-old to a new baby or about the aging process of an older adult with Alzheimer disease. This type of intervention targets the family's cognitive domain of functioning.
4. Recognize that persistent and intense emotions can often block the family's problem-solving abilities. ■ Families who predominantly experience emotions such as sadness or anger are often unable to deal with problems until the emotional constraint is removed.	4. Validate family members' emotional responses, when appropriate. ■ Family members suppressing grief over the loss of another family member may only need confirmation of the normal grieving process to work through their bereavement. This type of intervention targets the family's affective domain of functioning.
5. Recognize that suggesting specific tasks or assignments can often provide a new way for family members to behave in relation to one another that will improve problem-solving abilities. ■ Some tasks can facilitate changes in the structure of the family or family rules or rituals.	5. Assign tasks or assignments aimed at improving family functioning. ■ Suggest that the father and son spend one evening a week together in a common activity; suggest to the mother and father that one parent put the children to bed on odd days and the other on even days. This type of intervention influences the family's behavioral domain of functioning.

Continued

TABLE 5-3	Family Interviewing Skills for Nurses—cont'd

STAGE 4: TERMINATION

If Consultation or Referral Is Necessary:

Perceptual/Conceptual Skills	*Executive Skills*
1. Recognize that families appreciate additional professional resources when problems are quite complex. ■ Nurses cannot be expected to have expertise in all areas.	1. Refer individual family members or the family for consultation or ongoing treatment. ■ Say: *"I feel that your family needs professional input beyond what I can offer for Tracey's learning disability. Therefore, I would like to refer you to the learning center in the city. The center has more expertise in dealing with these types of problems."*

If Family Interviewing With Nurse Continues:

Perceptual/Conceptual Skills	*Executive Skills*
1. Recognize the importance of evaluating the family interviews or meetings at regular intervals. ■ Evaluating the progress of family interviews leads to more focused and purposeful time spent with the family.	1. Obtain feedback from family members about the present status of their problems or level of suffering, and initiate termination when the contracted problems have been resolved or sufficient progress has been made. ■ Families normally do not lead problem- or suffering-free lives. Rather, what is important is their feeling of confidence to cope with life's challenges and stresses.
2. Recognize when dependency on the nurse inadvertently may have been encouraged. ■ Many interviews over a prolonged period can foster excessive dependency.	2. Mobilize other supports for the family if necessary, and begin to initiate termination by decreasing the frequency of sessions. ■ Nurses can inadvertently provide "paid friendship," with mothers in particular, unless they mobilize other supports such as husbands, friends, or relatives.
3. Recognize family members' constructive efforts to solve problems or ease suffering. ■ The family's perception of progress is more significant than the nurse's perception.	3. Summarize positive efforts of family members to resolve problems and lessen suffering whether or not significant improvement has occurred. ■ Say: *"Your family has made tremendous efforts to find ways to care for your elderly father at home while still attending to your children's needs."*

TABLE 5-3	Family Interviewing Skills for Nurses—cont'd

STAGE 4: TERMINATION

Perceptual/Conceptual Skills	*Executive Skills*
4. Recognize that backup support by professional resources is appreciated by individuals and families in times of stress.	4. End the family interviews with a face-to-face discussion when possible. If appropriate, extend an invitation for additional family meetings should problems recur or if the family desires consultation.

nurse should be aware of the importance of not following this outline rigidly. Rather, the outline serves as a "map of interviewing" that allows considerable flexibility in application. The cultural norms of a family for giving and receiving information can provide a guide for the pacing of the meeting and must be considered. We cannot emphasize enough the importance of the nurse and the family developing a collaborative working relationship during the interview.

FAMILY NURSING EDUCATION

In the education of nurses developing family nursing skills, emphasis should be placed first on the development of perceptual and conceptual skills. This can be accomplished by several methods. Lectures and readings are helpful. Role-playing, simulation, practicing reflective inquiry, and observing and analyzing videos or DVDs of actual family interviews are all useful and effective ways to increase perceptual and conceptual skill accuracy.

Increasing use of technology to teach family nursing is occurring as a means to have learners become active participants and expand their knowledge and encourage reflection. Table 5-4 provides examples of the use of technology to teach family nursing.

Undergraduate and Graduate Nursing Education

Application of family nursing interview skills is one of the most meaningful skill-development opportunities for both graduate and undergraduate nurses. The literature indicates that there is a lack of evidence to support how family nursing is taught at the baccalaureate level and in master's and doctoral programs, and this is an area that requires further research.

In 2013, the IFNA released a document entitled "Position Statement on Pre-licensure Family Nursing Education." This document identifies that

TABLE 5-4	The Use of Technology to Teach Family Nursing	
AUTHOR/TITLE	**TARGET POPULATION**	**IMPLICATIONS**
Eggenberger, S. K. & Sanders, M. (2016). A family nursing educational intervention supports nurses and families in an adult intensive care unit. *Australian Critical Care, 29*(4), 217–223. doi: 10.1016/j.aucc.2016.09.002	Practicing nurses in critical care	Digital storytelling used as an educational intervention to measure nurses' attitudes and confidence in providing family care and families' perceptions of support from nurses in an adult critical care setting. Nurses reported increased confidence, knowledge, and skill following the educational intervention, and the intervention encouraged empathic understandings.
Fernandes, C. S., Martins, M. M., Gomes, B. P., Gomes, J. A., & Gonçalves, L. H. T. (2016). Family Nursing Game: Desenvolvendo um jogo de tabuleiro sobre Família [Family Nursing Game: Developing a board game]. *Esc Anna Nery, 20*(1), 33–37.	Practicing nurses in a hospital setting	Board game developed to teach family nursing, with the main purpose of showing nurses the possibilities to embrace when accompanying and visiting families of hospitalized individuals.
Smith, P. S., & Jones, M. (2016). Evaluating an online family assessment activity: A focus on diversity and health promotion. *Nursing Forum, 51*(3), 204–210. doi: 10.1111/nuf.12139	Registered nurse to Bachelor of Science in Nursing online transition course	Family assessment activity designed to emphasize diversity and health promotion utilizing the Family Health Systems approach to family assessment and *Healthy People 2020* as a framework for family health promotion. Constructivist strategies that emphasize active learning and the use of cinema to teach family assessment results in increased awareness of diversity and increased knowledge of opportunities for health promotion in families.

TABLE 5-4	The Use of Technology to Teach Family Nursing—cont'd	
AUTHOR/TITLE	**TARGET POPULATION**	**IMPLICATIONS**
Van Gelderen, S., Krumwiede, N., & Christian, A. (2016). Teaching family nursing through simulation: Family-Care Rubric development. *Clinical Simulation in Nursing, 12*(5), 159–170. doi: 10.1016/j. ecns.2016.01.002	Undergraduate nursing students	A research-based, family-focused simulation rubric, the Van Gelderen Family-Care Rubric (VGFCR) was developed to assist nurse educators with the evaluation of nursing student performance during a family-focused nursing care simulation. VGFCR assists students to recognize strengths and opportunities for improvement in supporting family health and to identify actions that facilitate family assessment and communication skills. Recommendations include utilizing the rubric with practicing nurses to discern the transferability to clinical practice.
Liebold, N., & Schwarz, L. M. (2014). WebQuests in family nursing education: The learner's perspective. *International Journal of Nursing, 1*(1), 39–50.	Undergraduate nursing students	The use of WebQuests as a teaching/learning strategy for family nursing content. WebQuests encouraged thinking about ways to interact with patients and families and organize and plan work with a family. More research is needed to address the use of WebQuests with family nursing content.

family-focused nursing education should build on foundational competencies in relational practice and provides examples of activities and outcomes to achieve this (IFNA, 2013, p. 4).

One example of an educational facility where family nursing education, practice, and research is growing in recognition is the Glen Taylor Nursing Institute for Family and Society (http://ahn.mnsu.edu/nursing/institute/). Established in 2010 at the School of Nursing at Minnesota State University, Mankato, Minnesota, it focuses on innovating nursing practice knowledge and providing leadership and expertise to influence the health of families in society.

Moules and Tapp (2003) offer some creative, innovative ideas and exercises for educators conducting family nursing labs for undergraduate students. They found that experiential and interactive, inquiry-based activities aimed at creating personal and meaningful relational family nursing practice, such as role-playing using a questioning exercise to emphasize reciprocity between the family and the nurse interviewer, received positive student feedback. They also developed a commendations exercise aimed at offering students the opportunity to genuinely look for, find, and then offer a sincere acknowledgment to a real student. The exercise was designed similarly to the questioning exercise, with one student receiving commendations offered by other group members. They reported that the experiential, personal component of these exercises enriched students' valuing of relational family nursing practice. This was further applied with students completing spontaneous, reflective writing exercises in which the value of personal reflections, commendations, and life-changing realizations for both students and faculty were reported (Moules & Johnstone, 2010).

Live supervision of clinical practice with families, particularly at the graduate level, is regularly provided in very few locations worldwide (Duhamel, 2010; Wright & Bell, 2009). Case discussion and process recording remain the predominant methods of supervision in the development of family nursing skills. However, live supervision is essential to developing and achieving therapeutic competence in nursing practice with families (Tapp & Wright, 1996; Wright, 1994; Wright & Bell, 2009). Observing peers as a mirror of one's own development and seeing one's own internal experience as normal were reported as helpful in increasing self-confidence. With the increasing use of high- and low-fidelity simulation, we believe that there is an opportunity to further explore live supervision as a teaching strategy at both an undergraduate and graduate level.

A useful study that examined the pedagogical practices in family systems nursing at the Family Nursing Unit, University of Calgary, revealed that feeling supported through live and video supervision, having competencies emphasized, and receiving feedback about specific in-session positive behaviors contributed to increased self-confidence and the development of advanced practice clinical skills (Moules, Bell, Paton, & Morck, 2012). However, the study also gleaned that the intensity of the learning process was reported to have both useful and limiting consequences by master's and doctoral students.

Registered Nurses and Advanced Practice Nurses

The Centre of Excellence in Family Nursing, Faculty of Nursing, University of Montreal, is an example of how the bridges between research, theory, and clinical practice are being addressed. The center was unique in that it combined family nursing education and research while providing counseling to families experiencing difficult health events. It provided opportunities for practicing nurses, as well as undergraduate and graduate students, to further develop family assessment skills while working with families in the university clinic setting.

If a nurse is unable to perform a specific executive skill, it is useful to find out whether the individual has developed a perceptual and conceptual base for that particular skill. This is the value of matching these skills in pairs. We encourage nurses to reflect on their practice to distinguish their areas of strengths and weaknesses in the conceptual, perceptual, or executive areas. Leahey and Harper-Jaques's (2010) work with practicing nurses demonstrates how this can be done in a relational clinical setting. Nurses were asked to create a clinical vignette of a client presenting to their setting and then discuss the conceptual, perceptual, and executive skills involved in that client's care. Nurses shared these vignettes and skill descriptions at their monthly team seminars. This contributed to advancing their personal skill development and increasing the team focus on clinical practice.

Learning-centered and outcome-based pedagogies in family nursing are part of the trend in multidisciplinary professional education, including marriage and family therapy, medicine and psychiatry, psychology, and social work (Gehart, 2011).

CASE SCENARIO: THE KAPPOR FAMILY

The Kappor family consists of Rahul (35 years old), Anji (33 years old), and their two children, an 18-month-old son, Sameer, and a 4-year-old daughter, Shaheena. Rahul completed his MBA and was working at an oil and gas company until recently, when the economic recession resulted in his being terminated from his job with only 1 month's notice. Anji works for a small law firm in the administrative department. The couple recently found out that they are expecting a new child. Anji is very excited, but Rahul worries about his family and is not happy. He becomes very irritated and agitated with his situation but does not want to worry or disappoint Anji. He has started to isolate himself from his wife and his children, and he has been staying out late at night.

Anji and Rahul are attending the prenatal clinic for their first appointment with the nurse. When the nurse asks Anji how she is doing, she responds, "I am worried about Rahul. I can't sleep because I don't know where he is going at night." When the nurse asks Rahul about what he thinks, he responds with, "She wouldn't understand, so why should I tell her? It's not going to change anything; she can't get my job back for me."

Reflective Questions

1. What questions should the nurse ask to gain an understanding of the relationship between the family and the health problem and attempted solutions?
2. What are two perceptual skills and two executive skills that the nurse can use during this initial interview with the Kappor family?

CRITICAL THINKING QUESTIONS

1. Consider your own clinical practice. Can you provide examples of how you implement perceptual, conceptual, and executive skills in each stage of family interviewing?
   a. Are there skills that you find challenging? If so, why? How might you overcome these challenges?
2. How are you developing your family interviewing skills?

Chapter **6**

How to Prepare for Family Interviews

Learning Objectives

- Identify concepts of the family-nurse relationship.
- Describe how to generate hypotheses.
- Discuss how to plan for an initial and subsequent interview, including the interview setting, who will be present, and contacting the family.
- Explain resistance and noncompliance in relation to family interviewing.

Key Concepts

Family-nurse relationship

Hypothesis

Resistance and noncompliance

Nurses who work in various types of settings often ask, "How do I prepare for a family interview?" For many nurses, family meetings happen by chance, such as when family members are visiting their loved one in the hospital. For others, family presence in emergency departments or intensive care units is an accepted practice, and nurses are expected to interact with family members as part of their usual practice and supported by institutional and/or administrative policy. A systematic review conducted by Bélanger, Bussières, Rainville, Coulombe, and Desmartis (2017) found that flexible visiting policies lead to greater patient satisfaction with care as perceived by patients, families, and staff. The review also found that some staff members view the presence of families and visitors as obstacles to care and fear increased workloads. The importance of adequately preparing staff members and supporting them is essential in order to overcome this resistance.

Some nurses must overcome the belief that they would be intruding on the family visit if they were present in the patient's room. For many nurses, tension caused by the time required to set up an interview, develop a relationship with the family, and intervene effectively is a major challenge to overcome. Time tension is something that health-care professionals need to learn to manage; otherwise, they can become immobilized by it.

For both the nurse and the family, the first interview or family meeting is often filled with anxiety due to lack of experience or skills, or both, regarding how to involve families. We find this to be a natural reaction of nurses who desire to expand their practice and include families as part of their relational practice and are committed to this goal. We believe that the less anxious the nurse is, the more the nurse invites confidence in family members, thereby reducing their anxiety.

IDEAS ABOUT THE NURSE-FAMILY RELATIONSHIP

Since the first edition of this book, there has been a steady increase in the attention paid to the relational aspect of nurse-family encounters. The relationship is actualized through the microcontext of "therapeutic conversations," meaning the nurse clinician acts *with,* rather than on, patients. We believe that nurses cannot avoid their influence on families, particularly the potential healing power of their words. Nurses need to be self-reflective and aware of current societal views and practice and their influence. Nurses and families inevitably influence each other, but not always with predictable results.

Bell (2011) has championed the idea that relationships are the heart of the matter in family nursing and asks:

- "What would happen if family nurses would continue to focus on families but with a keener interest and heightened sensitivity to relationships?" (p. 3)
- "What if, in nursing education, we were to begin instead (of teaching how to do an assessment) to teach about the ways we enter into relationships with the family?" (p. 5)

The idea of nurses increasing their attention, especially to the first few minutes of an encounter with a client, is a powerful one.

Nurses' positive attitudes toward families encourage them to engage more frequently in therapeutic conversations with families. Sveinbjarnardottir, Svavarsdottir, and Saveman (2011) support the notion that the attitude psychiatric nurses have is fundamental to the quality of interventions offered to families.

However, Luttik and colleagues (2017) conducted a study to describe the attitudes of nurses toward family involvement in the care of patients with cardiovascular disease. Their findings indicated that the attitudes of nurses were mostly positive but varied among nurses with lower education levels and novice nurses with limited experience with family care. Positive attitudes were the highest among nurses who had experience with family care because novice nurses often perceive families as burdensome, thus impacting their attitude toward the family. These findings further support the association between experience and education level and nurses' attitudes toward family care. Svavarsdottir and colleagues (2015) found that nurses who received training in family systems nursing reported having a more positive attitude toward family presence and involvement than those who did not receive the training.

We believe that families and nurses each have their own health-care system. Families provide diagnoses, advice, remedies, and support to their members in both sickness and health. They have constraining and facilitating beliefs about the illness experience (Wright & Bell, 2009). Nurses also have their own constraining and facilitating beliefs, theories, opinions, recommendations, and remedies about managing problems or illness that they share with families. Leahey and Harper-Jaques (1996) have outlined five assumptions relating to the family-nurse relationship and the clinical implications of each assumption. Emphasis is on both the nurse's *and* the family's contribution to establishing and maintaining the relationship. We believe that it is useful for a nurse to reflect on his or her potential contribution to the relationship *before* meeting with a family. It is also helpful for the nurse to reflect with the family about their working relationship at the end of their contract. More ideas on this topic are provided in Chapter 12. Five assumptions related to the family-nurse relationship are discussed in the following sections.

KEY CONCEPT DEFINED

Family-Nurse Relationship

The reciprocal relationship between the nurse and the family.

Assumption 1: The Family-Nurse Relationship Is Characterized by Reciprocity

The family and nurse are connected in a pattern that is quite distinct from the positivist-based idea of two separate components, either family or nurse. It is the "fit" between the family and the nurse that is important to fostering a collaborative partnership.

Questions the nurse might ask to foster a collaborative partnership include the following:

- "What are your thoughts on working together? Is it a good fit so far? What can you imagine will be your preferred way of contributing to our time together?"

- "What direction do you hope we move in over the next few meetings?"
- "Do you have any questions, or is there anything you'd like to know that would make the conversation easier?"

Trust is essential in the family-nurse relationship and is a process that evolves over time. A 2015 systematic review on patients' experiences of trust in patient-nurse relationships identified that good communication; nurses being open, competent, practical, interested, concerned, and confident; and nurses sharing control were necessary in order to facilitate and foster trust (Rortveit et al, 2015, p. 205).

Collaboration with trust and respect for each other's contribution is essential for action to be taken. Box 6-1 offers additional questions the nurse can use for self-reflection regarding reciprocity.

Assumption 2: The Family-Nurse Relationship Is Nonhierarchical

Each person's contribution is sought, acknowledged, and valued. A conversation is a co-construction of ideas and mutual discoveries. However, both the nurse and the family remain aware that they are bound by moral, legal, and ethical norms. Tapp's research (2000) identifies useful practices to counterbalance hierarchy and expert professional views: "offering commendations,

---

Box 6-1 Questions About Reciprocity

For the nurse's self-reflection:
  To what extent will I:

- Elicit the patient's and family members' expectations, hopes, questions, and ideas?
- Consider the patient's and family members' expectations, knowledge, experience, and desires when planning nursing care?
- Communicate information, ideas, and recommendations to patients and families on a regular basis?
- Involve the patient and family to their satisfaction in making decisions for the overall treatment plan?

To ask the family when evaluating care:
  To what extent do you feel that:

- I heard your opinions and ideas?
- I was available and approachable to answer your questions?
- I showed interest in your ideas and experience with illness?

Leahey, M., & Harper-Jaques, S. (1996). Family-nurse relationships: Core assumptions and clinical implications. Journal of Family Nursing, 2(2), 133–151. Copyright 1996 by M. Leahey and S. Harper-Jaques. Reprinted by permission of Sage Publications.

coevolving a description using the family's language, exploring the illness story and the medical story, asking questions that invite reflection, and initiating conversations about family members' preferences" (p. 69). In a study by Aston and colleagues (2015) exploring the power of relationships among public health nurses and mothers during postpartum visits, therapeutic relationships were identified as being central to the home visits because they enabled mothers to effectively work through their concerns in a nonhierarchical manner. Public health nurses were initially viewed by the mothers as professionals with power and judgment, and the mothers were fearful that they would be judged and told what to do. However, the majority of mothers experienced a reciprocal relationship that was respectful and calming. In addition, public health nurses identified their awareness of the power that mothers held and encouraged them to trust themselves as decision makers. This strategy allowed public health nurses to work with mothers to shift away from a hierarchal relationship to a strengths-based relationship (Aston et al, 2015, p. 26). Box 6-2 offers additional questions the nurse can use for self-reflection regarding hierarchy.

Assumption 3: Nurses and Families Each Have Specialized Expertise in Maintaining Health and Managing Health Problems

Families who live with chronic conditions develop expertise in managing symptoms, adapting their environments, and adjusting their lifestyles. They live "near illness," "alongside of illness," and "with illness" (Wright & Bell, 2009). When they meet with nurses, they bring a wealth of information and

---

Box 6-2 Questions About Hierarchy

For the nurse's self-reflection:

- To what extent am I imposing my beliefs on the family? Allowing the family to impose their beliefs on me?
- How well do the family's expectations and my expectations match?
- When there is a mismatch, whose opinion usually predominates?
- How frequently are decisions about the patient's health care made mutually by the patient, family, and me?

To ask the family when evaluating care:

- Overall, what percentage of the time were decisions about your health care made in a mutual way between you and me?
- To what extent did I help you feel more in control of your health?

Leahey, M., & Harper-Jaques, S. (1996). Family-nurse relationships: Core assumptions and clinical implications. Journal of Family Nursing, 2(2), 133–151. Copyright 1996 by M. Leahey and S. Harper-Jaques. Reprinted by permission of Sage Publications.

personal expertise to the encounters. Nurses, through their education and experience, also bring expertise to relationships with the families. Through these mutually respectful encounters, family members' confidence in their ability to self-manage diseases can be enhanced. Diabetes management, for example, depends largely on self-regulation.

We believe that more traditional compliance models relying on pressure to follow recommendations need to be replaced by patient-empowerment models. Nurses risk starting to believe they really know what the best answers are for a family or a particular problem. We agree with Tapp (2000) that "these beliefs can become oppressive when the expert has the expectation that their advice must be obeyed" (p. 81). Nurses can think about their own expertise and the family's expertise as they prepare to meet with the family to discuss managing a particular health problem. Developing and nurturing a kernel of appreciation and respect for the client is foundational to a therapeutic alliance. Box 6-3 offers additional questions the nurse can use for self-reflection regarding expertise.

Assumption 4: Nurses and Families Each Bring Strengths and Resources to the Family-Nurse Relationship

Nurses who use a resource-identification lens strive to draw forth the family's cultural, ethnic, spiritual, and other beliefs that have been helpful in dealing

---

Box 6-3 Questions About Expertise

For the nurse's self-reflection:

- What do I know about the family's ideas and plans for care during this course of treatment?
- What can I learn from this family about their experiences in living with this health problem?
- What knowledge and expertise do I have to offer this family?
- How does this family demonstrate its trust in my expertise?
- Who in the family has the most expertise in getting Grandpa to take his medications?

To ask the family:

- What are the things that you or other family members do to help you relieve the pain?
- What ways have you found most useful to invite your father to take care of his own personal needs?

Leahey, M., & Harper-Jaques, S. (1996). Family-nurse relationships: Core assumptions and clinical implications. Journal of Family Nursing, 2(2), 133–151. Copyright 1996 by M. Leahey and S. Harper-Jaques. Reprinted by permission of Sage Publications.

with the health problem. Nurses also bring to the relationship their own life experiences; clinical intuition; and cultural, ethnic, spiritual/religious, and educational backgrounds. Questions the nurse might ask the family to evaluate the effectiveness of their relational practice include the following:

- "What have I as a nurse done with you as a family that has made a difference? A positive difference?"
- "Looking back, what was your preferred way of contributing to our conversations? Is there something in particular that you feel pleased about with the outcome?"

Box 6-4 offers additional questions the nurse can use for self-reflection regarding strengths.

Assumption 5: Feedback Processes Can Occur Simultaneously at Several Different Relationship Levels

Nurses have often focused on family dynamics and interactional patterns within family systems. Rarely do nurses address the interactive patterns that can simultaneously occur at different relational levels. A 2016 umbrella review of evidence completed by Wiechula and colleagues on factors that influence the caring relationship between a nurse and a patient identified the following:

- Nurses need to be mindful of patients' expectations about the nurse-patient relationship and adjust their behavior to align with fitting values and attitudes.
- The need for the compassionate aspects of nursing care and technical care should be considered and provided together.
- Evaluation of the nurse-patient relationship should occur, and feedback should be used to improve the relationship, affecting both the nurse and patient.

Box 6-4 Questions About Strengths

For the nurse's self-reflection:

- Will my actions and comments acknowledge the strengths and abilities of this family?
- What interventions can I use to further enhance this family's strengths?
- How am I inviting this family to trust my knowledge and skill in helping them with this health problem?
- What are the strengths that I bring to this relationship?

Leahey, M., & Harper-Jaques, S. (1996). Family-nurse relationships: Core assumptions and clinical implications. Journal of Family Nursing, 2(2), 133–151. Copyright 1996 by M. Leahey and S. Harper-Jaques. Reprinted by permission of Sage Publications.

Box 6-5 offers additional questions the nurse can use for self-reflection regarding the family-nurse relationship.

HYPOTHESIZING

Before meeting the family for the first time, the nurse should develop an idea of the purpose of the interview and an understanding of the family's context. This will assist the nurse to develop one or more hypotheses about the presenting problem rather than making assumptions and quickly drawing conclusions. The process of hypothesizing requires nurses to pay close attention to the information that is presented to them.

KEY CONCEPT DEFINED

Hypothesis

A supposition or proposed explanation made on the basis of limited evidence as a starting point for further investigation; developed by the nurse prior to a family interview and related to the purpose of the meeting.

Nurses have always been encouraged to generate hypotheses related to the purpose of the meeting before the interview. In the past, Fleuridas, Nelson, and Rosenthal (1986) defined hypotheses as "suppositions, hunches,

---

Box 6-5 Questions About the Family-Nurse Relationship

For the nurse's self-reflection:
   To what extent did my relationship with the patient and family help to:

- Increase their knowledge? Insight? Coping?
- Increase *my* knowledge? Insight?
- Improve or enhance their emotional well-being? My emotional well-being?
- Improve the patient's physical health?
- Build stronger relationships between the patient and family members?

To ask the family when evaluating care:
   To what extent did our meetings together:

- Meet your needs?
- Contribute to your having an increased sense of confidence in living with your illness?

Leahey, M., & Harper-Jaques, S. (1996). Family-nurse relationships: Core assumptions and clinical implications. Journal of Family Nursing, 2(2), 133–151. *Copyright 1996 by M. Leahey and S. Harper-Jaques. Reprinted by permission of Sage Publications.*

maps, explanations, or alternative explanations about the family and the 'problem' in its relational context" (p. 115). For them, the purpose of a hypothesis is to connect family behaviors with meaning and guide the interviewer's use of questions. Today, the definition of a hypothesis remains the same: "a supposition or proposed explanation made on the basis of limited evidence as a starting point for further investigation" ("Hypothesis," 2018). The purpose of generating hypotheses is to provide order for the interviewing process. It offers a systemic view of the family and generates new views of relationships, beliefs, and behaviors. Preferably, the hypothesis should be circular rather than linear to maximize the therapeutic potential. For example, we know from stress theories and from our own personal and professional experiences that the time of diagnosis of an illness is generally stressful, and in many cases, symptoms temporarily become worse.

Using this as a hypothesis, the nurse can arrange a family interview to discuss the impact of the diagnosis on the family, the family's response to the illness, and the family's expectations of the nurse. In this way, the nurse can explore family patterns of adjusting to the diagnosis and also the family members' ideas of the types of relationships they would like to have with health-care providers. The hypothesis provides general direction for the nurse interviewer in exploring with this particular family their unique adjustment to a diagnosis.

The value of curiosity and naïveté for the nurse working with families, especially in immigrant and marginalized populations, cannot be overestimated. Cultural naïveté and respectful curiosity can be as significant as or more significant than knowledge and skill. It is important for us to point out how our thinking about hypotheses has changed as we work toward operating within a postmodernist paradigm and shift from a modernist point of view. Our attention has shifted from what *we* think about what patients and families are telling us to trying to grasp what *they* think about what they are telling us.

How to Generate Hypotheses

Hypotheses can be formulated from many bases. For example, they can be based on information the family provided or on ideas about the family gathered during hospital admission, during visiting hours, or from the other staff. The information may consist of opinions, observations of behavior or interactive patterns, and other data. In considering this information, we encourage nurses to ask themselves what they think the other staff thinks about what they are saying. We believe the most relevant hypotheses are generally based on information already provided by the family.

Hypotheses can also be based on the nurse's previous experience and knowledge. This experience and knowledge can involve families whom the nurse believes to have similar ethnic, racial, or religious or spiritual backgrounds. The nurse may recall similar problems, symptoms, or situations and similar interactive patterns noticed with previous patients and families. The nurse may generate a hypothesis based on knowledge about family development and life-cycle stages, research literature, or another conceptual framework that he or she finds most relevant. We encourage nurses to include in their hypotheses ideas about a family's strong spirit, generosity of heart, devotion to one another, deep caring, and commitment. These are enduring qualities that families can draw upon in times of stress.

In addition to formulating hypotheses based on information from or about the family or from previous experience and knowledge, nurses may develop hypotheses based on whatever is salient or relevant to them about the health problem or risk that is encountered at the time. For example, if a recent tragedy has occurred in the immediate community, the nurse may find such information relevant in generating a hypothesis about what might be most meaningful for this particular family at this point.

We believe that it is important for nurses to state (to themselves) their hypotheses explicitly and consciously before the interview. We do not concur with those who state that hypotheses are unnecessary. Our belief is that a nurse cannot *not* hypothesize or think about a family before the meeting. It is important for nurses to explicate their hunches so that these thoughts may be refined and made transparent as the nurse and family engage in the interview process. Hypothesizing before the family meeting is viewed as a way to start focusing on the family, churning up the gray matter, making connections, and generating questions. It should not involve preparing an agenda for the session that is imposed on the family regardless of what the family members desire and despite changes that may have occurred since the last meeting (see Chapter 11 for ideas on how to avoid these kinds of mistakes).

Guidelines for designing hypotheses, adapted from the work of Fleuridas, Nelson, and Rosenthal (1986), include the following:

- *Generate hypotheses that are useful; there is not one "correct" or "right" hypothesis.* The goal is to generate useful explanations that lead to desired outcomes. We believe that stories are authored through conversations. The story that is co-constructed between the nurse and the family is uniquely personal. We cannot know which hypotheses will fit for a particular family or where people's stories will go. We can only attune ourselves one piece at a time to the story as it unfolds.
- *Develop hypotheses that are circular rather than linear.* A hypothesis that includes all the components of the system (e.g., the family *and* the nurse) is most likely to be more circular than one that includes *either* the nurse *or* the family. (See Chapters 2 and 3 for a more in-depth discussion regarding circularity.)
- *The hypothesis should be related to the family's concerns.* This is important because, as previously stated, a hypothesis guides the interview. For example, if the nurse develops a hypothesis that is unrelated to the family's concerns, the nurse will ask questions that do not relate to the

family's reason for coming to the interview or health-care facility. The nurse who is attuned to the family's concerns will listen for openings, through questions and reflective discussion, of problem-saturated stories and unique outcomes (see Chapter 7). These outcomes, or "sparkling events," would not have been predicted in light of the problem-saturated story. We remind ourselves that it is the clinician's certainty about his or her beliefs and opinions that can oppress and constrain opportunities to hear the patient's and family's story as they experience it.

- *Develop a hypothesis that is different from the family's explanation or hypothesis.* For example, a family may have the explanation that Heather is a "bad daughter" who is shirking her responsibility by not caring for her elderly mother in her own home. The nurse, on the other hand, may develop an alternate hypothesis that fits the same data. The nurse's hypothesis might be that Heather is overwhelmed by having to take care of her two preschool children while maintaining a full-time job. Thus, she is stretched to the limit in also trying to take responsibility for her elderly parent. Furthermore, Heather's elderly mother may be sensitive to her stress and thus may be reluctant to live with her.

Box 6-6 provides a brief at-a-glance summary of the guidelines for generating hypotheses.

Once hypotheses have been designed, the nurse can use them to guide the interview. The nurse can ask questions of each member and note the responses to questions, thus confirming, altering, or rejecting a hypothesis. In conversation with families, the nurse should be sure to pay attention to the small and the ordinary. We agree somewhat with the notion that the starting point for hypotheses is arbitrary and intuitive but that hypotheses

---

Box 6-6 Guidelines for Generating Hypotheses

- Choose hypotheses that are useful.
- Generate the most helpful explanations of the family's behaviors for this particular time.
- Understand that there are no "right" or "true" explanations.
- Include all participants in the "problem-organizing system" to make the hypothesis as systemic as possible.
- Relate the hypothesis to the family's presenting concerns so that the interview can proceed along the lines most relevant to the family (versus those relevant to the nurse).
- Make the hypothesis different from the family's hypothesis to introduce new information into the system and avoid being entrapped with the family in solutions that are not working.
- Be as quick to discard unhelpful hypotheses as you are to generate new ones.

are either validated or invalidated by evidence (i.e., they may be confirmed, rejected, or modified). We remain acutely aware that our notion of validation and evidence is just from our "observer perspective."

Hypothesizing and interviewing constitute a reciprocal cycle and are interdependent. The nurse develops a hypothesis, asks questions, converses with the family about the "problem" and its influence on their lives, and gathers evidence that either confirms or refutes the nurse's hypothesis. Box 6-7 illustrates questions that invite hypothesizing about the system and the problem. As new information is generated, the nurse modifies the previous hypothesis and evolves a more useful one. The goal of the interview is to bring forth the family's resources to deal with the presenting issue.

Box 6-7 Questions That Invite Hypothesizing About the System and the Problem

Who

Who is in the system? Who are the key players?
Who first noticed the problem?
Who is concerned about the problem?
Who is affected by the problem? (most, least)
Who is interested in keeping things the same? (most, least)
Who referred the system?

What

What is the problem at this time?
What is the meaning that the problem has for the system and for different
    members of the system?
What solutions have been attempted?
What question(s) do I feel obliged to ask?
What beliefs perpetuate the problem?
What beliefs might be identified as core beliefs?
What beliefs are perpetuated by the problem?
What problems and solutions perpetuate the beliefs?

Why

Why is the system presenting at this time?

Where

Where has the information about this problem come from?
Where does the system see the problem originating?
Where does the system see the problem and the system going if there is no
    change or if there is change?

> ## Box 6-7 Questions That Invite Hypothesizing About the System and the Problem—cont'd
>
> ### When
>
> When did the problem begin?
> When did the problem begin in relation to another phenomenon of the system?
> When does the problem occur?
> When does the problem not occur?
>
> ### How
>
> How might a change in the problem affect other parts of the system (key players, relationships, beliefs)?
> How does a change in one part of the system affect another part of the system or the problem?
> How will I know when my work with this system is over?
> How might my work with this system constrain the system from finding its solution?

More information about how to conduct family interviews is provided in Chapters 7 to 11.

Leahey and Wright (1987) provide an example of how alternative hypotheses can be generated before the first family meeting:

> A nurse working in an extended-care facility noted that the family, especially the 9- and 10-year-old children, avoided visiting their 41-year-old mother who had Huntington disease and that the patient's symptoms worsened around visiting days. The children seemed depressed and withdrawn every time they came to the nursing unit on their monthly visits. During case conferences, the staff wondered whether there might be a connection between the family's avoidance and the patient's flailing and head banging. They generated several hypotheses to explain why the family might be avoiding the patient and why the patient's symptoms seem to exacerbate around the time of the family visits.

- One hypothesis pertained to the children's belief that head banging and flailing were controllable. Perhaps the children felt that their mother was not trying to control herself so she would not have to return home to care for them. This made them angry, and they avoided her.
- An alternate hypothesis concerned the children's conflicting loyalties toward their mother and the aunt who took care of them. Perhaps they felt that if they visited too often, their aunt might think they did not appreciate her care. Thus, they spaced out their visits and seemed depressed and withdrawn. They demonstrated both loyalty to their aunt and affection for their mother.

- A third hypothesis involved the children's fears of developing Huntington disease themselves. They avoided visiting and showed sadness because of their own expectations of contracting the disease. (p. 60)

Having generated several hypotheses about the family and the problem in its relational context, the nurse arranged a meeting with the family. The purpose of the interview was to clarify how the family members wanted to be involved with the patient and how the staff could be most helpful to them. The nurse's hypotheses were relevant to the purpose of the interview. She did not know if the frequency of the family visits was a "problem" for either the children or the patient. Rather, the staff had identified the problem. Thus, the nurse chose to frame the purpose of the meeting as one in which the staff wanted to know how they could be most helpful to both the family and the patient during the patient's hospitalization. The patient and family were collaborating with the staff rather than the family being the object of care.

INTERVIEW SETTINGS

A family interview or meeting can take place anywhere: in the home (e.g., kitchen, living room, patient's bedroom), in an institution (e.g., bedside, urgent care center, nurse's clinic or office, treatment room), or in the community (e.g., interviewing room, school, office, health clinic, on the street where a homeless family "resides," on Skype for patients/families in remote areas). Depending on the purpose of the clinical interview, some settings are more conducive to beginning a therapeutic conversation than others. Nurses and families, therefore, need to consider the advantages and disadvantages of various settings. They should be flexible in choosing a setting that is appropriate for the specific purpose of the interview. Families should be offered a choice of setting whenever possible.

Home Setting

Many nurses interview families in their home setting. There are some concrete advantages to interviewing in the home:

- Infants, children of all ages, and older family members are able to be present more easily.
- Chances are increased for meeting significant but perhaps elusive family members, such as boarders, adolescents, or grandparents.
- Firsthand assessment of the physical environment is also possible. For example, the presence of staircases and the display of family photographs can be observed.
- Firsthand experience of the family's social environment is possible. For example, rituals of eating, challenges with mobility, or who answers the doorbell can be noted.

In addition to the concrete advantages to interviewing in the home, there are also other advantages. These are particularly important if the nurse is from a different socioeconomic or ethnic background than the family. Articulate middle-class parents may report only the most exemplary family interactions in the office or school. The nurse may thus have difficulty understanding how the apparent competence of the parents and the banality of the reported parent-child incidents are in such sharp contrast to the degree of behavioral upset manifested by the child.

Disadvantaged families sometimes have difficulty bridging the gap and explaining their situation to middle-class nurses who are unfamiliar with their home milieu. For example, a nurse suggests that an older woman prepare her husband several small meals a day rather than one very large meal, which he is unable to consume. The nurse did not know (and the family members were too embarrassed to mention) that the family shared cooking facilities with other people in their apartment building. A home interview can thus give the nurse a clearer direction for therapeutic suggestions and can enhance the relationship between the family and nurse.

However, there are also disadvantages to using the home setting for family interviews:

- Increased administrative and personal costs are involved in the nurse's travel.
- The meeting may have far more disruptions and may require the nurse to structure the interview flexibly.
- Nurses should be aware that a family's home is their sanctuary. If family members are asked in their own home to share intense and deep emotions, they are often left without a retreat. For example, if abuse is an issue, the nurse should anticipate that the family's affective disclosure would be quite intense. Perhaps they will need more physical and psychological space to deal with the issues than their home permits. On the other hand, if the purpose of the interview is to facilitate shared grieving over the loss of a family member, the home setting might be ideal.
- Ideas about therapeutic boundaries and hierarchy, confidentiality, and the timing and pacing of interventions can sometimes be challenged during home interviews. Doubts and confusion about the usefulness of intervention are not uncommon. Experiencing families in their homes can teach nurses that there are small opportunities even when a client's world seems to go under. It can make them more confident and comfortable in facing clients' hopelessness and helplessness and being with them to develop strategies to get unstuck, rather than trying to rescue them.

Before setting up a home visit, the nurse should consider the following:

- Explain to the family that you would like to have an interview in the home "to get a better feel for their situation."

- Explain that, in your experience, there are frequently interruptions to an interview in the home (e.g., telephone calls, texting, neighbors dropping in, children wanting to put on the television or play computer games). Ask, *"How should we handle this if it comes up?"* In this way, you have already set the stage for work, rather than for visiting, and for a specific purpose to the interview.
- Handle social offerings, such as coffee or a cold drink, by saying, *"Thanks, but maybe we could work first and then have coffee afterward."* The work and social boundaries are thus clearly identified. Keep in mind that although this boundary might be useful for some nurses working with certain ethnic groups, such a boundary might be offensive to families from other ethnic groups or from rural areas.

Office, Hospital, or Other Work Setting

Advantages of using the work setting are as follows:

- The setting is the nurse's base or territory. Therefore, the nurse can capitalize on the opportunity and adapt the setting to the needs of the interview.
- Fewer telephone calls, mobile phones, and visitor interruptions are also possible.
- The nurse has a greater opportunity to obtain consultation from colleagues when interviewing the family in the work setting.

Disadvantages of using the work setting are as follows:

- Issues of context may arise; for instance, a family might be intimidated by the professional trappings (e.g., large institution, plush furniture, complicated equipment) of the office and therefore may display anxiety or reluctance to talk. Suggestions for how beginning interviewers can maximize privacy in hospital settings are given later in this chapter.
- Inadvertent fostering of the belief that pathology resides in the individual. For example, *"Mom's the sick one. We're only coming to help Mom get over her depression."* This attitude is particularly evident if the mother has been hospitalized in a psychiatric unit. This disadvantage can be handled by using the family's willingness to "help Mom." The interviewer can reframe or discuss the mother's hospitalization in a positive light, for example, by saying, *"Perhaps your mother's hospitalization has provided the family with an opportunity to all work together in a new way."*

How to Use the Work Setting

Some hospitals, clinics, or universities have elaborate interviewing rooms, but most nurses must make do with the usual hospital or clinic facilities.

Therefore, they may have to negotiate with coworkers for space and privacy. The nurse should consider the following:

- Choose a private place where you will not be interrupted. For example, an unused patient room or an office is often more quiet and private than a four-bed room with curtains, a visitor's lounge, or a waiting area.
- Remove any important or intimidating equipment (such as machines and monitors). The discussion area should ideally be sparsely furnished with movable chairs and no big desks, couches, or examining tables. This allows family members to control their own space, move closer or farther away from someone, and not worry about children touching hospital equipment. A few quiet toys, such as rubber or cloth hand puppets or paper and crayons, are useful to have readily available in the room.
- Books and magazines should not be available during the interview because they give a mixed message to the family, especially to adolescents. The participants should expect to discuss issues; they should not expect to read during the interview.
- Acquaint yourself with the physical layout of the room before the session. This is likely to increase your feelings of comfort when first meeting the family.
- At the beginning of the interview, if children are present, you can say to the parents, *"I'd like you to handle the children in whatever way you usually do. That will give me a better idea of how things go at home."* If the baby starts to cry, observe who comforts the baby. If the noise level gets beyond your tolerance, notice what tolerance level the family has.
- Unless absolutely necessary, try to avoid giving behavioral directives (e.g., *"Watch out for that plant,"* or *"Don't touch Dad's chest tube"*) during the first interview unless they are required for safety. Valuable information can be lost if you impose your standards of behavior upon family members. At the same time, be sure to structure the interview to avoid chaos and thereby the potential to lose your therapeutic leverage.

At the end of the session, assess the influence of the work setting. Ask family members if they behaved differently than they usually do:

- "Did the children behave better or worse today than they usually do at home?"
- "Were family members more or less talkative than they are at home?"

WHO WILL BE PRESENT

Deciding who will be present for the first and subsequent interviews is important. The decision is generally determined together by family members and the nurse. In our early days of working with families, we thought it imperative that *all* family members be present for family interviewing.

However, we have significantly changed in our thinking about who should come to the meetings. We now believe that a nurse can develop hypotheses, assess, and intervene with a family regardless of who is in the interviewing room. The number of family members sitting in front of a nurse does not constitute family nursing. Rather, what is more important is how the nurse conceptualizes human suffering, problems, and solutions. See Chapter 10 for a clinical vignette where Dr. Lorraine Wright interviews an individual to gain a family perspective about chronic illness.

We believe that nurses who are beginning to interview families will generally find it easiest to invite everyone living in the household to be present for the first interview. In this way, the nurse can more easily elicit information from members who most likely have a description of the problem, concern, or illness. To begin family work by interviewing just one person reduces the number of perspectives on the concerns, but it is still possible to inquire about family functioning even if seeing only one family member. If the problem concerns a couple, we usually try to have both spouses together for the first meeting. Similarly, if the issue is parenting-related, then both of the parents and the child should be invited to the meeting.

The more family members present, the more information it is possible to gather. In addition, the more viewpoints and descriptions by family members of the influence of the problem or illness on their lives and relationships can then be considered by the nurse. Family members at the first interview might include the young children, the grandparent "who never has much to say," and the nephew "who just moved in for the weekend." Sometimes the most significant thing that the nurse is able to accomplish in a family interview is just to bring the whole family together in one spot at one time to discuss an important issue. When deciding whom to invite to the first meeting, we believe it is very useful to consider the network of professional resources involved with the family as well as the family members themselves. We believe that relational family nursing is best practiced in context.

Nurses frequently question whether they should include in the first interview family members who are psychotic, those who are mentally or cognitively disabled, or elderly family members who are experiencing dementia or Alzheimer disease. Generally, the answer is yes. Including these family members provides the nurse with an opportunity to talk with the family about the impact of the psychosis, mental disability, or dementia on the family. In addition, it shows the nurse how the family and individual interact to deal with the presenting problem.

> *Example:* A family requested help for their 6-year-old daughter, who was *"regressing, having imaginary friends, and refusing to play with peers or go to school."* During the initial interview, the little girl walked over to the door and turned the doorknob. The nurse asked her not to leave the room. In response, the girl's siblings said that she was not leaving but rather *"was letting the cat out the door."* The nurse looked a

bit startled because there was no cat in the room. The nurse then asked the other children how they knew that this was what the little girl was doing and proceeded to inquire if this was how they usually responded to the child's behavior. Had the "psychotic child" not been present, the nurse would have been unaware of the siblings' contribution to perpetuating the presenting problem.

Deciding who should be present for the first meeting is an important indicator of the collaborative nurse-family relationship. It is important for the nurse to be aware of who is in relevant conversation with whom about the problem or illness outside the interview room. Given the ever-increasing use of telecommunication devices such as e-mail, chat rooms, Skype, Facebook, and text messaging, it is useful for nurses to inquire not just about the family contacts in the immediate vicinity but also those online. We must respect family members' ideas about *what* is germane to the conversation and *who* should be involved in it. We recommend that all decisions about *who* should be involved in meetings, *when*, and *what* is talked about are determined collaboratively, one conversation at a time.

FIRST CONTACT WITH THE FAMILY

The way in which the nurse makes the first contact with the family conveys an important message to the parents and the children. We believe that the quality of the nurse's relationship with the family and the nurse's manners and etiquette are important ingredients for accountable and effective therapeutic engagement. Good manners and etiquette may help manage deep currents of tension and ease potentially awkward situations. Showing good manners, such as respect, tact, and humility, can go a long way in establishing the nurse-family relationship. (See Chapter 9 for more ideas about using good manners in relational practice.) By inviting each person in the household to the family meeting, the nurse implicitly states that each family member is significant and has a role to play in understanding, describing, and dealing with the problem.

The rationale for involving as many family members as possible can be explained in several ways. If a baby is in the intensive care nursery, the nurse might use the following explanation:

"When a baby is in the intensive care nursery, we frequently find that family members are concerned and often anxious as well. Bringing family members together results in more information for the whole family on how best to help the baby."

Another idea is for the nurse to say:

"Years ago, fathers and family members were kept out of the delivery room and out of the hospital units. We've learned, though, how important it is to have family members present for special events such as the birth of a baby. Now we recognize that it is even more important for family members to be

present and involved in health care when there is some type of illness. Family members know and care about each other. In many cases, they have a lot to offer each other."

With a family experiencing a crisis, such as the diagnosis of a stage 4 glioblastoma in a previously healthy 62-year-old father, nurses may want to focus on providing physical information relating to the patient. Nurses can also see if the family is interested in hearing about services for families coping with the sudden onset of a life-threatening illness. They may state that in times of crisis, families often find comfort in meeting with health professionals so that they can gain accurate, up-to-date patient information. Nurses are aware from their knowledge of crisis theory that the time frame for intervention is limited because crises are self-limiting. Assertiveness and a calm demeanor are generally useful postures for nurses to take when a family is overwhelmed by a crisis.

Spouses sometimes agree to come for an interview but object to having the children present or taking the children out of school. One way to handle the latter problem is to have meetings before school, during the lunch hour, after school, or in the evening. If this is not possible because of the nurse's work schedule, the nurse may say:

"I understand your concern about the children missing school. In my experience, however, children have a tremendous amount to contribute to a family interview. They generally feel quite relieved when they see that the family is dealing with an issue about which they may have been worrying. Schools also are usually quite agreeable to children missing an hour."

How to Set Up an Appointment

On an outpatient basis, the purpose of the initial telephone contact with the family is to set up an appointment for an interview, explain the rationale for involving family members, and determine with the family who will be present at the interview. Naturally, both nurse and family gather much useful information about each other over the telephone. Telephone contact is therefore part of the development of a collaborative working relationship, and the nurse should treat it as such.

Generally, the first telephone contact sets the stage for subsequent interviews. Our advice is to pay careful attention to this contact, whether you call the family to set up an appointment or a family member calls you. The following is a sample first telephone contact:

Mother: Hello.

Nurse: Hello, Erin. This is Kaiya Wilson. I'm the community health nurse in your neighborhood.

Mother: Yes.

Nurse: I understand that you have a new baby girl. It's our practice to come out and visit all families with new babies.

Mother: Oh, I didn't know that.

Nurse: Yes, we usually do a physical examination of mom and the baby and answer any questions or concerns you may have.

Mother: Oh, that seems like a good idea. The doctor didn't tell me much about feeding.

Nurse: Sure, we can talk about that during our visit. I was just calling to set up a time that would be convenient for your family and for me. It would be great to meet the whole family and see how you are all doing.

Mother: Well, my partner is usually around in the afternoon, so that would be the best time to come. Also, I would like to ask you about my 2-year-old son, who usually seems to like his baby sister, but last night I saw him pinch her.

Nurse: Okay, how about tomorrow afternoon at 1 o'clock? The meeting will probably take about an hour. We can definitely discuss your questions about your 2-year-old further.

Mother: Tomorrow afternoon works well because my partner will be home at that time. Also, I want you know that we didn't have a very positive experience in the hospital this time, and my partner was very frustrated and angry with the whole experience; she is still really upset and has her doubts about receiving any supports at this point.

Nurse: Thank you for sharing that information with me beforehand. I would like you to know that I want to support you and your family in the best way possible; what do you think would be the best way for me to do this at this time?

Mother: I appreciate that, and I would really like you to come tomorrow to check on me and my baby.

Nurse: Okay, great. I look forward to seeing you and the whole family then.

Mother: Yes, me too.

Nurse: Goodbye.

Mother: 'Bye.

In this example, the nurse was clear, confident, focused, and accommodating. She set forth the purpose of the interview and who she thought should be involved. She invited all family members to be present by stating that this is the clinic's usual practice. She responded directly to Erin's concern about the difficult experience her family had in the hospital. Whether the nurse refers to her collaborative time with a family as a "meeting" or an "interview" is arbitrary; it is most important that the nurse use the most palatable language with families based on the context in which she encounters them. The nurse took charge by identifying and introducing herself without apologies and offered specific appointment times. Furthermore, the nurse received much information that can be useful in the family meeting:

"The doctor didn't tell me much about feeding."
"I saw [the 2-year-old] pinch her."
"My partner was very frustrated and angry with the whole experience; she is still really upset."

It is not possible to provide written guidelines to cover all the various situations that nurses will encounter in trying to set up a family interview. Some suggestions for involving families include the following:

- Emphasize the value and importance of all family members' perceptions and observations.
- Demonstrate respect for all of the family members' time by asking if the telephone call was made at a convenient time.
- Use positive verbal cues (e.g., common courtesies, personal titles, a cheerful and interested tone of voice, positive phrases, and affirming remarks) in order to maintain rapport.

Each family presents different challenges for the nurse, and vice versa. Therefore, each interview must be approached with flexibility. A unique approach is always the rule in clinical practice. Each telephone contact demands a slightly different plan of action to invite family members to an interview or to elicit the family's permission for a home visit. We strongly encourage nurses, especially community health nurses, to plan their telephone calls and appointments to maximize efficiency and the possibility of developing a collaborative partnership with the family. We generally do not recommend that appointments be set up by e-mail or text because there can be issues of confidentiality and ambiguity about how promptly the e-mail or text will be responded to and by whom. However, we do recognize that, in some rural or very remote areas, setting up and even offering family meetings may be done online via Skype, e-mail, or instant messaging. Online family meetings may prove to be very useful if a face-to-face meeting is not possible.

RESISTANCE AND NONCOMPLIANCE

Often in our clinical supervision with nurses, we have been asked how to deal with resistant, difficult, or noncompliant families. When nurses ask this, they are generally referring to families whom they perceive to be "in denial," oppositional, or noncompliant with ideas and advice that they have offered or could offer to promote, maintain, or restore health. The family is designated as noncompliant when they do not respond to particular nursing interventions; nurses often interpret this behavior as an unwillingness or a lack of readiness to change (Wright & Levac, 1992).

> **KEY CONCEPT DEFINED**
> ### Resistance and Noncompliance
> Resistance involves the client's reluctance to uncover or recover from some anxiety-filled experience. Noncompliance is a failure to act, or to be in denial, or to be oppositional.

We do not use the terms *resistance* and *noncompliance* because we have not found them clinically useful in relational family nursing practice. *Resistance* was initially used to describe a client's reluctance to uncover or recover from some anxiety-filled experience. Resistance is still generally viewed as "located" in the client and is often described as something the client "does." This is a linear view that implies that problems with adherence to treatment regimens reside within individuals and families, not in the interactions or relationships between individuals. However, we see the idea of resistance as a *product* of client-interviewer interaction. We believe that *resistance* and *noncompliance* are not terms describing a unilateral phenomenon but rather an interactional phenomenon.

Rather than using these terms, we have found the multidirectional terms *cooperation* and *collaboration* to be very useful clinically. When nurses think of how they work collaboratively with families, they are less likely to impose their will on them. They tend to open space for the family and to be more tentative and receptive to the family's point of view.

There has been an increase in a solution-focused, strengths-based, and resiliency orientation to family interviewing (Bell & Wright, 2011; Zhang, Franklin, Currin-McCulloch, Park, & Kim, 2017). With emphasis on a solution comes an increasing emphasis on change, cooperation, and collaboration. They open us to reflect on conversation, language, and possibilities rather than pathologizing labels.

How to Deal With a Hesitant Family Member

A family member may be hesitant to attend the family session for several possible reasons. Each requires a different approach on the part of the nurse. The following are a few common situations that interviewers encounter with possible strategies:

Situation:

"My partner would never come to a family interview. He thinks that my mother's stroke and how to handle it are my responsibility."

Strategies:
- Ask what the client thinks about her partner attending the interview.

- If the mother's chronic illness is believed to be the responsibility of the client, the client may not be interested in inviting her partner to a family interview. The nurse should engage in conversation with both individuals to see what domain of functioning the nurse may intervene at (see Chapter 4 for more about domains of functioning).

Situation:

"My partner wouldn't want to come to a family interview. Besides, I wouldn't know how to get him there."

Strategies:

- If this client feels uncertain about how to invite her partner, explore with her why she feels the partner might be hesitant. There could be several reasons:
  - The partner may view the problem as not his own.
  - The timing of the interview might be inconvenient.
  - The setting of the meeting may be intimidating (e.g., hospital or clinic with sick people around).
  - The partner may be afraid of being blamed for not taking a more active role in the mother's care.
- Ask the client if she thinks any of these feelings or thoughts might be stopping her partner from becoming involved. After considering the reasons for the partner's hesitance and the client's own desire for him to be present, discuss alternate ways to engage him:
  - Discuss with the client her need for her partner to help deal with her mother's illness.
  - Find out convenient times for each of them to come to a half-hour meeting.
  - Provide information about where the interview will be held (e.g., patient room, family meeting room, clinic).
  - Let both partners know the importance of each person's presence during the meeting in order to ensure inclusivity, promote understanding of relationships, and explain the purpose of the family interview.

It is important for nurses to recognize that family members may be at different stages in their desire to seek help. Some of this may be attributable to gender differences, orientation, values and beliefs, and culture.

Another strategy for inviting an anxious or threatened family member to an interview is to suggest that the person be asked to be present as an observer, just to see what is happening. Also, the person can come whenever he or she is "in the mood" and act as a historian, an accuracy checker, or a consultant. If these suggestions are followed, it is important to ask the "observer" or "historian" to react at the *end* of the interview to what the family has discussed in the session. Gradually, as the family member continues to observe sessions, the individual often becomes more comfortable and is willing to participate *during* the interview. This may be a particularly useful way of engaging some adolescents. Asking family members not to talk places no direct pressure on them to participate. Silent members are often closely attuned to the process, and when a sensitive area is broached, they forget their defensive stance and join in the process. Other times, they may remain silent but hear the information.

Box 6-8 summarizes points for nurses to consider in preparing for family interviews. These ideas are the result of striving toward a collaborative relationship between the nurse and the family.

Box 6-8 Helpful Hints for Planning a Family Meeting

Before initiating a family meeting, the nurse needs to:

- Ascertain the purpose and benefit of a family meeting from the family's perspective.
- Explain why a family meeting may be beneficial to the family.
- Determine who in the family agrees that a problem exists and who might be willing to come to a family meeting.
- Mutually determine with the family when and where a meeting could take place (home, office, school).
- Read literature about working with families experiencing similar health problems to better understand the issues, concerns, and lived experiences of that specific population.
- Begin to formulate hypotheses (explanations about the family's behaviors that connect the family system and the particular problem).
- Prepare linear and circular questions that will elicit relevant data about family structure, development, and function. (See the discussions of the CFAM in Chapter 3 and the CFIM in Chapter 4 for examples of questions.)

Levac, A. M. C., Wright, L. M., & Leahey, M. (2002). Children and families: Models for assessment and intervention. In J. A. Fox (Ed.), Primary health care of infants, children, and adolescents (2nd ed., pp. 10–19). St. Louis, MO: Mosby. Copyright 2002. Adapted with permission from A. M. C. Levac, L. M. Wright, & M. Leahey.

CASE SCENARIO: OLA AND ABI

Ola is a 20-year-old woman who has recently immigrated to Canada. She has a 3-year-old daughter, Abi, who is having temper tantrums that Ola is struggling to control. During a recent drop-in visit to the local public health clinic, Ola asks the community health nurse (CHN) for guidance. She tells the CHN that she is becoming increasingly frustrated and feels that she and her partner do not have the same beliefs about what to do about Abi. She tells the CHN that she always

Continued

CASE SCENARIO: OLA AND ABI—cont'd

attends the drop-in clinic each month, but it is difficult because she takes the bus and the weather is often very cold. The CHN observes that Ola appears very tired, and she yawns many times during their conversations. The CHN offers to call Ola tomorrow to set up an appointment to meet with the CHN the following week. Ola expresses great interest in meeting with the CHN and provides her contact information.

Reflective Questions

1. What should the CHN consider when setting up the appointment with Ola?
2. What hypotheses can the CHN generate prior to meeting with Ola?
   a. How might these be useful as the CHN prepares for the initial meeting with Ola and during the first meeting with Ola?
3. What questions can the CHN ask to ensure reciprocity during the first meeting with Ola?

CRITICAL THINKING QUESTIONS

1. Consider your practice area and identify an opportunity for you to conduct a family interview and answer the following questions:
   a. What might your potential contributions to the family-nurse relationship be?
   b. What questions would you ask to help generate hypotheses about the system and the problem?
   c. What is an appropriate setting to conduct the interview?
   d. How do you contact the family members?
   e. Who should be present at the family interview?
2. Reflect on an experience in which you encountered resistance and noncompliance with family members.
   a. How did you respond? What would you do differently?

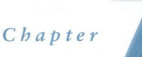

C h a p t e r 7

How to Conduct Family Interviews

Learning Objectives

- Summarize the guidelines for each stage of an initial family interview.
- Explain strategies used to engage and establish a therapeutic relationship with a family.
- Describe various types of questions used during the assessment phase to identify the problem, explore the relationship between family interaction and the health problem, and explore the attempted solutions for solving problems and achieving family goals.
- Discuss how to plan and deal with complexity during a family assessment.
- Identify factors to consider when deciding to intervene with a family.

Key Concepts

Assessment stage	**Intervention stage**	**Termination stage**
Engagement stage	**Miracle question**	

O nce a nurse and a family have decided to meet, the nurse can begin to consider how to conduct the meeting. Just as there is an interviewing procedure, there is also a process in initial family interviews. This process provides the nurse with an interview structure and can help to allay the nurse's anxiety. It is not uncommon to move back and forth between the stages of a family interview to obtain more clarity or additional assessment information about the concerns. Sometimes it is even necessary to return to the engagement guidelines to strengthen the therapeutic relationship before further intervention ideas can be offered. Thus, there should

211

be fluidity between these stages so that they remain true guidelines rather than a rigid prescription for how to conduct a family interview.

GUIDELINES FOR FAMILY INTERVIEWS

The stages that generally occur in initial interviews are briefly presented in Table 7-1 and discussed in detail in the following subsections.

KEY CONCEPT DEFINED

Engagement Stage

The stage during the family interview in which the family is greeted and made comfortable and the relationship continues; based on compassion, collaboration, and consultation.

Engagement Stage

During the engagement stage, or first stage of the interview, the nurse and the family begin to establish a therapeutic relationship. The goal is for

TABLE 7-1	Stages of Initial Interviews
STAGE	**OBJECTIVES**
Engagement	The family is greeted and made comfortable, and the relationship continues.
Assessment	**Problem identification**—the nurse explores the family's presenting concerns and/or suffering.
	Relationship between family interaction and health problem—the nurse explores the family's typical responses to the health problem and how the health problem is affecting their family life and relationships.
	Attempted solutions—the family and nurse talk about the solutions the family has tried and their effects on the presenting issues.
	Goal exploration—the nurse draws together the information, and the family members specify what goals, changes, or outcomes they are seeking. (Note: if family members are suffering from the impact of an illness, it is also important to clarify if they desire an alleviation or easing of their suffering in the emotional, physical, and/or spiritual domains).
Intervention	The nurse and family collaborate on areas for desired change.
Termination	The nurse and family conclude the interview.

family members and the nurse to develop a mutual alliance so that they can collaborate on the desired changes (Box 7-1).

In the beginning, the nurse is often perceived as a stranger, unknown, untrusted, and potentially helpful or unhelpful. Because family members do not know what to expect from the nurse, the nurse must establish a relationship with the members by demonstrating understanding, competence, and caring (Box 7-2). Family nursing is relational nursing practice, acknowledging the expertise and knowledge of families.

We encourage nurses to consider the type of relationship that they would like to establish with families. Research in the area of health-care professionals establishing relationships with families is minimal. Thorne and Robinson (1989) have described various stages of the evolution of relationships between families experiencing chronic illness and their health-care professionals: naïve trust, disenchantment, and guarded alliance. They propose that naïve trust among the chronically ill, their families, and health-care providers is inevitably shattered in the face of unmet expectations and conflicting perspectives. Anxiety, frustration, and confusion often result in disenchantment. Trust can then be reconstructed on a more guarded basis so that the chronically ill patient, the family, and the nurse can continue to engage in health-care activities. Wong, Liamputtong, Koch, and Rawson (2015) conducted a qualitative study about families' experiences of their interactions with nurses in intensive care units. The findings indicated that nurses facilitating communication and interacting in supportive ways helped alleviate anxiety and distress among families with a critically ill member. Examples of nursing responses included providing reassurance, responding to nonverbal cues, and being open and honest.

Reciprocal trust is a critical dimension to consider during the engagement phase of family interviewing. The nurse helps the patient and family to feel more confident in their own competence in managing illness. In order to develop a high degree of trust in the nurse, the patient and family are encouraged to explicitly state their expectations for health care.

Box 7-1 Purpose of Engagement

- Promote a positive nurse-family relationship by developing an atmosphere of comfort, mutual trust, and cooperation between the nurse and the family.
- Recognize that family members bring strengths and resources to this relationship that may have previously gone unnoticed by health-care professionals.
- Prevent potential nurse-family misunderstandings or problems later on in the therapeutic relationship.

Levac, A. M. C., Wright, L. M., & Leahey, M. (2002). Children and families: Models for assessment and intervention. In J. A. Fox (Ed.), Primary health care of infants, children, and adolescents (2nd ed., p. 11). St. Louis, MO: Mosby. Copyright 2002. Adapted with permission.

Box 7-2 The ABCs of Engaging Families

A	B	C
• Assume an active, confident approach.	• Begin by providing structure to the meeting (time frame, orientation to the context).	• Create a context of mutual trust.
• Ask purposeful questions that draw forth family assessment data.	• Behave in a curious manner, and take an equal interest in all family members, whether present or not.	• Clarify expectations about your role with the family.
• Address all who are present, including small children.	• Build on family strengths by offering commendations to the family.	• Collaborate in decision making, health promotion, and health management.
• Adjust the conversation to children's developmental stages.	• Bring relevant resources to the meeting (list of agencies, phone numbers, pamphlets).	• Cultivate a context of racial and ethnic sensitivity.
		• Commend family members.

Levac, A. M. C., Wright, L. M., & Leahey, M. (2002). Children and families: Models for assessment and intervention. In J. A. Fox (Ed.), Primary health care of infants, children, and adolescents (2nd ed., p. 11). St. Louis, MO: Mosby. Copyright 2002. Adapted with permission.

The nurse provides the opportunity for family members to express their desires. If the patient and family are to have a high degree of trust in their own competence, family members and health-care providers must acknowledge the family's resources. This is further supported by a literature review conducted by Dinc and Gastmans (2013) that suggests that the development of trust is important in establishing a nurse-family relationship; it is a process during which trust can be broken or reestablished depending on the nurse's competencies and interpersonal caring attributes (p. 501). Reeves and colleagues (2015) found that "family members noted that their experience on the intensive care unit was particularly positive when they felt they had a trusting relationship with the staff. Staff knowledge of patient's history, frequent communication regarding the patient's condition and informal communication with the family helped to facilitate this positive relationship" (p. 234).

One way of reminding ourselves not to fall into the trap of certainty, judgmentalness, and expertness on the family's situation has been to develop a strong sense of curiosity. When initiating engagement, we assume a position of neutrality or curiosity. Cecchin (1987) draws connections between neutrality or curiosity and hypothesizing. He maintains that curiosity is a delight in the invention and discovery of multiple patterns. "Curiosity helps us to continue looking for different descriptions and explanations, even when we cannot immediately imagine the possibility of another one ... hypothesizing is connected to curiosity. Hypothesizing has more to do with technique. Curiosity is a stance, whereas hypothesizing is what we do to try to maintain this stance" (p. 411). We believe that curiosity nurtures circularity and is useful in the development of hypotheses. We have found hypothesizing, circularity, and curiosity to be extremely important components of our clinical work.

We agree with Cecchin (1987), who states, "circular questioning can be understood as a method by which a clinician creates curiosity within the family system and therapy system" (p. 412). (See Chapters 2 and 3 for more information about circularity, and see Chapter 6 for additional ideas about hypothesizing.) By using hypothesizing, circularity, and curiosity, nurses become more open to families, and families, in turn, develop more reciprocal trust. The family perceives the nurse as inquisitive when he or she does not take sides with any one member or subgroup. Nurses who are inquisitive are seen as aligned with everyone and no one in particular at the same time. They are seen as nonjudgmental and accepting of everyone.

To enhance engagement, the nurse must provide structure, be active and empathic, and involve all members of the family. To provide structure, the nurse might say something such as, *"We'll meet now for about 10 minutes so that I can get a better sense of your expectations and any concerns you have about hospitalization. We can then talk about what I might be able to help you with. How does that sound to you?"* By stating the structure at the beginning of the meeting, the nurse reduces the family's anxiety about how long they will meet and also gives some direction for the conversation. Sundet's (2011) findings that families found it helpful when the clinician asked questions, gave time, and structured the work further support this idea.

One way in which the nurse can be active during the engagement phase of the interview is to find out who is present. Many times, we have found that "extra" family members attend interviews in the hospital. Leahey, Stout, and Myrah (1991) found that of families invited to meetings on an inpatient mental health unit in a Canadian community hospital, 94% attended. Extra family members attending interviews held constant over a 7-year period. In many cases, family members of whom the nurse was unaware showed up for the family meeting. For example, extended family members or former spouses might have been invited by the patient or other family members who believed it was important for them to be present.

Some nurses have found it useful to start an interview by working with the family in constructing a genogram or ecomap (see Chapter 3). Duhamel and Campagna's genograph (2000) is a particularly helpful educational tool that can assist nurses in drawing a genogram and determining what questions to ask. Families generally find that constructing a genogram is an easy way to involve themselves in giving the nurse relevant information. The genogram can be obtained reliably and accurately in a brief interview. Furthermore, genograms obtained by a health-care provider are likely to have more influence on care and health outcomes than those completed by the patient or health assistant and placed on file.

At the start of the interview, the nurse should ask questions of each member. This is particularly important for nurses working with families with adolescents. Engaging adolescents by asking what their favorite computer games or school subjects are and why, whether they play sports, what musical groups they like, and whether they have any special talents and hobbies can sometimes be useful. The purpose of these questions is to start establishing a shared habit (between the nurse and the young person) of discussion and banter about the young person's opinions about personal aspects of his or her life. However, we do not recommend that this type of conversation go on for longer than 5 minutes because it seems easier for families to engage around the presenting problem than to chat in a general nature. We believe it is important for the nurse to create an environment where the client expects to get down to business, work on the hard issues, and make the necessary changes to improve family functioning in the context of illness, loss, or disability. Box 7-3 provides tips on dealing with verbose clients.

Box 7-3 Tips for Working With Verbose Clients

- **Let** the person tell his or her illness story or particular concern.
- **Set** the time frame at the beginning, such as, *"We have 20 minutes to meet. What are the most important things that we need to discuss?"*
- **Say,** *"I know we only have time to skim the surface today in talking about your experiences, so what shall we focus on?"*
- **Explain,** *"I'm not connecting what you're telling me with the reason you've come in today. Could you help me out on this, please?"*
- **Take a break** to pull your thoughts together or to seek a consult.
- **Stop** the discussion and set limits, such as, *"We can spend 10 minutes talking about the poor addiction services in our city and 10 minutes on what you said your goals were and how you're addressing them. How does that sound as a plan for today?"*
- **Use humor and interrupt** by saying something such as, *"Seems like we could talk all day about this issue, but I'm mindful of the time."*
- **Determine** who is most interested in the client being seen if the client has been referred by another health professional: *"The note from your physician indicated she wants you to have ... Is this your understanding of why you are here today? Did you have another goal for our meeting?"*

Nurses should initially attempt to spend an equal amount of time with each family member. We suggest that the nurse ask the same or a similar question of each member to gather each person's ideas about a particular topic. We believe that when families answer questions, they are not retrieving particular experiences. Rather, in the conversation with the clinician, family members put forth their own storytelling of their unique experiences, suggest beginnings and endings for these experiences, and highlight portions of experiences while diminishing or excluding others.

If the engagement between the nurse and family does not proceed well or if a fit cannot be established, we recommend that the nurse stop and think about the relationship. We have found the following ideas about relationships with families helpful to keep in mind in our clinical practice:

- Both the health-care provider and patient and/or family members are experts. The patient is expert in the illness experience, and usually, but not always, the health-care provider is expert in the physiology of the disease process, illness management, and easing suffering.
- The health-care provider will try to facilitate change, but the ultimate agent of change is the patient/family.
- To construct a workable management plan, the patient/family and the health-care provider's interpretation of the symptoms must both be acknowledged.

The engagement stage is also the phase of the interview in which a context for change is created that constitutes the central and enduring foundation of the therapeutic process (Bell & Wright, 2011; McLeod, Tapp, Moules & Campbell, 2010; Wright & Bell, 2009). Wright and Bell suggest that all obstacles for change need to be removed during this stage so that a full and meaningful nurse-family engagement may be made. Examples of obstacles to change in working with families include a family member who does not want to be present or who attends the meeting under duress, previous negative experiences with health-care professionals, and unrealistic or unknown expectations of the referring person about treatment.

Most central to this stage, however, is that the family members should feel that the nurse is willing to listen and witness their voices, to "do hope," as Weingarten (2000) calls it. But hope does not reside within one individual; it is not solitary. Hope is something we do with others. "It is the responsibility of those who love you to *do hope* with you" (Weingarten, 2000, p. 402). One study sought to understand couples' experiences in nurse-initiated health-promoting conversations about hope and suffering during home-based palliative care. It was revealed that couples found these conversations with nurses to be a healing experience that also enabled them to learn and find new ways for managing daily life (Benzein & Saveman, 2008). Ward and Wampler (2010) suggest distinguishing categories of hope on a continuum from lost hope to ambivalent/low hope to solid hope. Parents of children suffering from cancer found that when health-care professionals went above and beyond in the care they provided, it increased the parents' connection to the health-care providers and strengthened the parents' hope for their children (Conway, Pantaleao, & Popp, 2017). This type of connection is considered essential if families are to experience comfort and hope (Angström-Brännström, Norberg, Strandberg, Söderberg, & Dahlqvist, 2010).

We find this notion useful in our clinical work. Especially during the engagement phase, nurses should follow the clients' lead, listening for and adopting their language, worldview, goals, and ideas about the problem and legitimizing their illness experiences to foster a trusting relationship nested in hope. We encourage nurses to get to know their clients outside of the influence of the problem and connect with them in their lives. For example, a nurse could appreciate the lived experiences of a family's past hardships (death, loss, illness, divorce, immigration, war, and other difficulties) and could wonder how this stamina might now serve the family as they stand together against illness.

Assessment Stage

During the assessment stage, the nurse and family explore four areas:

- Problem identification
- Relationship between family interaction and the health problem
- Attempted solutions to solving problems
- Goals

KEY CONCEPT DEFINED

Assessment Stage

A stage during the family interview when problem identification and exploration occurs, including delineation of strengths; an ongoing process.

Problem Identification: Exploration and Definition

During this phase of the family interview, the nurse asks family members about their main concerns, complaints, or suffering. The nurse could ask, for example, *"What is the concern that each family member would most like to see addressed or changed?"* A focus on change and expectation for something to happen is important for time-effective therapeutic meetings. Slive and Bobele (2011) have demonstrated this in their landmark work documenting single-session walk-in therapy. After exploring each family member's perception of the most pressing concern (once adequate engagement has occurred), we have found it useful to ask the "why now?"

question: *"What made you decide to come in today?"* We assume the family probably consulted others prior to meeting with the nurse and are curious about why, at this point in time, the client chose to seek help.

Another useful question is the "one-question question" suggested by Wright (1989): *"If you could have only one question answered during our work together, what would that one question be?"* (For more information about the one-question question, see Chapter 8.)

It is important to emphasize that an effective interview does not depend on the use of one type of question but on the knowledge of when, how, and to what purpose questions are used with particular family members at particular points in time. (For more information on various types of questions, see Chapters 4 and 8.)

Table 7-2 gives examples from Leahey and Wright (1987) of how to elicit the family's concerns by asking circular questions that focus on the present, past, and future.

One thing to consider is that children or adolescents may be reluctant to identify concerns in the family, and the nurse may need to ask the children alternative questions. Children may hesitate to disagree with their parents' description of the situation. A nurse can ask a child what he or she would like to see different in the family or how he or she would know if the problems went away. For example, one 8-year-old, Brian, repeatedly stated that

TABLE 7-2	**Circular Questions to Elicit a Family's Concerns**	
PRESENT	**PAST**	**FUTURE**
■ What is the family's main concern now about Shaheena's cyberbullying? ■ How is this concern a problem for the family now as compared with before? ■ Who agrees with you that this is a problem? Is this a problem that Mom believes she has control over? ■ What is your explanation for this?	■ **Differences:** How was Shaheena's behavior before her cyberbullying was noticed? ■ **Agreement or disagreement:** Who agrees with Dad that this was the main concern when the family lived in Uganda? ■ **Explanation or meaning:** What do you think was the significance of Shaheena's decision to stop using the family computer for her messaging?	■ If Rahim suddenly developed renal disease, how would things be different from the way they are now? ■ Does Rahim agree with you? ■ If this were to happen, how would you explain the change in Shaheena's relationship with Mom?

Leahey, M., & Wright, L. M. (1987). *Families and chronic illness: Assumptions, assessment and intervention.* In L. M. Wright & M. Leahey (Eds.), Families and chronic illness (pp. 55–76). Springhouse, PA: Springhouse Corp.

there were no difficulties surrounding his brother's diabetes and his mother's intense involvement with the sick child. However, when the nurse asked a future-oriented question about what differences he would notice in the family if his brother did not have diabetes, Brian said that he and his mother could go to basketball games after school. At the time of the interview, the mother had stated she was hesitant to leave the house after the boys returned from school for fear that her older son, Ray, would have an insulin reaction.

Whatever strategy is used to engage young people in conversation, we recommend nurses be aware of the importance of inviting active thinking by children and adolescents versus the expectation of compliance with adult thinking. This is foundational to relational practice. Box 7-4 presents ideas for involving children and adolescents in family interviews.

In exploring the presenting concern, the nurse should obtain a clear and specific definition of the situation. We recommend that nurses pay attention only to the concern as defined by the family, setting aside their own definition of the problem. We believe it is helpful to coevolve a problem description using the family's language and to initiate conversations about family members' preferences. Table 7-3 lists some factors for the nurse to consider when defining the problem.

In our conversations with families, we try to remember that each family expresses its pain and suffering in a unique way. For example, nurses need to consider how culture, ethnicity, religion, gender, age, personal coping practices, life experiences, and education could all impact how individuals and families may express pain and suffering. When differences among family members exist, the nurse should clarify the issues further to help define the problem for which the family is seeking change. The nurse can also ask questions of each member about his or her own explanation for the current situation. It is important for nurses to attend to *how* clients talk about the concerns that prompted them to show up for a meeting. Box 7-5 provides questions the nurse could ask to bring a family focus to situations.

Wright and Bell (2009) believe that exploring the family's illness beliefs in the first meeting and at times of crisis is particularly important. If the

---

Box 7-4 Ideas for Involving Children in Family Interviews

- Art techniques (drawing a family picture)
- Verbal techniques ("Columbo" strategy of taking a position of not knowing)
- Role-playing or make-believe
- Storytelling techniques to allow families to personify, reframe, and externalize problems
- Puppet and doll techniques to ask the family about interactions
- Video games
- Experiential techniques (family sculpture)

TABLE 7-3	Factors to Consider in Defining the Problem	
PRESENTING PROBLEM	**PROBLEM IDENTIFICATION**	**PROBLEM EVOLUTION**
▪ Specify	▪ Who in the family was the first to identify the problem? And then who? ▪ When was the problem identified? ▪ What were the concurrent life events or stressors at the time of identification of the problem? ▪ Who else (family members, friends) agrees that it is a problem? Who disagrees? ▪ How does the family understand that this problem developed (beliefs)?	▪ What behaviors became problematic? ▪ Pattern of development ▪ Frequency of problem emergence ▪ Time intervals of quiescence ▪ Factors aggravating ▪ Factors alleviating ▪ Who in the family is most and least concerned?

Adapted from Family Nursing Unit records, Faculty of Nursing, University of Calgary.

Box 7-5 Questions to Bring Family Focus to the Situation

- Has anyone else in the family had this problem?
  Rationale: Addresses family history.
- What do other family members believe caused the problem or could treat the problem?
  Rationale: Explores the individual's explanatory model and health beliefs.
- Who in the family is most concerned about the problem?
  Rationale: Helps to understand the relational context of the concern.
- Along with your illness and symptoms, have there been any other recent changes in your family?
  Rationale: Addresses family stress and change.
- How can your family be helpful to you in dealing with this problem?
  Rationale: Focuses on family support.

---

family members think that their beliefs or explanations about the illness are not acknowledged, they may feel marginalized. The nurse can ask them to explain, for example, why they believe this problem exists at this point in time. We believe it is also important to ask if the client and family have any control over the problem. The simplest way to do this is to ask direct, explanation-seeking questions such as, "*What do you think is the reason for your son's violence toward his peers? Do you think Sara has any control over the problem?"*

Another idea is to ask clients to use their imagination to discuss an explanation. The interviewer can also offer a variety of alternative explanations or "gossip in the presence" by asking triadic questions such as, *"William, what do you think is Zack's explanation for your mother's depression?"* In exploring the family's preexisting explanations, it is essential for the interviewer to be curious and to avoid agreeing or disagreeing with the explanation.

There are several advantages to exploring the family's causal explanations, including improving cooperation between the interviewer and the family, developing systemic empathy with all family members versus selective empathy with one or two, detaching oneself from explanations provided by other professionals, recognizing and avoiding coalitions, loosening firmly held explanations, diluting negative explanations, and developing an ability to speculate with the clients about the effects of believing in one explanation or the other.

The problem-defining process, or "co-evolving the definition," is a critical aspect of family work. Cecchin (1987) warns clinicians to accept neither their own nor the client's definition too quickly, and Maturana and Varela (1992) caution clinicians to adopt an attitude of permanent vigilance against the temptation of certainty. By remaining curious, a clinician has a greater chance of escaping the "sin of certainty," or the sin of being too invested in one's own opinion. As clinicians, nurses need to avoid being preoccupied with their own brightness or ideas. Rather, each nurse should ask, *"What does the client need from me? What are the client's beliefs, thoughts, hunches, and theories about the problem? About the extent of their control over the problem? Their solutions?"* We try to always "keep the problem on the table" as we engage with families.

Relationship Between Family Interaction and the Health Problem

Once the main problems have been identified, the nurse asks questions about the relationship of family interaction to the health problem. Box 7-6 lists some factors to consider in exploring family interactions related to the presenting problem. The nurse conceptualizes the information that has already been gathered from the family in light of the meaning it has for the family and the hypotheses generated before the interview. For example, a home-care nurse talking with parents caring for a technology-dependent child at home might be mindful of the parents' new role as care specialists, the transformation of family space and privacy with the introduction of multiple health-care professionals, and the financial drain on their resources.

The nurse then begins to develop additional questions that focus on interactional behaviors dealing with the three time frames of present, past, and future. Within each time frame, the nurse once again explores differences, agreements and disagreements, and explanations or meanings. It is

---

Box 7-6 Factors to Consider in Exploring Family Interaction Related to the Problem

- Current manifestations of the problem
- Typical responses of family members and others to the problem
- Other current associated problems, challenges, or concerns
- How the problem influences family functioning
- What family members appreciate about how they have coped with this challenging situation
- How family members understand that they have not been successful in conquering this problem (beliefs)

Adapted from Family Nursing Unit records, Faculty of Nursing, University of Calgary.

---

important to emphasize that the purpose of asking these questions is not merely to gather data—that is, by asking circular questions, the nurse generates new ideas and explanations for the nurse and the family to consider.

Present

In exploring the present situation, the nurse could ask, *"Who does what, when? Then what happens? Who is the first to notice that something has been done?"* The nurse should steer away from asking about traits that are supposedly intrinsic to a person, for example, being shy. Rather, the nurse might ask, *"When does Ari act shy?"* or *"To whom does he show shyness?"* Then, *"What does Jennifer do when Ari shows shyness?"* The nurse can explore areas of difference, inquire about areas of agreement or disagreement, and explore the family's explanation for the sequence of interaction. The following example questions might be used.

Difference:
- "Who is better at getting Grandmother to make her meals, Shanghi or Puichun?"
- "Do your ex-husband and José fight more or less than your ex-husband and Nadiya?"
- "Do you worry more, less, or the same about your wife's health since her emergency surgery?"

Agreement/Disagreement:
- "Who agrees with you that Brandon is most likely to forget to give your mother her eye drops three times per day?"
- "Who disagrees with you?"

Explanation/Meaning:
- "How do you understand Brandon's tendency to be most forgetful about the eye drops?"

- "Are there times when he does remember?"
- "What seems to be different about the times when he remembers?"

Past

In exploring the past, the nurse should use similar questions to explore difference, agreement or disagreement, and explanation or meaning.

Difference:
- "How was Brandon's caregiving different before he had high-speed Internet?"
- "How does that differ from now?"

Agreement/Disagreement:
- "Who agrees with Murdock that Dad was more involved in Genevieve's exercise program?"

Explanation/Meaning:
- "What does it mean to you that, after all this time, things between your wife and her mother have not changed?"

In addition to exploring how the family members saw the problem in the past, we have found it extremely useful to explore how they have seen changes in the problem. Change in the problem situation frequently occurs before the first meeting with the interviewer. If prompted, family members can often recall and describe such changes. It is important to note that in many cases, the family must be prompted to emerge from their problem-saturated view of the situation. For example, a man may tell the nurse at the community mental health center that his male partner drinks very heavily and has done this "until recently." If the nurse is attuned to inquiring about pretreatment changes, the nurse will ask questions about the differences that the man has noticed recently. For example, the nurse might inquire, *"Is his recent behavior the kind of change you would like to continue to have happen?"* The idea of noticing exceptions to problems is one that we have used frequently in our clinical work, and we are indebted to de Shazer (1991) and White (1991) for emphasizing it.

Future

By focusing on the future and how the family would like things to be, nurses instill hope for more adaptive interaction regarding the presenting concern. They also co-construct a reality between family members and themselves for a system in which the problem has dissolved. Example questions nurses could ask include the following:

Differences:
- "How would it be different if your grandfather did not side with your mother against your father in managing Paola's Crohn disease?"

Agreement/Disagreement:
- "Do you think your mother would agree that if your grandfather stayed out of the discussions, things would be better?"

Explanation/Meaning:
- "John, if your wife stopped phoning her father for advice about Paola's Crohn disease, what would that mean to you?"

We believe it is especially important to ask future-oriented questions when working with families dealing with a new diagnosis or a change in health status because the changed expectations and possibilities for the future may be disrupting to family life transitions.

During this stage of the interview, the nurse does the following:

- Attempts to gain a systemic view of the situation and a description of the cycle of repeated interactions. Interactions may be between family members or between family members and the nurse. The nurse does not have to understand or agree with the problem but instead be curious about the family's description of its positive and negative impact. Appreciative inquiry is questioning that elicits and builds on appreciated practices and engages family members in discussion with each other about what works for them. In this way, families can take a "both/and" position.
- Describes the sequence of the problem's development over time, the current contextual problem interaction, whether the family believes it has some control over the problem, the times when the problem does not show itself, and what the family members appreciate about their personal and cooperative efforts to work together.

What happens with clients who don't see themselves as having a problem and yet are referred to the nurse? They may be mandated for treatment or present under duress. In situations where individuals and families have different agendas for a meeting and different definitions of the problem, we believe it is important for the nurse not to rigidify the interaction, however inadvertently. By insisting too early that it is *definitely* a problem, the nurse can invite a rigid no-problem response from the client. We do not use the word *denial* because this generally fosters an antagonistic relationship over the question of who is "right." Although we sometimes find ourselves tempted to give advice and confront the situation head-on, we have found that this typically invites defensiveness and promotes shame. (Additional ideas on how not to give advice prematurely are given in Chapter 11.)

Attempted Solutions for Solving Problems

During the next phase of the assessment, the nurse explores the family's attempted solutions to the problem. The process can begin with general questions related to the problem. For example, *"What improvements have you noticed since you first contacted our clinic?"* This type of question conveys the idea to families that they have the strengths and resources to change, and it assumes that changes have already occurred, which can help set in motion a positive self-fulfilling prophecy for them. Another example might be, *"How have you tried to obtain information from physicians and nurses about Mandy's condition in previous hospitalizations?"*

Box 7-7 lists some factors to consider when exploring the family's attempted solutions.

More specific questions should then be used to identify the least and most effective solutions for achieving what the family desires. The nurse can ask when these solutions were used. For example, *"What was least helpful in trying to get information from the nurses about Surjit's resuscitation? What was most effective?"* The nurse can ask if any successful elements in the solutions are still being used, and if not, why. Similar types of sequences of interaction questions that focus on difference, agreement or disagreement, and explanation or meaning can be used to explore the family's attempted solutions to the presenting concerns.

When nurses are told that no solutions have been attempted or that "nothing has worked," it is useful to ask the following questions:

- "How come things aren't worse?"
- "What are you doing to keep this situation from getting worse?"

The nurse can then amplify these problem-solving strategies by asking about their frequency, effectiveness, and so forth. The nurse should also try to expand the family's view of typical solutions to include complementary and alternative medical and health approaches.

We also find it useful to draw on the concept of resilience in these situations. In talking with families about their resilience, we use such terms as *endurance, withstanding, adaptation, coping,* and *survival* and try to draw forth other qualities surfacing in the face of hardship or adversity. We talk about the ability to "bounce back" or make up for losses. We believe resilience is forged *through* adversity, not *despite* it. Bouncing back is not the same as "breezing through" a crisis. Resilience involves multiple recursive

---

Box 7-7 Factors to Consider in Exploring the Family's Attempted Solution

- How has the family tried to resolve the problem?
- Who tried?
- With whom?
- What were the results?
- What were the events precipitating the search for professional help?
- Who is most in favor of agency help? Most opposed?
- What are the client's thoughts about the nurse's role in the change process?
- What was the sequence of events resulting in actual contact with the agency?

Adapted from Family Nursing Unit records, Faculty of Nursing, University of Calgary.

processes over time. It is this layering and recursiveness that we inquire about when we ask families about their coping and attempted solutions.

In working with families dealing with life-threatening or chronic illness, the nurse should also be aware of additional "helping agencies" involved in health-care delivery. A nurse may ask questions such as the following:

- "Have any other agencies attempted to help you with this problem?"
- "What has been the most useful advice that you have received?" "Did you follow this advice?"
- "What has been the least helpful advice?"

It is useful to explore the differing ideas espoused by the helping systems. If there is unclear leadership or a confused hierarchy within the helping systems, the family can be placed in a conflictual situation that is similar to that of a child whose parents continually disagree. Confusion among helping agencies can exacerbate the family's concerns. In this way, the attempted solution (assistance by helping agencies) can become an entirely new problem for both the family and other agencies. It is important for the nurse to be aware of whether this situation exists before attempting to intervene.

Having consolidated a shared view of the problem and elicited some relevant solutions, it can simply be stated to the family that the nurse would like to work with them to achieve their goals. This small but profound acknowledgment is an opportunity for the nurse to show compassion to the client and enter into a deeper relationship and collaboration.

Goal Exploration

At some point during the interview, the nurse and family establish what goals or outcomes the family expects as a result of change. Families are pragmatic: They are seeking practical results when they come to a health-care provider; they are "in pain" or "suffering," and their desire is to get rid of a problem. The problem may be between themselves as family members or between the family and the nurse (e.g., the family desires practical information about the acceptable level of physical activity after a myocardial infarction [MI], and the nurse has not provided such concrete information). Family members may expect a large change (e.g., *"My brother Sheldon will be able to walk without the aid of a cane"*) or a small but significant change (e.g., *"We will be able to leave our handicapped daughter, Kayla, with a babysitter for 1 hour a week"*). In many cases, a small change is sufficient. We believe that a small change in a person's behavior can have profound and far-reaching effects on the behavior of all persons involved. Experienced nurses are aware that small changes lead to further progress. Box 7-8 lists some factors for nurses to consider when exploring goals.

Goals describe what will be present or what will be happening when the complaint or concern is absent. We believe that unidimensional behavioral

---

Box 7-8 Factors to Consider When Exploring Goals

- What general changes does the family believe would improve the problem?
- What specific changes?
- What are the expectations of how the agency may facilitate change in the problem?

Adapted from Family Nursing Unit records, Faculty of Nursing, University of Calgary.

---

goal statements such as *"I will be eating less"* are not as desirable as multidimensional, interactional, and situational goal statements that describe the "who, what, when, where, and how" of the solution. Such a multidimensional goal statement might be, *"I will be eating a small, balanced meal in the evening at the dinner table with my partner and our children; the television and computer will be off, and we will be talking to each other."* Examples of future-orientated questions nurses could ask to clarify family goals include the following:

Difference:
- "What would your parents do differently if they did not stay at home every evening with Sanna?"
- "How would your parents' relationship be different if your dad allowed your uncle to take care of Sanna one evening a week?"

Agreement/Disagreement:
- "Do you think your dad would agree that your parents would probably have little to talk about if they went out one evening a week?"

Exploration/Meaning:
- "Tell me more about why you believe your parents would have a lot to talk about when they went out that one evening a week."
- "What would that mean to you?"

We sometimes find it useful to combine past and future questions. For example, *"If you were to tell me next week (or month or year) that you had done X, what could I find in your past history that would have allowed me to predict that you would have done X?"* The questions capitalize on the "possibility to probability" phenomenon while also inviting a richer account of the history of the new/old story.

Another useful strategy that has been shown to be beneficial in eliciting family goals is the "miracle question" that de Shazer (1988) describes this way:

> Suppose that one night there is a miracle and while you are sleeping the problem ... is solved: How would you know? What would be different?
>
> What will you notice different the next morning that will tell you there has been a miracle? What will your spouse notice? (de Shazer, 1991, p. 113)

The miracle question elicits interactional information. The person is asked to imagine someone else's ideas as well as his or her own. The framework of the miracle question (and others of this type) allows family members to bypass their causal explanations. They do not have to imagine how they will get rid of the problem but instead can focus on results. Thus, the goals developed from the miracle question are not limited to just getting rid of the problem or complaint. Clients often are able to construct answers to this "miracle question" quite concretely and specifically. For example, *"Easy, I'll be able to say no to cocaine,"* or *"She'll see me smile more and come home from work with less tension."*

KEY CONCEPT DEFINED

Miracle Question

A question asked by a nurse during a family interview that elicits interactional information; a person is asked to imagine someone else's ideas as well as his or her own; allows family members to bypass their causal explanations.

McConkey (2002) suggests strategies for solution-focused meetings that we believe are particularly useful if a family is angry and the nurse is feeling defensive. The nurse can shift the meeting from the problem picture to the future solution picture by engaging in conversation (p. 192). Here is an example of the nurse's strategies in such a dialogue:

- "Obviously, you want things to be better for your child, and so do I."
  Purpose: Validating the parent
- "In order to make the most of this meeting, I'm going to ask you an unusual question."
  Purpose: Bridging statement
- "How will you know, by the time you leave here today, that this meeting has been helpful?"
  Purpose: Shifting to the future
- "When things are better, what will your son be doing? What will I be doing? What will you be doing?"
  Purpose: Including all the stakeholders in the solution picture

Nurses working with families of a patient who has a chronic or life-threatening illness commonly find family members vague about the changes they expect. For example, parents might say, *"We would like Attila to feel good about himself even though he has a colostomy."* Experienced clinical nurses know that "feeling good about oneself" is very difficult to describe or measure. In this example, we recommend that the nurse ask the family members to describe the smallest concrete change that Attila could make to show that he "feels good about himself." By asking for this degree of specificity about desired change early in the nurse-family relationship, we believe it is more likely that the family and nurse can accomplish the desired change.

Planning and Dealing With Complexity

After an initial assessment is completed, a beginning nurse interviewer frequently worries about whether to intervene with a family. The following questions often arise: *"Am I the appropriate person to offer intervention? Is the situation too complex? Do I have sufficient skills, or should another professional, such as a social worker, psychologist, or family therapist, be called in? Does every family that is assessed need further intervention?"* This is not to say that interventions begin only at the intervention stage. Rather, they are part of the total interview process from engagement to closure. For example, just by asking the family to come together for an interview, the nurse has intervened. Each time the nurse asks a circular question, the nurse influences the family, generates new information, and intervenes. For nurses, the decision to offer interventions, refer the family to others, or discharge them is a complex one. Several factors need to be examined before making the choice: the level of the family's functioning, the level of the nurse's competence, and the work context.

KEY CONCEPT DEFINED

Intervention Stage

The stage during a family interview in which the nurse and the family collaborate on areas for desired change.

Level of the Family's Functioning

The nurse should recognize the complexity of the family situation and the family's level of functioning. Some clinicians have advocated that treatment begin if the referring problem has been detected early and clearly defined procedures for management have been published. Most nurses would agree with this position but would find it very idealistic.

Desire to Work on Issues

Nurses need to carefully assess the family's level of functioning and its desire to work on specific issues, such as management of hemiplegia after a stroke, impact of cystic fibrosis on the family, negotiation of services for elderly family members, or caring for a child with special needs. If the family is at all amenable to working on an issue, it is incumbent on the nurse either to offer intervention or to help them get appropriate assistance by referring them to others. (Guidelines for the referral process are provided in Chapter 12.)

Ethical Decisions

Nurses must consider ethical issues in deciding who should be treated and weigh two opposing positions when they decide to intervene with, refer, or discharge a family (potentially dangerous to self or others). They must also have the knowledge and skills of ethical principles, such as autonomy and beneficence, and adhere to their code of ethics and standards of practice.

Values and Beliefs

Nurses need to be aware of the values and beliefs held by the family and its members as well as their own and be cognizant not to impose personal values and beliefs.

Nurse's Level of Competence

Nurses need to consider their personal and professional capacity prior to making the decision to intervene with a family. It is important to note that we believe that a nurse does not have to personally have dealt with a situation (e.g., raising teenagers) to help a family.

Personal Capacity

- *Personal Experiences:* Nurses need to be aware of how their life experiences may impact their ability to intervene appropriately and effectively with families (recent loss, new diagnosis, life transition).
- *Values and Beliefs:* Nurses need to be aware of their own values, beliefs, assumptions, and judgments.

Professional Capacity

- *Competence Level:* Nurses need to evaluate their competence by asking self-reflective questions, such as the following:
  - "Am I at the beginning or the advanced level of family interviewing skill?"
  - "Can I obtain supervision to aid in dealing with families who present with complex issues?"

- *Scope of Practice:* Nurses need to be aware of their roles and responsibilities and provide interventions that they are authorized, educated, and competent to perform, including legal obligations.
- *Evidence Informed:* Nurses need to be well informed, with up-to-date information and resources, and not just offer advice that might or might not be helpful.

Work Context

- *Workplace Structure:* Considerable controversy is sometimes raised about the issue of who is competent to assist clients when working in an interdisciplinary team. This controversy involves issues of definition and professionalism. How a "family problem" and a "medical problem" are defined in a particular work setting can fuel the controversy. Nurses often work as mediators, advocates, case managers, and navigators as a way to manage these controversies.
- *Health-care System:* Changes in health-care reimbursement have required all nurses and health-care providers to examine and adapt their practices to account for the provision of timely, efficient, and cost-effective services. Managed care in its many varieties, health insurance reform, increased focus on primary care, and other complex issues have changed the face of nursing practice.

The increase in the consumer movement, health economics, and technology has huge implications for practice that are more apparent than ever. Nurses must consider these practice implications when they decide to provide interventions. Nurses have to do more than just heal their patients. Day after day, they must also attend to the socioeconomic and political context of health care and to the survival of their careers. We believe that it is vital for nurses to find ways to thrive professionally and for families to receive optimal care.

Intervention Stage

Once a family intervention has been decided on, we recommend that the nurse review the Calgary Family Intervention Model (CFIM; see Chapter 4). This model, which stimulates ideas about change, can help the nurse design interventions to work with the family to address the particular domain of family functioning affected: cognitive, affective, or behavioral. Helpful hints about interventions are offered in Box 7-9.

In choosing interventions, we encourage nurses to attend to several factors to enhance the likelihood that the interventions will focus on change in the desired domain of family functioning. Interventions, offered within a collaborative relationship, are not a demand but rather an invitation

---

Box 7-9 Helpful Hints About Interventions

- They are the core of clinical work with families.
- They should be devised with sensitivity to the family's ethnic/cultural/religious background.
- They can only be *offered* to families; the nurse cannot direct change but can create a context for change to occur.
- They are offered in the context of collaborative conversations; nurse and family together devise solutions to find the most useful fit.
- When the nurse's ideas are not a good fit for the family, the nurse should be open to offering other ideas rather than becoming blameful of self or the family.

Levac, A. M. C., Wright, L. M., & Leahey, M. (2002). Children and families: Models for assessment and intervention. In J. A. Fox (Ed.), Primary health care of infants, children, and adolescents (2nd ed., p. 18). St. Louis, MO: Mosby. Copyright 2002. Adapted with permission.

---

to change. Factors to consider when devising interventions include the following:

- What is the agreed-upon problem to change?
- At what domain of family functioning is the intervention aimed?
- How does the intervention match the family's style of relating?
- How is the intervention linked to the family's strengths and previous useful solution strategies?
- How is the intervention consistent with the family's ethnic/cultural/religious beliefs?
- How is the intervention new or different for the family?

We do not believe that there is one "right" intervention. Rather, there are only "useful" or "effective" interventions. In our experience, we have found that a nurse sometimes reaches an impasse, with a family not changing, when the nurse persists in either using the same intervention repeatedly or switching interventions too rapidly. Sometimes we find that clients fail to notice responses containing possible solutions. The same can be said of nurses. Interventions are successful when constraints are lifted and important aspects of life change are noticed. The result is a clearer image of how things can be different in the future.

We have also found that sometimes the nurse is too constrained and fails to consider alternate system levels for intervention. For example, if a family does not want to hear or discuss the possibility of older adults having sexual activity at a residential care center, then the nurse may design an intervention not with the family but rather with the care center. Such an intervention with a residential care center could be to plan an in-service around the topic of HIV and older adults. The outcome may be that condoms are available in the center and clients have the information they need to keep themselves safe.

With the availability of computers, smartphones, tablets, e-readers, instant messaging, Twitter, and Facebook, we believe that nurses have become increasingly creative in finding electronic means to facilitate intervention. Just as the use of computers, e-mail, chat rooms, Listservs, blogs, and smartphones for business and education has had dramatic effects on family interaction, we believe their use in health care has also profoundly affected nurse-family interaction. The following list highlights examples of the use of technology as an intervention:

TITLE	AUTHOR
Study Protocol: Pragmatic Randomized Control Trial of an Internet-Based Intervention (My Tools 4 Care) for Family Carers (2017)	Williams et al
The Use of Information and Communication Technologies to Support Working Carers of Older People—A Qualitative Secondary Analysis (2016)	Andersson, Magnusson, & Hanson
The Effectiveness of an Internet Support Forum for Carers of People With Dementia: A Pre-Post Cohort Study (2014)	McKechnie, Barker, & Stott
The Provision of Social Support to Single, Low-Income, African-American Mothers via E-mail Messages (2009)	Campbell-Grossman, Hudson, Keating-Lefler, & Heusinkvelt

Note: Full citations can be found in the Reference list.

Once an intervention has been devised, the nurse must attend to the executive skills (see Chapters 5 and 10) required to deliver it. Part of the success of any intervention is the manner in which it is offered. The family must feel confident that the intervention will promote change. The nurse also needs to show confidence in the intervention or task requested and believe that it will benefit the family.

However, interventions need to be tailored to each family; therefore, the preamble or preface to the actual intervention will vary. For example, if family members are feeling very hopeless and frustrated with a particular problem, the nurse may say: *"I know this might seem like a hard thing that I'm going to ask you to do, but I know your family is capable of…"*

On the other hand, if the nurse is making a request of family members who tend to be quite formal with one another, then the nurse might preface it with: *"What I'm going to ask you to do may make you feel a little foolish or silly at first, but you'll notice that, as you do it a few times, you will become more comfortable."*

A good example of a generic intervention is the *"What are you prepared to do?"* question. The term *prepared* suggests a voluntary decision to participate in the change process.

When giving a particular assignment for a family to do between meetings, the nurse should try to include all family members. The nurse must review the particular assignment with family members to ensure they understand what is being requested. Reviewing the assignment is a good idea, whether it is carried out within the interview or between interviews. If assignments or experiments are given between sessions, the nurse should always ask for a report at the next interview. If the family has not completed or only partially completed the assignment, the reason should be explored.

We do not subscribe to the view that families are noncompliant or resistant if they do not follow our requests. Rather, we become curious about their decision to choose an alternate course and try to learn from their response. We believe that family interviewing is a circular process. The nurse intervenes, and the family responds in its unique way. The nurse then responds to this response, and the process continues. See Chapter 2 for more ideas about circularity.

During the intervention stage, the nurse must be aware of the element of time. How useful or effective an intervention is can be evaluated only after the intervention has been implemented. With some interventions, change may be noted immediately. However, more commonly, changes will not be noticed for a lengthy period. Just as most problems occur over time, problems also need an appropriate length of time to be resolved. It is impossible to state how long one should wait to ascertain if a particular intervention has been effective, but changes within family systems need to filter through the various system levels. Families themselves offer useful observations and feedback about what interventions are most useful. Robinson and Wright (1995), identified interventions within two stages of the therapeutic change process that they thought were critical to healing: (1) creating the circumstances for change and (2) moving beyond and overcoming problems. (For further elaboration on these stages, see Chapter 1.) More information about devising interventions is provided in Chapters 4, 8, 9, 10, and 12.

Termination Stage

The last stage of the interviewing process is known as *termination* or *closure*. It is critically important for the nurse to conceptualize how to end treatment with the family to enhance the likelihood that changes will be maintained. In Chapter 5, we outline the conceptual, perceptual, and executive skills useful for the termination stage. In Chapter 12, we address in depth the process of termination and focus on how to evaluate outcomes.

> **KEY CONCEPT DEFINED**
>
> ## Termination Stage
>
> The stage during the family interview when the therapeutic relationship between the nurse and the family is ended.

CLINICAL EXAMPLE

The following is an example of how a nurse conducted interviews with a family using the guidelines we have given in this chapter and in Chapter 6. An example of a 15-minute interview is given in Chapter 9.

Pre-Interview

Heinz Auerswald, 51, is a paraplegic and in a wheelchair because of a multiple trauma suffered in an industrial accident. He is unemployed. Eva Auerswald, 49, a homemaker, is the primary caregiver. She is reported to be depressed. A home health agency has received a referral on the Auerswald family for home nursing services, physiotherapy, nutrition counseling, and mental health counseling.

Developing Hypotheses

The home-care nurse hypothesized that Mrs. Auerswald's depression could be related to feeling overly responsible for caring for her husband. The nurse wondered if the husband's role and beliefs might be perpetuating this. She was also curious to know what other social and professional support systems were involved and what their beliefs were about the family's health problems. During the course of the family interview, the nurse gained much evidence from both the husband and wife to confirm the usefulness of her initial hypothesis. She used this hypothesis to provide a framework for her conversation with the couple.

Relation to the CFAM

The nurse generated her hypothesis based on knowledge of and clinical experience with other families in similar situations in addition to the following categories of the Calgary Family Assessment Model (CFAM):

- **Structural:** Internal and external family structure, ethnicity, gender
- **Developmental:** Middle-aged families
- **Functional:** Roles, power or influence, circular communication, beliefs

Arranging the Interview

Mrs. Auerswald stated that she did not want to discuss her depression with the nurse while her husband was awake. For the first home visit, the nurse requested that the husband and wife be interviewed together. The couple agreed to this.

Relation to the CFAM

The nurse thought about family roles and gender and speculated that Eva may be protecting her husband, Heinz, from her problem. The nurse considered the following category of the CFAM:

* **Functional:** Verbal communication (clear and direct communication between Heinz and Eva might be absent or infrequent)

Interview

Engagement

The genogram data revealed the following:

* Heinz and Eva are alone in the city; extended families and children live in other cities and visit infrequently.
* Eva had been married previously and had stayed with her first husband for 18 years, although he physically abused her. She thought it was her responsibility to protect her children.
* This is Heinz's first marriage.

Relation to the CFAM

The preceding information added some support for the nurse's initial hypothesis in terms of Eva's beliefs about responsibility and an isolated family structure.

Assessment

Problem Definition

* *Eva:* "Heinz has had such a hard tragedy, but now I'm the one who is depressed. It doesn't make sense."
* *Heinz:* "Eva is worrying too much."

Relationship Between Family Interaction and Health Problem

The nurse asked circular questions and discovered the following:

* Eva had not allowed herself a break from caregiving for 2 years.

- Heinz encouraged her to "go out and meet people," but she stated that she was fearful he might be too lonely if she met other people.
- Heinz stated that this would not be a problem for him.
- They both reported that Eva had recently become depressed. She cried frequently and had difficulty sleeping.
- Eva takes excellent physical care of Heinz and bathes him daily.
- Heinz is appreciative of all her nursing care.
- Eva feels guilty about asking for help from Heinz's parents.

Attempted Solutions

- Eva had recently visited her family doctor and was prescribed an antidepressant.
- Eva had requested home-care services once before, but she discontinued treatment with the nurses because their schedule was unreliable and she never knew when they were coming.
- On the advice of her physician, Eva agreed to try home care again.

Relation to the CFAM

- **Functional:** Problem solving

The Auerswalds' problem-solving approaches involved either self-sufficiency or professional resources outside the family. They sought help from the family doctor and from the home-care agency only infrequently, and they were reluctant to call on extended family for assistance.

Goals

- *Eva:* To not feel depressed and feel good about herself; to be able to go out one afternoon a week without feeling guilty
- *Heinz:* In agreement with Eva's goals

Intervention

Consideration of the CFIM

Having developed a collaborative relationship with the couple and a workable hypothesis that fit the data from the family assessment, the nurse began to consider interventions with Eva and Heinz in the *cognitive, affective, and behavioral* domains of family functioning. The focus of intervention was Eva's depression. Table 7-4 shows the interventions the nurse used with Eva and Heinz and their outcomes.

TABLE 7-4	Interventions and Outcomes
INTERVENTIONS	**OUTCOMES**
The nurse did the following: ■ Asked questions about beliefs and feelings of responsibility ■ Encouraged change in Eva's beliefs by asking both husband and wife behavioral effect, triadic, and hypothetical questions about responsibility ■ Asked the couple to engage in behavioral experiments to try new ways of being self-responsible	Both Eva and Heinz challenged their own beliefs about depression being a solely biological problem and began to take more responsibility for their own lives.
■ Eva requested caregiving help from her mother-in-law; this was arranged in addition to help from a home-care agency.	Eva was able to leave her husband alone for 2 hours, three times per week, while she played cards with friends. The couple reported significant improvement in Eva's depression.
■ The home-care agency continued to provide nursing and physical therapy services for the family. ■ The nurse and home health aide focused on supporting the couple's new beliefs about responsibility.	The couple reported significant improvement in her depression.

CASE SCENARIO: JULIA

The primary care clinic nurse meets Julia for the first time when she attends the clinic for her annual well-woman check. Julia is 31 years old and married to Kate. She has a very demanding, high-stress job as a second-year medical resident in a large hospital. During her physical assessment, Julia mentions that she has been feeling defeated lately. When the nurse questions her about these feelings, she explains that she has always been a high achiever and graduated with top honors in both university and medical school. She says that she has very high standards for herself and can be very self-critical when she fails to meet them. Lately, she has struggled with significant feelings of worthlessness and shame due to her inability to perform as well as she always has in the past. For the past few weeks, she has felt unusually fatigued and found it increasingly difficult to concentrate at work. Julia's wife, Kate, is in the waiting room. Kate has driven Julia to the clinic today because Julia says that she felt too tired to drive.

Continued

CASE SCENARIO: JULIA—cont'd

Reflective Questions

Engagement Phase

1. What strategies can the nurse use to establish a relationship with Julia?

Assessment Phase

2. What questions can the nurse ask Julia and Kate to explore the following issues?
   a. Problem identification
   b. Relationship between family interaction and health problem
   c. Attempted solutions to solving problems
   d. Goals

CRITICAL THINKING QUESTIONS

1. Identify a situation from your clinical practice and reflect on how you completed the following stages of a family interview:
   a. Engagement
   b. Assessment
      • Problem identification
      • Relationship between family interaction and health problem
      • Attempted solutions
      • Goal exploration
   c. Intervention
   d. Termination
2. What worked well, and what did not? What would you do differently based on your experience?

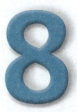

Chapter **8**

How to Use Questions in Family Interviewing

Learning Objectives

- Compare the difference between linear and circular questions, and explain when to use them.
- Describe how to apply questions to achieve the following:
  - Engage all family members and focus the meeting.
  - Assess the impact of the problem or illness on the family.
  - Elicit problem-solving skills, coping strategies, and strengths.
  - Intervene and invite change.
  - Request feedback about the meeting.

Key Concepts

Assessment questions   **Interventive questions**   **One-question question**

Throughout our book, we have discussed the usefulness of asking questions in family interviewing. We believe questions are useful for family assessment, and they are one of the most helpful family interventions nurses can offer. We have found the research of Healing and Bavelas (2011) to be encouraging in this regard. Their "controlled experiment confirmed that interview questions on the same topic but with a different focus can affect the interviewee, producing different attributions and even different behaviors" (p. 43). This is an important finding for clinical work. Through the use of examples of clinical interviews in this text, we demonstrate and reveal how questions are used in relational practice.

> **KEY CONCEPT DEFINED**
>
> ## Assessment Questions
>
> Types of questions that inform the nurse; often investigative questions, such as asking a family member to describe the illness experience or problem.

QUESTIONS IN CONTEXT

First, we discuss a few ideas about asking questions in the context of clinical practice, specifically in the context of a therapeutic conversation between a nurse and a family. We believe that useful or helpful questions have the potential to provide information to *both* the family and the nurse, invite family members to reflect on their illness experience, and can be potentially healing when the nurse asks them in a manner of sincere inquiry or curiosity. Questions are not effective in and of themselves; rather, it is only through a therapeutic conversation that questions help nurses be effective. (See Chapter 7 for more ideas about therapeutic conversation.) Questions also enhance a nurse's understanding of family members' experiences with a particular illness or problem. Answers to questions can help the nurse and the family appreciate the family's coping strategies, unique strengths, and resources. These types of conversations are very different from ones that a family may have with an intake worker or data clerk. We frequently have found that just telling the story can be therapeutic.

> **KEY CONCEPT DEFINED**
>
> ## Interventive Questions
>
> Questions asked by the nurse during a family interview that invite reflection and effect change; questions may encourage family members to see their problems in a new way and subsequently to discover new solutions.

There are numerous and various types of questions, such as difference questions, triadic questions, hypothetical questions, and behavioral-effect questions (see Chapter 4). In this chapter, we offer a simple dichotomy of questions that a nurse can ask: assessment and interventive questions.

- *Assessment (linear) questions:* The purpose is to inform the nurse; these are often investigative questions, such as asking a family member to describe the illness experience or problem.
- *Interventive (circular) questions:* The purpose is to invite a reflection and effect change; these questions may encourage family members to see their problems in a new way and subsequently to see new solutions.

The important difference between these two categories of questions is in their *intent*. Thus, as the family's answers provide information for both the family and the nurse, the nurse's questions may provide information for the family.

At the start of the family meeting, it can be helpful for the nurse to explain to the family members that various kinds of questions will be asked in order to obtain a thorough understanding of their situation. Also, this gives the family an opportunity to familiarize themselves with the nurse. In a social conversation, it is often considered rude to interrupt someone to ask a question while that person is speaking. However, in a time-limited family interview, it could be considered rude not to obtain each family member's perception of the health concern. Sometimes interrupting one family member to include the perspective of another is most appropriate.

It is also appropriate in therapeutic conversation for nurses to understand that they are not invading a family's privacy by asking questions. In training our students to overcome such a mental barrier, we have found it helpful to teach them to say to clients or patients, *"I don't know you very well, so can I trust that if I ask you something too sensitive, or something you would prefer not to talk about, that you will let me know?"* In this way, the nurse obtains the family's permission to have a wide-ranging discussion. If conflict among family members erupts as a result of the nurse's questions, we encourage our students not to be frightened or intimidated by this. Rather, the nurse could say, for example, *"Is this typically what happens when the two of you do not agree on an issue?"* The nurse's tone is also important when asking questions so as not to convey judgment or criticism but rather to convey a message of the nurse's desire to seek a sincere understanding of the illness or issue and invite the family to a reflection that may result in a new perspective and new behaviors. (See Chapter 7 for additional ideas about engagement and assessment.)

Useful, effective, and time-efficient questions are part of relational practice in that they aid in relationship building and collaboration between nurses and families. Most important, questions can be very effective in creating a safe context for the family to describe their illness experience and, hopefully, glean ideas for how to soften or diminish their suffering. Through the asking of interventive questions as well as other useful interventions, the nurse can invite, encourage, and support families to change.

Example 1: Engage All Family Members and Focus the Meeting

In this first example, Dr. Lorraine Wright is meeting with a couple, Nicholas and Bev. Nicholas had a heart attack recently, and this is a follow-up clinic visit. Dr. Wright asks the "one-question question": *"What one question would you most like to have answered during our meeting together?"* The one-question question is a term that Dr. Wright coined (Wright, 1989), and themes of answers to this question have been explored in a study by Duhamel, Dupuis, and Wright (2009). This question emphasizes a *specific* concern and also asks the couple to prioritize their concerns; she asks what they would *most* like to have answered. The question also includes a time frame (i.e., "during our meeting together").

KEY CONCEPT DEFINED

One-Question Question

A question asked by the nurse during a family interview that emphasizes a specific concern and helps family members to prioritize their concerns.

When Dr. Wright asks the one-question question of both Nicholas and Bev, she does not ask Bev to comment on Nicholas's answer. Rather, she engages each family member and elicits their primary concern. Dr. Wright paraphrases and clarifies each person's response so that both she and the person are in agreement about what has been said. In this example, the nurse and the client collaborate to set the focus for the meeting. Notice how the nurse, Dr. Wright, persists in obtaining an answer from Bev. Gentle persistence can be an important skill in establishing a meeting's focus.

> *Dr. Wright:* I'm wondering, then, in the brief time we have, is there any particular question you would most like to have answered during our meeting today?
>
> *Nicholas:* I'd like for her *(looking at his wife)* to deal differently with her anxiety. Me … I'm fine.
>
> *Bev:* Hmm … Oh yes, he wants me to go on tranquilizers. So … sure … *(Turning away)*
>
> *Dr. Wright:* *(Looking at the husband)* So you want to know how to help your wife deal with her anxiety?
>
> *Nicholas:* Oh yeah…
>
> *Dr. Wright:* And for you, Bev, what is the one question you would most like to get answered?
>
> *Bev:* I would like to get him to start exercising more, watch his diet, spend some time with the family, and stop worrying so much about work…
>
> *Nicholas:* *(Looking down)*
>
> *Dr. Wright:* Is there one question you'd like answered, Bev?
>
> *Bev:* Well, how can we get him to change his lifestyle?
>
> *Dr. Wright:* Okay…

We want to emphasize that there is no single, "correct" question to ask. Rather, by engaging in purposeful conversation with patients and their families, nurses will choose and select the most helpful questions in the context of each particular family along with their unique concerns and issues.

Example 2: Use Questions to Assess the Impact of the Problem/Illness on the Family

Asking questions about the impact of the illness or problem is essential to understanding the effect, impact, and changes caused by illness in family members' lives and relationships. By inquiring in this manner, we are giving the family an opportunity to talk about their illness experience or illness story. Families have reported to us that telling their illness story or narrative was helpful in their emotional, physical, or spiritual healing because the illness is understood, listened to, acknowledged, and witnessed. Too often, families have not been given this opportunity to tell their illness story through useful and skillful questions posed by a caring nurse.

In the next example, Dr. Leahey is meeting with a middle-aged couple that is experiencing multiple chronic illnesses. In particular, Phyllis is coping with osteoarthritis and uses a scooter for mobility. Both Ken and Phyllis are 59 years old. They have two sons: the elder, age 26, is married, while the younger, age 22, lives in the family home.

Dr. Leahey explores the impact of osteoarthritis on the couple. Notice how initially, the husband says it has not had an impact on them but then does talk about the impact of his wife's pain upon him. Phyllis commends her husband for his support and assistance with household chores but then offers, with sadness, her decision to leave the teaching profession, which she loved, because her energy is being depleted by her illness. Phyllis believes she needs to save her energy for her family but openly admits that it is a huge adjustment to being a full-time homemaker. This one question about the impact of the illness upon them as a couple opened up a very useful discussion about how osteoarthritis has dramatically changed their lives, careers, and relationships and offered a window into their suffering, coping, and healing experiences. These types of questions address the suffering the family may be enduring and the systemic effects of that suffering.

> **Dr. Leahey:** What has been the impact of these illnesses on the two of you?
>
> **Ken:** I don't know if there has really been an impact ... I know that I feel at times ... I wish I could take some of the pain away. It is very hard on me to see ... especially someone I love so much, suffering with pain.
>
> **Phyllis:** *(Looking at husband)*

Dr. Leahey: *(Nodding)*

Ken: And it's a continual, chronic pain…

Dr. Leahey: Yes. *(Nodding)*

Ken: But I try to be as supportive as I possibly can, but…

Phyllis: He is just so helpful and so wonderful … When I think about the impact … I was a teacher, an elementary teacher, and when my arthritis got to bother me so badly, I decided to take a leave of absence because at school, I had to be cheerful and bubbly. I had to put myself forward, but when I came home I was not *(turning toward husband and laughing)* quite as bubbly. I thought this is not really fair to my own children. So I thought if I am at home, I will be able to do more for them with less effort. So actually, it did impact our lives because I stopped teaching … and when I was teaching, I was really quite independent, I think…

Ken: *(Nodding)* You were … It took you a long time to adjust…

Phyllis: It did. Away from school, from being a teacher at school to just being at home, it was really difficult for me, but Ken adjusted really quickly with helping me with things I needed help with. Also, our boys, I think, were very aware of the change in our family … how things changed, because truly they were different.

Dr. Leahey: It sounds like the two of you made tremendous changes.

It is helpful to remember that talking can be healing, and these kinds of questions have the potential for simultaneously assessing and intervening. If Ken and Phyllis expressed a desire to work on changing or modifying a particular coping strategy, Dr. Leahey could then have asked them a variety of other questions to foster change.

Example 3: Use Questions to Elicit Problem-Solving Skills, Coping Strategies, and Strengths

Families coping with chronic or life-threatening illness or psychosocial problems can commonly feel defeated, hopeless, or failing in their efforts to overcome the illness or live alongside it. Asking questions about the family's problem-solving abilities and their coping strategies and strengths not only serves as assessment but also can be considered interventive. Exploring these areas of problem-solving skills and coping strategies can often remind families of forgotten or suppressed skills and strengths. Through interventive questioning, families can rediscover and reclaim their own abilities to solve problems and bring back to their hearts and minds their inherent strengths. McGoldrick, Carter, and Garcia-Preto (2011, p. 451) offer some questions to help clients look beyond the stress of their current situations and access the strengths of their heritage. For example, the nurse could ask:

- How might your grandfather, who dreamed of your immigration but never made it himself, think about the problem you are having with your children?
- Your great-grandmother immigrated at age 21 and became a pieceworker in a sweatshop but managed to support her six children and had great strength. What do you think were her dreams for you, her daughter's daughter's daughter? What do you think she would want you to do now about your current problem?

In this next example, Dr. Wright is meeting with a family with young children: Chris, age 36; Carleen, age 28; Reuben, age 5; Mariah, age 2; and Rebecca, age 9 months. Chris, an immigrant from Zimbabwe, is employed full-time; Carleen, who grew up in a small, rural town in western Canada, is the resident manager in their building. The health concern for this family is Carleen's thyroid condition.

In the first section of the example, Chris comments on the many changes in his life with three preschoolers, in addition to his working full-time and taking evening courses. Notice how Dr. Wright empathizes with the many demands upon Chris but then asks the couple an interventive question: *"What have you learned that works to assist you with all of these demands?"* This interventive question invites Carleen to talk about how things are more organized for her family when she mobilizes resources such as friends to assist them. This solution gives her an opportunity to do her own work as resident manager plus gives her husband more time for his studies. Notice that after Carleen shared her thoughts about "what works" in the family to assist with all of their demands, Dr. Wright commended the couple for their very good idea of friends taking turns caring for each other's children.

> **Chris:** The accounting program is very demanding time-wise … and then the kids … I'm finding it … I am having a hard time finding time to study because we have three of them … to feed them, get them ready for bed sometimes and then to help clean up the house. By the time … I am so tired…
>
> **Carleen:** *(Looking over at him)*
>
> **Dr. Wright:** Well, sure … you are pooped yourself.
>
> **Chris:** I do not put in as much time as I should into studying. This has been one of the biggest changes from my point of view.
>
> **Dr. Wright:** So many demands upon yourself … and so what have you learned to handle this? What have you learned that works or does not work?

> *Chris:* Mmm…
>
> *Carleen:* If I can get things ready, have them all fed, have the place cleaned, have my work done … 'cause often when he comes home, I have to go out and do some of my work. I have friends who help me out and I help them out. We babysit for each other.
>
> *Dr. Wright:* Oh really … that is good…
>
> *Carleen:* That allows me to get work done during the day.
>
> *Dr. Wright:* That's a good idea … a good arrangement.
>
> *Carleen:* It gives me more time in the evening.

In this next section of the example, Dr. Wright normalizes the difficulty of time pressures for mothers and fathers; she asks if Carleen has been able to work out finding any time for herself. An important conversation unfolds with Carleen illustrating her problem-solving skills. She talks about involving her son to watch the youngest child while she does yoga in their home. This sparks Chris to remember how he gives his wife some time for herself when he takes all three children to the park. Once again, Dr. Wright is able to commend the family for these efforts.

> *Dr. Wright: (To Carleen)* Have you been able to find any time for yourself?
>
> *Carleen:* Yeah, I have. I try to get up before the kids … that does not always work, though. This one *(turning toward 5-year-old Reuben)* gets up, and then the baby is up … I'll go downstairs and I'll do yoga, and Reuben will just watch me. Or I'll do aerobics…
>
> *Dr. Wright: (Looking at Reuben)* So you watch Mommy do yoga … Do you ever join in and do it with her?
>
> *Reuben: (Looking at Dr. Wright)* … when the baby's awake … watching her…
>
> *Carleen:* He watches the baby.
>
> *Dr. Wright:* Very nice.
>
> *Chris:* Sometimes what I do is take the kids out to the park so she can have the day to herself. I still try to do it, but some days she'd rather be doing her work.

Asking about a family's problem-solving skills, coping, and strengths can set the stage for further interventions, if needed. For example, if Carleen had stated she wanted to increase her problem-solving skills, Dr. Wright could have pursued this with her. For instance, they could have discussed possible playgroups in the area, available community resources, and so forth.

Example 4: Use Questions as Interventions and to Invite Change

The intervention process represents the core of clinical practice with families. Myriad interventions are possible, but nurses need to tailor their interventions to each family they encounter. Openness to certain interventions is profoundly influenced by the relationship between the nurse and the family and the nurse's ability to help the family reflect on their health problems.

Questions in and of themselves can provide new information and answers for the family; thus, they become interventions. Interventive questions can encourage family members to view their problems or illness experience in a new way or to change their beliefs and subsequently discover new solutions. Some clinicians and authors recognize how questions can introduce alternative possibilities, theories, beliefs, and views, simply in their posing (Bell, 2016; McGee, Del Vento, & Bavelas, 2005; Östlund, Bäckström, Saveman, Lindh, & Sundin, 2016; Wright & Bell, 2009).

The next example is with a couple, Al and Benz. This is Benz's first marriage and Al's second marriage. Benz is close to being discharged from the hospital following surgery for breast cancer. The first interventive question in this example is, *"And who would you say, between the two of you, was the most upset with this diagnosis and news when you got it?"* This leads to a very poignant therapeutic conversation about Benz's future. In this therapeutic conversation, Benz is very concerned about her prognosis. Dr. Wright asks about Benz's beliefs about her prognosis when she says to Benz, *"What are your thoughts about your future?"*

> *Dr. Wright: (Looking at Benz)* Have there been any other kinds of cancer in your family?
>
> *Benz:* No … we are all pretty healthy.
>
> *Dr. Wright: (Looking at Al)* … and what about for you, Al—has there been any history of cancer in your family?
>
> *Al:* No … I cannot think of any … I had an aunt and uncle who got lung cancer. Both were heavy smokers.
>
> *Dr. Wright:* So this was something very new for both of you, dealing with cancer. And who would you say, between the two of you, was most upset about this diagnosis and news when you got it?
>
> *Al:* Oh, Benz was, I think.

Benz: I would say so, too. I cried and cried. I just could not handle it.

Dr. Wright: Yes…

Al: … and I just don't see what a lot of crying accomplishes. I think you have to really think positively and know in your heart that you can beat this thing.

Dr. Wright: That's how you've been trying to encourage Benz?

Benz: Yeah, he kept telling me that. I just felt I needed to cry. That's the only thing I needed to do…

Dr. Wright: Yes…

Al: Well, a certain amount of this is understandable, and I have tried to be sympathetic, but you have got to get onto the positive-thinking path and really believe you're going to beat this thing.

Dr. Wright: *(Nodding)*

Al: I really do believe that. I really do believe that.

Dr. Wright: *(Looking at Al)* … You do. *(Looking at Benz)* And what are your thoughts for the future? Because I've met other women with breast cancer who worry … What are your thoughts?

Benz: Some days I am pretty good about it. I am in good hands; my doctor is good. And some days, I just do not know. It fluctuates. Some days are good and some are bad.

Dr. Wright: So some days you are more optimistic about your future and other days you…

Benz: I think the worst.

Dr. Wright: And what do you think about when you think the worst?

Benz: That Al and our child, Bryan, would be alone without me. I care about them so much.

Al: And this is the kind of thinking I try to discourage. I do not think it is good.

Dr. Wright: So when you hear your wife talking this way and I am not here, do you try to cheer her up and get her off of this topic?

Al: Oh yeah. I allow her a little bit of it. She has to express herself and express her feelings, but once she has got that out, she has to get back to being hopeful.

Dr. Wright: *(Looking to Benz)* And do you like that approach Al takes? He tries to get you off of this topic and to think optimistically. Or do you want to be able to say more about the other side, the "worry side"?

Benz: Well, I know he is being kind and wants me to do well. But sometimes, that is just the way I feel. Maybe if he would just listen to me...

These are not easy conversations when a nurse "speaks the unspeakable" by introducing a conversation about a family's beliefs about prognosis (Wright & Bell, 2009). Knowing the family's beliefs about various aspects of their illness assists the nurse in knowing if their beliefs are constraining or facilitating. We believe that nurses have a socially sanctioned role and thus can talk about such delicate and intimate topics with families. In our clinical experience, we have found that families rarely mind any question if it is asked in a kind, nonjudgmental, purposeful, and thoughtful manner. We have encouraged our students to be curious and pursue hard topics with families. If the nurse working with the family cannot address potentially difficult areas with them, then we encourage the nurse to transfer the family to another nurse, if possible, or request that another nurse continue the conversation.

Dr. Wright's question invited a very useful disclosure about this couple's differences in beliefs about how to cope with worries and face the future. Benz wanted to talk about her fears for the future, whereas Al preferred to deal with worry by being optimistic. Instead of Dr. Wright taking sides with either Al or Benz about the best way to handle fears, she asked Benz, *"And do you like that approach Al takes* (her husband's optimism)? *Or do you want to say more about the other side, the 'worry side'?"*

This simple, but powerful, interventive question had the potential for inviting healing change in one or both spouses. Benz offered very clearly that she would prefer that her husband listen to her. It is very understandable that Al wanted to cheer her up, but it was not Benz's preferred way for her husband to comfort her.

In this example, interventive questions invited family members to explore and reflect on their beliefs about the illness experience, the prognosis, and how best to manage their illness. Reflections are invited through very deliberate, thoughtful, and purposeful interventive questions.

Example 5: Use Questions to Request Feedback About the Family Meeting

We seek to ask questions that are in keeping with our philosophy of fostering collaborative relationships between nurses and families. These kinds of questions imply to family members that their satisfaction with the meeting, or lack thereof, matters and that we want to improve our care to families.

Collaborative questions also give the family the chance to voice concerns about what specifically was helpful to them.

In the following example, at the end of the meeting with Al and Benz, Dr. Wright asks if the conversation has been helpful to them. Benz gives a short answer and comments on the relationship with Dr. Wright by saying, *"You are kind."* Notice how Dr. Wright's question invites much more pondering from Al. He reflects back on Benz's suggestion about wanting him to listen more. This is a lovely example of how an interventive question invited a reflection and how Al decides on his own that he could make a behavioral change that would be more in tune with his wife's preferred way to be comforted. This is always the most desirable and sustaining kind of change—that is, when a family member initiates the change rather than being instructed to do so.

> **Dr. Wright:** *(Looking at the couple)* Well, just before we end, was there anything about this conversation that has been useful or helpful for you or not helpful?
>
> **Benz:** … I think you are very kind.
>
> **Dr. Wright:** *(Nodding to Benz and then looking to Al)* Anything that was helpful for you, Al?
>
> **Al:** Yeah … it made me think. It made me think. Perhaps I need to listen a little bit more and not be so free with the advice.
>
> **Dr. Wright:** *(Looking at Benz)* I think it is wonderful to have a husband who wants to cheer you up and make you feel better…
>
> **Benz:** I'm lucky.
>
> **Dr. Wright:** But there are times when you want him to hear you out about what you are thinking and feeling.

Of course, families do not always convey positive feelings about the meeting with the nurse. If the family members express dissatisfaction or discontent, we encourage the nurse to explore their reasons for being dissatisfied and accept the feedback nondefensively. The nurse can thank the family members for their insights and ask for their suggestions for how she could be more helpful to other families. If the nurse takes a sincere "one-down" position when receiving feedback, it encourages the family to maintain a collaborative relationship. It also permits the nurse to reflect on her practice and potentially alter her actions for future family meetings.

CASE SCENARIO: MEHRZA, ZOYA, AND SHAILA

Mehrza and Zoya moved from Afghanistan to Canada in 1991 with their two children, Ali and Rahmaan. Mehrza worked hard in retail while completing his studies in accounting. Zoya stayed home for the first 10 years and then went back to work to provide additional financial support for the family. Both of their children are now young adults attending university. Mehrza recently sponsored his younger sister, Shaila, who is a trained physician, and her two young children, Akbar (26 months old) and Zeeya (6 months old), to come to Canada. They are currently living with Mehrza and Zoya.

Shaila's childhood was very difficult; her family was always moving from one area to another due to conflict and safety concerns in Afghanistan. She is struggling with the transition to living in the West and speaks very little English. She feels overwhelmed and is always worried about her children's safety. Mehrza and Zoya take Shaila to the nearest walk-in clinic because she does not have a family doctor and they are concerned about her. When the nurse begins to ask Shaila questions, she is hesitant to answer and begins to get teary. Mehrza and Zoya are very vocal regarding their concerns about Shaila and her children, and they wonder if she is experiencing posttraumatic stress disorder.

Reflective Questions

1. What types of questions could the nurse ask to assess the impact of the problem on the family?
2. What types of questions could the nurse ask to elicit the problem-solving skills, coping strategies, and strengths of the family?
3. What questions can the nurse ask to assess the family's emotional and verbal communication?

CRITICAL THINKING QUESTIONS

1. What are some questions that a nurse could use to engage all family members and focus the conversation?
2. Reflecting on your own clinical practice, what questions could you ask that foster change in relation to the impact of an illness or problem with a family?
3. Consider your clinical practice and reflect on the conversations you have had with patients and families. What questions have you asked about problem-solving skills, coping strategies, and strengths?
4. What questions can invite feedback about the usefulness of the therapeutic conversations that nurses have with families?

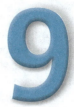

Chapter **9**

How to Do a 15-Minute (or Shorter) Family Interview

Learning Objectives

- Discuss the purpose of completing a 15-minute interview.
- Summarize the key ingredients of a 15-minute family interview.
- Identify possible constraining beliefs nurses might have for not including family members in their practice.
- Explain how to provide a brief family interview without family members present.

Key Concepts

15-minute family interview	Manners
Art of listening	Therapeutic conversation
Commendations	Therapeutic questions
Genogram	Therapeutic relationships

F amily nursing *can* be effectively, skillfully, and meaningfully practiced in just 15 minutes or less. We have listened to and read in professional journals the many stories and reports by nurses of how these ideas have been implemented in their practice and thus how their practice with patients and families has changed in rewarding ways (Duhamel, 2010; Duhamel, Dupuis, Turcotte, Martinez, & Goudreau, 2015; Goudreau, Duhamel, & Ricard, 2006; LeGrow & Rossen, 2005; Moules, Bell, Paton, & Morck, 2012; Moules & Johnstone, 2010). Bell (2012) offered the compelling thought that the 15-minute family interview is one of the most "sticky" ideas in family nursing. By "sticky," she is referring to ideas that are unexpectedly introduced, credible, efficient, and subsequently have had an enthusiastic worldwide implementation in family nursing teaching, research, and practice.

One of our goals in developing these ideas was to address head-on the perception among nurses that they lack the time to involve families in their practice, and this effort seemed to resonate with many nurses. *"I don't have time to do family interviews"* is the most common reason nurses offer for not routinely involving families in their practice. In numerous undergraduate and graduate nursing courses, professional workshops, and presentations, we have encountered this statement as the resounding reason for the exclusion of family members from health care. With major changes in the delivery of health-care services through managed care, emphasis on providing more care in the community, budgetary constraints, increased acuity, and staff cutbacks, time is of the essence in nursing practice. However, it is our belief that families need not be banned or marginalized from health care. To involve families, and especially in a time-limited conversation, nurses need to possess sound knowledge of family assessment and intervention models, interviewing skills, and questions. We have witnessed and conducted enough interviews to know that family nursing knowledge can be applied effectively even in very brief family meetings. We also claim that a 15-minute family interview, or even a shorter family interview, can be purposeful, effective, informative, and even healing. Any involvement of family members, regardless of the length of time, is better than no involvement.

KEY CONCEPT DEFINED

15-Minute Family Interview

A condensed version of the core elements of conducting family interviews that is based on the theoretical underpinnings of the Calgary Family Assessment Model (CFAM) and the Calgary Family Intervention Model (CFIM).

But what is time? And what exactly can be accomplished in 15 minutes or less with a family? We have noticed that much of nursing practice time is socially and culturally coordinated, highly ritualized, and therefore honored. Nurses clearly articulate the start and end of their shifts, their schedules, and so forth. We propose that ritualizing and coordinating meeting time with families, even if it is only 15 minutes, can also become part of nursing practice.

However, for nurses' behaviors to change, they must first alter or modify their beliefs about involving families in health care. We have discovered that when nurses do not include family members in their practice, some very constraining beliefs usually exist (Wright & Bell, 2009). Some of these beliefs are as follows:

- If I talk to family members, I will not have time to complete my other nursing responsibilities.
- If I talk to family members, I may open up a can of worms, and I will have no time to deal with it.
- It is not my job to talk with families; that is for social workers and psychologists.
- I cannot possibly help families in the brief time I will be caring for them.
- If the family becomes angry, what would I do?
- What if they ask me a question and I do not have the answer? What would I do? It is better not to start a conversation.

Another constraining belief that nurses and other health-care professionals often have is that nothing meaningful can be accomplished in one meeting with a client. Slive and Bobele (2018) challenge this belief in their landmark book documenting clinical success with clients who use walk-in single-session therapy. The significance of having an opportunity to converse with a professional at the time most meaningful to the family cannot be overestimated. Research on time-effective single-session therapy has demonstrated its effectiveness and client satisfaction with the outcome (Green et al, 2011; Harper-Jacques & Leahey, 2011; Hopkins, Lee, McGrane, & Barbara-May, 2017). See Research Highlight: Single-Session Family Therapy in Youth Mental Health.

Research Highlight

Single-Session Family Therapy in Youth Mental Health

This research used quantitative analysis to assess the effectiveness of single-session therapy in young people and their families when presenting to a mental health service. Data were collected using self- and family-member-reported outcome rating scales. Findings indicated young people and their families found that single-session therapy intervention improved the mental health and well-being of the young people.

Source: *Hopkins, L., Lee, S., McGrane, T., & Barbara-May, R. (2017). Single session family therapy in youth mental health: Can it help?* Australasian Psychiatry, 25(2), 108–111.

Uncovering these constraining beliefs makes it more comprehensible why nurses may shy away from routinely involving families in nursing practice. We postulate that if nurses were to embrace only one belief, that "illness is a family affair" (Wright & Bell, 2009), it would change the face of nursing practice. Nurses would then be more eager to know how to involve and assist family members in the care of loved ones. They would appreciate that everyone in a family experiences an illness and that no one family member *has* diabetes, multiple sclerosis, or cancer. By embracing this belief, they would realize that, from initial symptoms through diagnosis and treatment, all family members are influenced by and influence the illness. They would also come to realize that our privileged conversations with patients and their families about their illness experiences can contribute dramatically to healing and the softening or alleviation of suffering (Wright, 2015, 2017; Wright & Bell, 2009). Our evidence for this belief comes from our clinical and personal conversations as well as from reading numerous blogs and books about illness narratives.

We also believe that nurses will increase their caring for and involvement of families in their practice, regardless of the practice context, if such behavior is strongly supported and advocated by health-care administrators (Leahey & Harper-Jaques, 2010; Leahey & Svavarsdottir, 2009). One powerful and visual way for health-care administrators to show their commitment to family-centered care is to involve nurses in the creation, development, and implementation of family-friendly policies and services (International Council of Nurses, 2002). Table 9-1 offers some examples of family-friendly policies and actions at various levels.

The following are some specific ideas for conducting a 15-minute (or shorter) family interview. These ideas are the condensed version of the core elements previously presented in Chapters 5 through 7 about conducting family interviews. The ideas honor the theoretical underpinnings of the

TABLE 9-1	Implementation of Family-Friendly Policies and Services
SYSTEM LEVEL	**DEPARTMENT/UNIT LEVEL**
■ Including family members as advisory-board or task-force members ■ Having family members as focus-group participants ■ Inviting family members to be program evaluators ■ Making family members participants in quality and safety initiatives ■ Providing parking at health-care facilities for families with limited income	■ Providing family-friendly visiting hours ■ Providing family-friendly spaces such as a play area for children or offering a quiet room for retreat or for family discussion of difficult situations or moments ■ Lobbying for routine provision of family nursing therapeutic conversations when families are suffering ■ Inviting family members to participate in new staff orientation ■ Volunteering to orient new families to the inpatient unit and mentor other families ■ Inviting families to patient conferences ■ Accompanying patients to tests ■ Supporting patients during procedures ■ Assisting patients with personal care

Calgary Family Assessment Model (CFAM; see Chapter 3) and the Calgary Family Intervention Model (CFIM; see Chapter 4) and highlight some of the most critical elements of these models.

KEY INGREDIENTS

The key ingredients of a healing, productive, and effective 15-minute family interview are presented in Figure 9-1.

The overall framework for ritualizing a 15-minute (or shorter) family interview consists of the following:

- Begin a therapeutic conversation with a particular purpose in mind that can be accomplished in 15 minutes or less.
- Use manners to engage or reengage. Introduce yourself by offering your name and role. Orient family members to the purpose of a brief family interview.

KEY CONCEPT DEFINED

Manners

A way of behaving toward others.

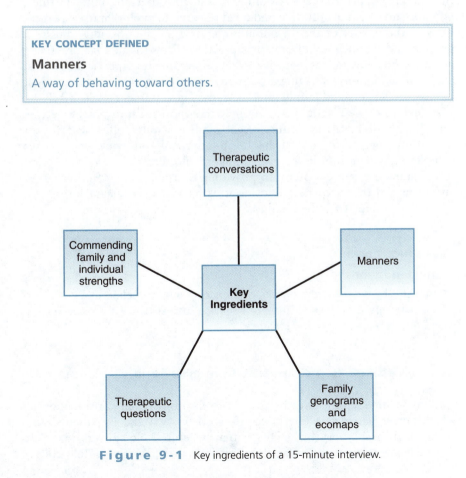

F i g u r e   9 - 1   Key ingredients of a 15-minute interview.

- Assess key areas of internal and external structure and function—obtain genogram information and key external support data.
- Ask three key questions of family members.
- Commend the family on one or two strengths.
- Evaluate usefulness and conclude.

All of these elements can be involved only within the context of a therapeutic relationship between the nurse and family.

KEY CONCEPT DEFINED

Genogram

A structural assessment tool that shows a diagram of the family constellation.

Holtslander (2005) described how the 15-minute family interview was successfully applied to the needs of families in a postpartum unit. Martinez, D'Artois, and Rennick (2007) conducted research to explore nurses' perceptions of the impact of the 15-minute interview on the hospital admission process and on their family nursing practice. They found that practicing pediatric hospital nurses perceived the genogram, therapeutic questions, and commendations as having a positive impact on their ability to conduct family assessments and family interventions. These nurses concluded that a 15-minute interview should be routinely incorporated into practice at the time of a child's admission. More recently, Silva, Moules, Silva, and Boussa (2013) investigated the use of the 15-minute family interview with nurses completing postpartum home visits in Sao Paulo, Brazil. The nurses found the 15-minute interview useful in providing a broad range of information and identified their experiences using it as having a significant impact on their relationships with the families.

KEY CONCEPT DEFINED

Commendations

Comments by the nurse during family interviews and counseling that emphasize observed positive patterns of behavior, such as family and individual strengths, competencies, and resources.

Key Ingredient 1: Therapeutic Conversations

All human interaction takes place in conversations. Each conversation in which nurses participate effects change in their own and in patients' and family members' biopsychosocial-spiritual structures. No conversation that a nurse has with a patient or family member is trivial (Wright & Bell, 2009).

Nurses are always engaged in therapeutic conversations with their clients without perhaps thinking of them as such.

KEY CONCEPT DEFINED

Therapeutic Conversation

Conversation in which nurses' participation effects change in their own and in patients' and family members' biopsychosocial-spiritual structures. Such conversations are purposeful and time-limited and have the potential for healing through the very act of bringing the family together.

The conversation in a brief family interview is therapeutic because, from the start, it is purposeful and time-limited, as is the relationship between the nurse and the family. Therapeutic conversations between a nurse and a family can be as short as one sentence or as long as time allows. All conversations between nurses and families, regardless of time, have the potential for healing through the very act of bringing the family together (Hougher Limacher & Wright, 2003, 2006; McLeod, 2003; Robinson & Wright, 1995; Svavarsdottir & Sigurdardottir, 2013; Sigurdardottir, Svavarsdottir, Rayens, & Adkins, 2013; Wright & Bell, 2009). One study evaluated the usefulness of short therapeutic conversations with families (15 to 50 minutes, with an average of 30 minutes) with a child/adolescent experiencing chronic illness. The study yielded both expected and unexpected results (Svavarsdottir, Tryggvadottir, & Sigurdardottir, 2012). A positive, expected result was that parents in the experimental group perceived significantly higher family support after the intervention compared with the parents in the control group. An unexpected result was that these same parents in the experimental group perceived significantly lower expressive family functioning (e.g., emotional communication, collaboration, problem solving, and verbal communication) after the intervention of a short therapeutic conversation.

Svavarsdottir and colleagues (2012) offer possible explanations for the lower expressive family functioning following the therapeutic conversation intervention. One might be that parents with children with acute illnesses were generally younger and may not have had the instrumental or emotional resources to adequately cope with this illness crisis. Another explanation might be that the parents may have trusted the nurse more during and after receiving the therapeutic conversation intervention and therefore offered more of their "real" experience of family functioning in the context of illness. These results point the direction that additional studies will need to examine further what happens "inside" the intervention and in the nurse-family relationship.

It is not only the length of the conversation or time that makes the most difference but also the opportunity for patients and family members to be acknowledged and affirmed in their illness experience that has tremendous healing potential (Bell & Wright, 2011; Hougher Limacher, 2003; Hougher Limacher & Wright, 2003, 2006; Moules, 2002; Moules & Johnstone, 2010; Wright & Bell, 2009). Nurses are socially empowered and privileged to bring forth either health or pathology in their conversations with families.

Another pretest/posttest research study that illustrates the possibility of healing within families was conducted in four acute psychiatric units with patients and family members (Sveinbjarnardottir, Svavarsdottir, & Wright, 2013). The experimental group received two to five short therapeutic conversations. A control group of patients and families received traditional nursing care. The family members in the group who received the short therapeutic conversations intervention perceived higher cognitive and emotional support than those receiving traditional care. As more research studies examine the short therapeutic family interviews, they will add to the knowledge base about the effectiveness of short interviews and thus what needs to be implemented into practice.

The art of listening is also paramount. The need to communicate what it is like to live in our individual, separate worlds of experience, particularly within the world of illness, is a powerful need in human relationships (Wright, 2017). Frank (1998) suggests that listening to families' illness stories is not only an art but also an ethical practice. Nurses commonly believe that listening also entails an obligation to do something to "fix" whatever concerns or problems are raised. However, in many cases, the most therapeutic move, intervention, or action the nurse can perform is showing compassion and offering commendations (Bell, 2016; Bell & Wright, 2011, 2015; Bohn, Wright, & Moules, 2003; Hougher Limacher, 2003, 2008; Hougher Limacher & Wright, 2003; Moules, 2002; Moules & Johnstone, 2010; Wright & Bell, 2009).

KEY CONCEPT DEFINED

Art of Listening

Listening to families' illness stories while showing compassion and offering commendations.

It is the integration of task-oriented patient care with interactive, purposeful conversation that distinguishes a time-effective 15-minute (or shorter) interview. The nurse makes information giving and patient involvement in decision making integral parts of the delivery process. He or she takes advantage of opportunities and searches for ways to engage in purposeful, healing conversations with families. These practices differ from social conversations and can include basic ideas such as the following:

- Families are *routinely* invited to accompany the patient to the unit, clinic, or hospital.

- Families are *routinely* included in the admission procedure.
- Families are *routinely* invited to ask questions during the patient orientation.
- Nurses acknowledge the patient's and family's expertise in managing health problems by asking about routines at home.
- Nurses encourage patients to practice how they will handle different interactions in the future, such as telling family members and others that they cannot eat certain foods.
- Nurses *routinely* consult families and patients about *their* ideas for treatment and discharge.

Key Ingredient 2: Manners

Good manners have always been the core of common, everyday social behavior and interaction. However, in the last several decades in North America, social behavior has dramatically shifted from formal to casual social interaction. Style of dress has been altered from "Sunday best" to "casual Friday." Martin's (2011) *Miss Manners' Guide to Excruciatingly Correct Behavior* offers her perspective and humor on manners. Miss Manners, as Martin is known, comments on what is missing in social interactions and thus what is missing in society. Manners are simple acts of courtesy, politeness, respect, and kindness. Culture as a whole seems to be undergoing an erosion of manners and thus civility. This erosion has spilled over into the nursing profession.

Nursing has not been immune to the changes in social behavior. In some situations, we can argue that formal nursing behaviors (such as dressing in starched uniforms and caps) perhaps inhibited our relations with clients and families. Countless nurses still maintain respectful, polite, and thoughtful relations with their clients. However, we have witnessed and listened to far too many professional and personal encounters between nurses, patients, and families in which manners were absent.

One of the most glaring examples of the absence of manners in nursing is in the basic social act of an introduction. Numerous stories have been told of nurses who do not introduce themselves to their patients, let alone the patients' family members. For example, Pablo, a 23-year-old man, was seen in an outpatient clinic in a large metropolitan hospital after open-heart surgery. He reported that the nurse did not introduce herself but began touching his body and adjusting his intravenous peripherally inserted central catheter (PICC) line without telling him what she was doing or why. He found this experience very invasive, frightening, and rude.

This clinical anecdote is consistent with what nurses have told us about nurse-family relationships in the intensive care unit. We believe that one of the nursing strategies that inhibit the establishment of therapeutic relationships is the depersonalization of the patient and family. Examples include not referring to the patient by name, labeling the patient or family difficult, providing care without encouraging participation by the patient or family, and not talking or making eye contact.

KEY CONCEPT DEFINED

Therapeutic Relationships

Helping relationships based on mutual trust and respect, the nurturing of faith and hope, and being sensitive to self and others; assisting with the gratification of patients' physical, emotional, and spiritual needs through the nurse's knowledge and skills.

Therefore, introduction is obviously an essential ingredient of a successful family interview and relational family nursing practice. However, introductions by nurses have changed from overly formal to overly casual. Just a few years ago, a nurse might introduce herself as *"Miss Garcia,"* whereas now a more typical introduction is *"Hello, my name is Sasha, and I'm your nurse today."* Any introduction is better than no introduction, but as one client remarked to us, *"Nurses don't introduce themselves any differently from a server who says, 'Hi, my name is Josh, and I'm your server tonight.'"* We encourage nurses always to introduce themselves by their full names, except in unique circumstances when there might be concerns about safety.

An equally serious omission is the lack of introduction by nurses to their patients' family members. What inhibits or prevents nurses in hospitals, community health clinics, and home care from introducing themselves to the people at a patient's bedside or to those accompanying the patient at a clinic? What prevents nurses from inquiring about their relationships to the patient? Worse yet, what precludes nurses from making eye contact with family members or friends, one of the most expected social norms in our North American culture? We have discussed this phenomenon with our nursing students and professional nurses. It has been revealed to us that the belief of "lack of time" constrains many nurses from talking with anyone but their patients for fear that family members or close friends may "ask questions" or "require time from me that I just don't have." We would like to counter this belief by suggesting that, in the end, nurses would *save* time if they would use a few manners with family members or friends. Nurses who did so would not be pursued at even more inopportune times by family members or friends inquiring about their loved ones. Nurses who have involved family members in their practice have reported that they have enjoyed greater rather than less job satisfaction (Leahey, Harper-Jaques, Stout, & Levac, 1995). Nurses who practice good manners also instill trust in family members. Box 9-1 provides some examples of manners.

> **Box 9-1 Examples of Manners**
>
> - Always call patients and family members by name.
> - Always tell the patient and family members your name.
> - Explain your role for that shift or meeting or any encounter with the patient and/or family.
> - Explain a procedure before coming into the room with the equipment to do it.
> - If you tell the patient or a family member that you will be back at a certain time, attempt to keep to that time or provide an explanation about why it didn't occur.

Key Ingredient 3: Family Genograms and Ecomaps

Nurses need to make it a priority to draw a quick genogram (and sometimes, if indicated, an ecomap) for *all* families but particularly for families who will likely be part of their care for more than a day. Extensive details for the collection of genogram and ecomap information are given in Chapter 3 in the discussion of the "structural assessment" category of the CFAM. In a brief interview, the collection of genogram and ecomap information needs to be brief also. This information can be gleaned from family members in a couple of minutes.

The most essential information to obtain includes data about the age, occupation or school grade, religion, ethnic background, immigration date, and current health status of each family member. Begin by asking "easy" questions (e.g., ages, current health) of the household family members. Drawing out information relating to, for example, siblings' divorces or grandchildren is not necessary or time-efficient unless this information immediately relates to the family and health problem. Once the genogram information is obtained, if indicated, expand the data collection to obtain external family structure information in the form of an ecomap. It may be useful to ask questions such as, *"Who outside of your immediate family is an important resource to you or is a stress for you?"* and *"How many professionals are involved in treating your husband's current heart problems?"* Obtaining structural assessment data through the genogram and ecomap also serves as a quick engagement strategy because families are usually very pleased that a nurse is asking about their entire family rather than just the person experiencing the illness. It quickly acknowledges to the family the nurse's underlying belief that illness is a family affair.

Ideally, the genogram should become part of any documentation about the family and patient. In one cardiac unit, genogram information is collected on admission, and the genogram is hung at the patient's bedside. Emergency telephone numbers for family members are listed on the genogram. In this way, the genogram acts as a continuous visual reminder for all health-care professionals involved with the patient to "think family."

Key Ingredient 4: Therapeutic Questions

Therapeutic questions are a key, defining element in a therapeutic conversation. Many ideas about and examples of linear, circular, and interventive questions were given in the presentation of the CFIM (see Chapter 4), in the discussion of family nursing skills (see Chapter 5), and in the vignettes demonstrating the use of questions (see Chapter 8). When nurses attempt to have a very brief family meeting, they can ask key questions of family members to involve them in family health care. We encourage nurses to think of at least three key questions that they will routinely ask all families.

KEY CONCEPT DEFINED

Therapeutic Questions

Questions that focus on the key, defining element in a therapeutic conversation and include linear, circular, and interventive questions.

Of course, these questions need to fit the context in which the nurse encounters families. For example, the questions that a nurse may ask family members in an emergency or oncology unit in a hospital might differ from the questions that a nurse might routinely ask family members in an outpatient diabetic clinic for children or in primary care. However, some basic themes need to be addressed, such as the sharing of information, expectations of hospitalization, clinic or home-care visits, challenges, sufferings, and the most pressing concerns or problems. Table 9-2 provides examples of questions that address these particular topics.

Key Ingredient 5: Commending Family and Individual Strengths

The important intervention of offering commendations (Bell, 2016; Bell & Wright, 2011, 2015; Hougher Limacher, 2003, 2008; Hougher Limacher & Wright, 2003, 2006; Moules & Johnstone, 2010; Wright, 2017; Wright & Bell, 2009) is fully discussed in the presentation of the CFIM (see Chapter 4). In each session, we routinely commend families on the strengths observed during the interview. In a brief family interview of 15 minutes or less, we endorse the practice of offering at least one or two commendations to family members on individual or family strengths, resources, or competencies that the nurse directly observed or gathered from another

TABLE 9-2	Therapeutic Questions
QUESTIONS	**PURPOSE**
How can we be most helpful to you and your family (or friends) during your hospitalization?	Clarifies expectations and increases collaboration
What has been most and least helpful to you in past hospitalizations or clinic visits?	Identifies past strengths and problems to avoid and successes to repeat
What is the greatest challenge facing your family during this hospitalization, discharge, or clinic visit?	Indicates actual or potential suffering, roles, and beliefs
With which of your family members or friends would you like us to share information? With which ones would you like us not to share information?	Indicates alliances, resources, and possible conflictual relationships
What do you need to best prepare you or your family member for discharge?	Assists with early discharge planning
Who do you believe is suffering the most in your family during this hospital-ization, clinic visit, or home-care visit?	Identifies the family member who has the greatest need for support and intervention (Wright, 2017)
What is the one question you would most like to have answered during our meeting right now? I may not be able to answer this question at the moment, but I will do my best or will try to find the answer for you.	Identifies most pressing issue or concern (Duhamel, Dupuis, & Wright, 2009; Wright, 1989)
How have I been most helpful to you in this family meeting? How could we improve?	Shows a willingness to learn from families and to work collaboratively

source. Remember that commendations are observations of behavior that occur across time. Therefore, the nurse is looking for patterns rather than a one-time occurrence that is more likely going to elicit only a compliment. An example of a commendation is *"Your family is showing much courage in living with your wife's cancer for 5 years."* A compliment would be *"Your son is so gentle despite feeling so ill today."*

Families coping with chronic, life-threatening, or psychosocial problems commonly feel defeated, hopeless, or failing in their efforts to overcome the illnesses or live with them. In our clinical experience, we have found that most families who are experiencing illness, disability, or trauma also suffer from "commendation-deficit disorder." Therefore, nurses can never offer too many commendations.

Immediate and long-term positive reactions to commendations indicate that they are powerful, effective, and enduring therapeutic interventions (Bell, 2016; Bell & Wright, 2011, 2015; Bohn, Wright, & Moules, 2003; Hougher Limacher, 2003, 2008; Hougher Limacher & Wright, 2003, 2006; Moules, 2002; Moules & Johnstone, 2010; Wright & Bell, 2009). Benzies (2016) identified implementing relational communication strategies, including the use of commendations, as a useful tool for negotiating role boundaries and shared decision making for nurses in their day-to-day practice in neonatal intensive care units (p. 233). Hougher Limacher's 2003 study, which specifically focused on understanding more about the intervention of commendations, lends even further validation to the power of commendations. Families who internalize commendations offered by nurses appear more receptive to and trusting of the nurse-family relationship and tend to readily take up ideas, opinions, and advice that are offered.

By commending families' resources, competencies, and strengths, nurses offer family members a new view of themselves. When nurses change the view families have of themselves, families are commonly able to look at their health problem differently and thus move toward more effective solutions to reduce any potential or actual suffering.

PERSONAL EXAMPLE OF INVOLVING FAMILY IN NURSING PRACTICE

To illustrate how involving family members in health care can be effective and healing—or ineffective and resulting in a needless increase of suffering—Dr. Wright offers a personal story to illustrate the best and worst of family nursing. These experiences occurred during two very brief interactions with nurses in the emergency unit of a large city hospital while accompanying her mother for a possible admission.

> Over the last 5 years of my mother's life, she experienced several major exacerbations of multiple sclerosis (MS), with frequent hospitalizations. Each exacerbation left my mother more physically disabled. The extreme exacerbations of the last year of her life left her a quadriplegic. With each exacerbation, she never returned to the level of either physical or cognitive functioning that she previously enjoyed. Despite all of these setbacks, there was tremendous courage on the part of both my mother and my father. Amazingly, my mother's moments of complaining, sadness, or grief were minimal, which of course buffered other family members' suffering. I saw my father become a very caring caregiver and "nurse" while his own life became very constrained.
>
> On one of my mother's admissions to the hospital, I encountered two very brief but powerful conversations with nurses in the emergency department (ED). One I prefer to call "Naughty Nurse" and the other "Angel Nurse." Both of these nurses had a profound impact on my emotional

suffering. Both of these nurses interacted with me for a very brief time, not more than 5 minutes each.

Before our arrival at the hospital ED, I spent a few very exhausting hours with my mother. My father, mother, and I were enjoying a day at our cottage about an hour out of the city. As the afternoon unfolded, it became apparent that my mother was becoming more wobbly when walking (at that time she was still able to walk a few steps with assistance). As we were packing to leave, she became unable to bear weight. With great difficulty, my father and I lifted her into her wheelchair and headed down the ramp of our cottage to the car. The greater challenge lay ahead of us: to get her from the wheelchair into the car. It took all of our strength and ingenuity to accomplish this task, with my mother, of course, frightened that we would drop her. After some 30 minutes and lots of perspiration, we realized our goal, with my mother safely in the car. On the way into the city, we made a mutual decision to take her to the hospital where she had been admitted on previous occasions to have her assessed for possible admission. We all believed that she was having another severe exacerbation.

When we arrived at the ED, I was very relieved. It had been a very worrisome and arduous few hours. I now looked forward to my mother's receiving nursing and medical assessment and treatment to assist her and us. My father waited with her in the car at the curb of the ED while I entered to seek assistance to lift my mother out of the car. On arriving at the nursing station, I encountered Naughty Nurse. I explained the current situation to her and requested assistance to lift my mother out of the car and into the ED. Naughty Nurse responded in a curt, mistrusting tone by saying, *"How did you get her into the car?"* This initial brief interaction was shocking to me; it was accusatory, blaming, and mistrusting of one another. No therapeutic relationship was being developed. This nurse's response invited me to counter with an equally rude, impolite response. I said, *"With great [difficulty], so we will need help to lift her out of the car."* Our conversation now escalated in terms of accusations and recriminations as Naughty Nurse retorted, *"Well, I can't lift her out of the car."* I suggested that perhaps one of her male colleagues could assist us. As Naughty Nurse and a male colleague approached the car to assist my mother, they did not introduce themselves to my mother nor did they discontinue their conversation with each other. This was an extreme example of what family nursing should not be. By now, I was very distressed and upset about our treatment by this particular nurse. Of course, she was completely unaware that, in my professional life, I teach, practice, research, and write about family nursing.

However, all was not lost. Within a short while, we were placed in a room in the ED, and after a brief wait, "Angel Nurse" appeared. First, she introduced herself to my mother, explained that she would be taking her blood pressure and temperature and that blood work had been ordered. Angel Nurse competently and kindly attended to my mother, inquiring about both her medical history and her illness experiences with MS. In a very impressive manner, she reassured my mother that she would probably be admitted for another round of intravenous steroids and that everything would be done to keep her comfortable.

Then she came to me, reached out her hand to shake mine, introduced herself, and warmly inquired about the nature of my relationship to the patient. I was softened by this nurse's kind and competent approach. I offered the information that I was the patient's daughter and that I was visiting from another city. Then the nurse offered a possible hypothesis in the form of a statement: *"This must be very upsetting for you."* In that one sentence, this nurse assessed and acknowledged my suffering. Angel Nurse provided comfort and understanding through her very brief interaction with me in probably less than 2 minutes. However, in just those 2 minutes, she had involved me in her practice and some of my emotional suffering had healed.

Later, on reflection, I realized that my reaction to this nurse's encounter with me was to make every effort to assist her in caring for my mother because I could see that she was overloaded with patients in the ED. Angel Nurse's particular nursing approach had encouraged me to want to be more helpful to her. Kindness invites kindness; accusations invite accusations. In this very brief interaction, Angel Nurse had entered into a therapeutic conversation with me, my mother, and my father. She also showed good manners by shaking my hand, introducing herself, eliciting some genogram information, and validating my suffering. Perhaps not all the key ingredients that we have suggested for a brief family interview are evident in this interaction with Angel Nurse; however, it exemplifies how the context and the appropriateness of the situation determine how much family members can be involved. This nurse beautifully demonstrated that family nursing can be done, even in busy EDs, in just 2 minutes and still effect healing.

CASE SCENARIO: KAREN NELSON

Karen Nelson is a 68-year-old woman who lives with her 70-year-old husband, Vern, in a small town 20 minutes outside of the city. Karen is at a hospital waiting to see an orthopedic surgeon; a few hours earlier, she fell in her apartment, broke her upper arm, and was transferred to the emergency department (ED) in the city. Presently, her son, Andrew, and daughter-in-law, Louise, are with her at the bedside in the ED. Karen tells Andrew and Louise that she is concerned about how Vern is managing at home alone and what they will do if she needs to stay in the hospital overnight or for a few days.

After 5 hours of waiting for the surgeon with Karen, Andrew and Louise decide to go home; they have left their 2-year-old son with Louise's parents, and Karen is becoming very tired and would like to sleep since it is 1 o'clock in the morning. Karen has not yet been seen by the orthopedic surgeon, and Louise and Andrew are very uncertain about whether Karen will have to stay in the hospital and how they will manage everything with Vern at home alone. As they begin to leave,

CASE SCENARIO: KAREN NELSON—cont'd

they realize that they have had very minimal interaction with the nurse who came in and out of the room in the ED all evening, and they are not sure of the nurse's name. Louise rings the call bell and asks for the nurse to come to their room. When the nurse arrives, Louise asks the nurse to write down Andrew's cell phone number in Karen's chart in case of an emergency or if Vern does not answer the phone during the night. The following conversation ensues:

Nurse: *"Well, who are you, anyway, and why would we need this number?"*

Louise: *"I am Louise, Karen's daughter-in-law, and this is her son, Andrew. We live close to the hospital, and Karen's husband, Vern, lives 20 minutes outside of town and has very poor mobility."*

Reflective Questions

1. What would be the benefits of the nurse conducting a 15-minute family interview with Karen, Andrew, and Louise?
2. How could the nurse use therapeutic conversation to provide Karen, Andrew, and Louise with the opportunity to share their feelings about their current situation?
3. What are three key therapeutic questions the nurse could ask Karen, Andrew, and Louise to gain an understating of their expectations during their time in the emergency department and the most pressing concerns or problems they currently have?

CRITICAL THINKING QUESTIONS

1. Identify barriers to involving family in your nursing practice area. What are potential solutions to these barriers?
2. Consider how you would complete a 15-minute family interview in your practice area. What are the benefits? What are the challenges?
3. Consider the key ingredients of therapeutic questions and commendations. Can you provide an example of how you would apply each of these specifically to your nursing practice?
4. What influences the manners of individuals or families? Consider values, beliefs, culture, age, society, and technology. How might this impact your therapeutic relationship?

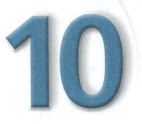

Chapter **10**

How to Move Beyond Basic Family Nursing Skills

Learning Objectives

- Compare the difference between basic and advanced skills in family nursing.
- Summarize the distinguishing features of advanced skills in family nursing.
- Describe advanced skills used when interviewing families of the elderly at times of transition.
- Describe advanced skills used for interviewing an individual to gain a family perspective on chronic illness.

Key Concepts

Advanced family nursing skills

Relative influence questioning

Basic family nursing skills

Moving beyond basic family nursing skills requires increased knowledge, increased clinical practice, and greater attention to the uniqueness of each practice context. It also involves an appreciation of the circularity between knowledge and practice.

Entering into therapeutic conversations with families can increase our understanding of and knowledge about families while simultaneously offering interventions to promote health and/or to address concerns or ease suffering. Our research efforts can augment the efficacy of our interventions with families, and this new knowledge is extended back into practice. Thus, both clinical practice and research operate in a continuous feedback loop for one another, with promising benefits for both families and nurses. Experienced nurses realize that it is always an interactional process of "evidence-based practice" and "practice-based evidence" that enhances the care offered to families.

KEY CONCEPT DEFINED

Basic Family Nursing Skills

Generalist-level nursing skills used when caring for families.

A major challenge in determining core competencies for family work is to distinguish what can be called "general skills and knowledge"—which are needed by all nurses working with clients or patients—from unique, advanced practice skills and knowledge, particularly those of family nurses. Another challenge is to delineate sufficient competencies to cover the range of practice settings and yet not specify so many that the practitioner is overwhelmed.

In Chapter 5 we discuss basic essential skills and stages in family nursing interviews. In this chapter we discuss the more advanced family nursing skills that we have identified and labeled as vital in interviewing families in various settings. Two clinical vignettes are offered to highlight advanced practice skills. In particular, we present sample skills for interviewing families of the elderly at times of transition and advanced skills for interviewing an individual to gain a family perspective on chronic illness. We also offer tips for advanced practice with these populations and delineate advanced micro-skills. Ideas for how to integrate family nursing into various practice contexts are also offered.

KEY CONCEPT DEFINED

Advanced Family Nursing Skills

An expanded range of nursing skills that improve health outcomes for patients and families in the larger discipline of nursing; these skills require increased knowledge, increased clinical practice, and greater attention to the uniqueness of each practice context.

FAMILY NURSING SKILLS IN CONTEXT

The importance of specifically tailoring family nursing interviewing skills to the relational practice context cannot be overstressed. We have found in our review of the literature that the contextual and clinical competence application is often overlooked. Leahey and Svavarsdottir (2009) advocate that knowledge translation and exchange are a shared responsibility requiring the involvement of researchers with potential knowledge users such as practicing nurses. Astedt-Kurki and Kaunonen (2011) recommend making family nursing more visible through intervention studies involving skilled nurses.

However, awareness of research findings does not necessarily mean adoption. Rather, interventions must be adapted to local settings that are inevitably varied, complex, and idiosyncratic. Duhamel (2010), who developed a Center of Excellence in Family Nursing at the University of Montreal, advocates "engaged scholarship" to create knowledge and application into practice in unique clinical settings. Svavarsdottir and Sigurdardottir (2011) have provided excellent examples of knowledge exchange in pediatric settings. In an ambitious and innovative project, Moules, Laing, Morck, and Toner (2011) have undertaken a program connecting family research in pediatric oncology to practice; they are devising interventions in an effort to reduce family suffering in the experience of childhood cancer.

The new knowledge created must be useful for nurses and families in the unique relational practice setting. McLeod, Tapp, Moules, and Campbell (2010) found that the skill of addressing specific family concerns in the oncology unit was particularly helpful. Gathering family members and opening space for conversation allowed the nurse to feel he or she "knew" the families. Coming to know the families as individuals with histories was an important skill identified by the researchers. Vandall-Walker, Jensen, and Oberle (2007) found that in the intensive care unit (ICU), skills identified as important in this setting included engaging with family members, sustaining them, and disengaging from them.

Leahey and Harper-Jaques (2010) created a method for integrating family nursing into practice settings and used a mental health urgent care context in a Canadian community health center as an example (Southern et al, 2007). Leahey and Harper-Jaques (2010) developed a grid and listed the main four elements of clinical practice in the setting: mental health/psychiatric assessment, physical health assessment, family nursing, and integrated behavioral health care. Alongside these practice framework elements, they listed Benner's (2001) skill levels from novice to advanced beginner to competent to proficient to expert. See Table 10-1 for mental health urgent care practice framework elements and ladders.

Staff had identified the need for a practice framework specific to their setting and participated in generating the skills relevant for each section of the grid. Through team discussion, observation of clinical work, reviews of the literature, clinical documentation audits, supervision, and feedback from clients and families, family nursing practice took hold in the setting. Family nursing grew to be seen as an integral part of practice rather than as an "add-on" or "one more thing to do." The value of this tool is that it can be adapted to various settings by tailoring the practice framework elements and specifying the unique family nursing skills for the context.

TABLE 10-1	Mental Health Urgent Care Practice Framework Elements and Ladders			
LADDERS	MENTAL HEALTH/ PSYCHIATRIC ASSESSMENT	PHYSICAL NURSING ASSESSMENT	FAMILY NURSING	INTEGRATED BEHAVIORAL HEALTH
1 Novice				
2 Advanced/Beginner				
3 Competent				
4 Proficient				
5 Expert				

Leahey, M., & Harper-Jaques, S. (2010). Integrating family nursing into a mental health urgent care practice framework: Ladders for learning. Journal of Family Nursing, 16(2), 200. Copyright 2010 by Maureen Leahey and Sandy Harper-Jaques. Reprinted by permission of SAGE Publications.

Duhamel and Dupuis (2011) believe that utilizing family systems nursing knowledge in clinical practice requires more administrative and educational support than is usually offered. They advocate a circular process among education, research, and practice, especially favoring the idea of having facilitators or coaches in the clinical setting to advance practice skills and implementation. The work of Litchfield (2011) in New Zealand similarly supports the value of a mentor and the inclusivity of stakeholders.

Nevertheless, Svavarsdottir et al (2015) identify the need for further research at an institutional level focusing on effective strategies to implement family systems nursing into practice.

BEYOND BASIC SKILLS

Differentiating basic and advanced skills in family nursing is a challenge. We believe that education, experience, practice time, and deliberate practice are considered to be distinguishing features between basic and advanced skills in family nursing.

Education

Education can be thought of as a differentiation point, with higher nursing education implying advanced skill level. Moules, Bell, Paton, and Morck

(2012) stress that "teaching graduate family nursing students the important and delicate practice of entering into and mitigating families' illness suffering signifies an educational practice that is rigorous, intense, and contextual, yet not articulated as expounded knowledge" (p. 1). More conceptual knowledge aims to lead to a more advanced skill level, but as Chesla (2008) points out, awareness of information does not necessarily lead to implementation or executive skills.

Experience

Experience can be another delineator of levels. For example, the novice interviewer typically talks with the family to obtain information *for the nurse,* whereas the more experienced nurse invites the family to ask questions and designs interventions *for the family's needs*. This is an important distinction. The more proficient nurse demonstrates curiosity about the family's needs, styles of coping, and so forth, in an effort to maximize the family's and nurse's ability to care for their loved one. In this situation, the nurse and family collaborate on a plan of care instead of the nurse controlling and directing the interview process with less regard for the needs and concerns of the family.

Practice Time

Another way to conceptualize expert or advanced practice skills is the "10,000-hour rule" popularized by social science commentator Malcolm Gladwell (2008). He claims that to be an expert and successful in any field requires 10,000 hours of deliberate practice. The 10,000-hour rule is usually attributed to the research done by Anders Ericsson (2006). He and his team divided students into three groups ranked by excellence at the Berlin Academy of Music and then correlated achievement with hours of practice. They discovered that the elite had all put in about 10,000 hours of practice, the good 8,000 hours, and the average 4,000 hours. This rule was then applied to other disciplines, and Ericsson found that it proved valid.

Deliberate Practice

More recently, Ericsson's work on deliberate practice has been geared toward application in established domains of expertise, such as nursing and medicine (Ericsson, Whyte, & Ward, 2007). It is our belief that the 10,000-hour rule could be one useful guideline to determine when nurses have become expert in their clinical skills when working with families.

Recognition and the ability to make relevant observations are factors in increasing perceptual skill development. Benner's ladders (2001) are another way of differentiating various skills by the changes in familiarity, integration, flexibility, and efficiency that accompany each skill level. We believe that whatever method one chooses to differentiate basic and advanced skills is less important than the compassionate application of these skills with unique families in specific relational practice contexts.

CLINICAL EXAMPLE 1: INTERVIEWING FAMILIES OF THE ELDERLY AT TIME OF TRANSITION

Setting, Family Composition, and Purpose of the Interview

Ross, age 72, and Myrna, age 70, are siblings whose mother has recently moved into a long-term care facility. They have two younger sisters, ages 69 and 60, who live in different cities. Ross is retired and separated from his wife. He has four children and four grandchildren. Myrna is a widow with two sons and four grandchildren, and she continues to work 3 days a week. Ross and Myrna's father died 15 years ago. Myrna and Ross have a photo of their mother at her 99th birthday party.

The purpose of this example is to offer tips for collaborating with senior children at the time of their elderly parents' transition to a care facility and to demonstrate the advanced micro-skills for quickly engaging with family members, obtaining a brief relevant history, discussing caregiver impact and burden, and responding to senior children's suggestions about their parents' care. The necessary clinical skill or skills are listed before each example.

Clinical Skills:

- *Engagement*
- *Creating welcoming context for collaboration*
- *Involving all family members*
- *Obtaining brief relevant history by co-constructing an illness narrative versus a medical narrative*

> **Dr. Leahey:** First of all, let me introduce myself. I'm Maureen. Glad to meet you. Myrna, is it?
>
> **Myrna:** Yes, it is.
>
> **Dr. Leahey:** And Ross? Glad to meet you, hi. So thanks very much for coming in this afternoon. I understand that this is the third facility that your mom has been in. And so one of the routine practices that we have here is that when our patients have been in other facilities, we like to meet with the family as soon as possible.
>
> Maybe one way we could start is for me to ask you, how did it come to be that your mom came to this facility?

Ross: Do you want to start, Myrna?

Myrna: Mom has lived at home until this year. She's been very independent, and she feels independent, but that's partly because the family's protecting her. But she was getting to a point where she really couldn't look after herself. She was getting quite forgetful, and we had several caretakers at different times in the home, but they didn't seem to work out. Things would go fine for a little while, and then Mom would not like something they did. So we went through a succession of those people but decided that we just really couldn't keep Mom in her home. So we have talked about it for years and finally really encouraged her last year that we just had to find a place for her and started looking.

Dr. Leahey: So what…

Ross: And it was trying because she's so independent. She's a tough old Norwegian, and independence is most important to her, so she was very resistant. We eventually did get her to look at two or three facilities, and she kind of gave in to it in a way. She was in her own home, multilevel, a lot of steps and preparing her own meals. She was not eating properly. We had to do something, so we did find a seniors' living residence. That was the first place that she moved into.

Dr. Leahey: Yes.

Ross: And she was … started to have some falls, so they … at one point they thought she had broken some bones and she had to be admitted to the hospital. In the hospital, she was assessed and told that she could not go back to her…

Myrna: Assisted living.

Ross: Her assisted living.

Dr. Leahey: Okay. So this has been a long haul for your family in getting your mom to this facility.

Ross: Very, very long.

Clinical Skill:

- *Eliciting impact of illness on family members*

Dr. Leahey: What do you think has been the impact of that on you, Ross?

Ross: Oh, the impact? I went through 14 years of always being there and available, and it just got more intense as time went on. The impact? By the time when we finally got her into a facility last August until December, I lost 18 pounds. I mean, my weight was dropping. It was really, really a big thing because when she was in the assisted living, I'd be getting phone calls every day. What do you want to do about this? What are you going to do about that?

Dr. Leahey: You look sad just talking about it. It's okay with me if you cry.

Ross: Oh, I'm not going to cry.

Dr. Leahey: Okay.

Ross: It's … but it is a fact of life, and this is—

Dr. Leahey: Yes.

Ross: Unfortunately, the way it went.

Dr. Leahey: And what do you think the impact has been on Myrna of looking after your mom?

Ross: She'll have to answer that. (*Smiles and nods*)

Myrna: I think it's … there's been much less impact on me partly because Ross has taken the major role. Having worked and not being available has made me less accessible to care.

Ross: It's that, but the other fact is that Mother is from a…

Myrna: A patriarchal viewpoint.

Ross: She has a patriarchal viewpoint that the girls cannot do the job as well as a man, and that's unfortunate because they can do better than I could probably. But it always has to be me who makes the final decision.

Clinical Skills:

* *Demonstrating curiosity*
* *Inquiring about the biopsychosocial-spiritual factors when asking about the impact of stress on family members.*

Dr. Leahey: Do you have some health problems, Myrna?

Myrna: I do. I was diagnosed with Parkinson's almost 7 years ago, and one of my main symptoms is tiredness. So I just find it hard to cope with any extra requests or demands of Mom. I think it's kind of settled down now. We've each got kind of our own jobs, and that's what we do.

Dr. Leahey: And how did you manage as a group of siblings to figure out your own jobs?

Ross: It just fell into place.

Dr. Leahey: Fell into place?

Ross: I mean, we each have our own strengths.

Dr. Leahey: Yes.

Ross: And we are close and we just ... we back each other up, and if we need help in an area, we ask the others for help or thoughts. It's cooperation. That's the big thing.

Dr. Leahey: And how about for you, Ross? Do you have any health problems?

Ross: No, my health is pretty good, basically.

Myrna: Although your blood pressure has—

Ross: Well, that was the other thing. My blood pressure shot up last fall, too, because of all the extreme stress that we were going through. But it's under control.

Clinical Skill:

- *Asking for other family members' noticings or ideas*

    Dr. Leahey: What impact would you say your sons would have noticed, Myrna, on you?

    Myrna: I think they're aware that it creates a strain for me, but day to day I don't think it really affects our relationship. I think they are more concerned about me than they are about their grandmother.

    Dr. Leahey: And what do you think they're most concerned with about you?

    Myrna: Tiring out. Just, you know, the Parkinson symptoms increasing, but I think they feel that Grandma is now in place.

    Ross: She's being looked after.

    Dr. Leahey: She's being looked after?

    Myrna: Yeah.

    Ross: It's not a concern.

    Myrna: Yeah.

Clinical Skills:

- *Summarizing*
- *Using the patient's language*
- *Commending*
- *Asking for other's advice to patient*

    Dr. Leahey: It sounds like your mother has been very fortunate to have the two of you and your sisters who have looked after her as well as you have. And sometimes it sounds like at the expense of your own health. I mean, your blood pressure, your weight loss, the tiredness and stress on your Parkinson's. And if your boys were here, what advice might they want to give to you, Myrna, about your health?

Myrna: That I shouldn't stress myself. I should take it easy. They really are very sensitive about it.

Dr. Leahey: And would you take their advice?

Myrna: I think I do. Yeah.

Dr. Leahey: What do you think? Does she take it enough?

Ross: I don't know.

Myrna: They don't put a lot of demands on me.

Clinical Skill:

- *Inviting conversation about various family members' beliefs and coping styles*

  Dr. Leahey: One of the things I did want to ask you is, if your mom were here with us today, what might she say has been the most challenging part of coming into this facility?

  Myrna: I think leaving her home.

  Dr. Leahey: Leaving her home. And what do you think, Ross?

  Ross: Well, leaving her home is a very big thing to her. I'd say it was her anchor. Also leaving her cat.

  Myrna: Yeah.

  Dr. Leahey: Oh.

  Ross: And her pet was a very big thing in her life.

  Myrna: And actually, that was one of the ways we were able to move her initially because they allowed pets where she moved, so she could take her cat.

  Dr. Leahey: I see. And is her cat still alive?

  Ross: It was this morning. (*Laughs*)

  Dr. Leahey: Okay, good. (*Smiles*)

  Myrna: Ross inherited the cat.

  Dr. Leahey: And you know that you can bring the cat into the facility here?

  Ross: Yes, we're aware, and we have plans to do that. We also realize that the shots have to be up to date, and that's taken care of.

Dr. Leahey: Good, and your mom, does your mom know that the cat can come and visit her?

Ross: Yes.

Dr. Leahey: Okay.

Myrna: She asks about the cat all the time.

Dr. Leahey: Okay.

Myrna: More so than the family members.

Dr. Leahey: And how's that for the family members?

Myrna: It's fine.

Ross: We understand. She's focused on certain things, more things that have immediate meaning to her.

Clinical Skill:

- *Asking patients what others might appreciate about them*

Dr. Leahey: So if your mom were here with us now, what might she say that she most appreciates about the two of you?

Ross: I don't know. Probably looking after her affairs.

Dr. Leahey: Looking after her affairs.

Ross: Yeah. Being the house and her monetary things.

Myrna: Well, it's an interesting question because sometimes I wonder if Mom appreciates what we're doing for her, really truly appreciates. There's not a lot of, well, she'll say thank you for doing this or that, but there's … to me, there's not a sense of real appreciation.

Ross: I don't think she grasps the amount of effort that is involved, and to her, well, it's just you do it, and that's the way it is.

Myrna: She knows. She gets upset if we don't visit every day, but she doesn't appreciate what that does to our lives.

Ross: She's become quite self-centered.

Myrna: Which I think is normal.

Dr. Leahey: So that can be very hard when you're caregiving as much as you have been to feel like your mom, although appreciative, is not really aware of the impact that it has on your lives. How do you both cope with that?

Ross: Well, I understand that her health is deteriorating. Her mental abilities are deteriorating, and that just goes with age. We'll all reach that point and just try and understand that this is not the person you knew, and they can't help it.

Dr. Leahey: So that's your belief ... she can't help it and...

Ross: For the most part. Sometimes she uses it, but for the most part, yeah.

Dr. Leahey: And how about for you, Myrna?

Myrna: I think I have the same attitude. It really hurts when she uses it or goes off into a tantrum, which is unfair, really.

Dr. Leahey: Yes.

Myrna: But you very quickly come around to the realization that's how she's feeling, and that's the only way she can demonstrate it. I mean, I try to put myself in her place, and it must be horrible. I don't know what you wake up every morning looking forward to, so I can certainly understand some of her comments and criticisms. But I think she's getting much better.

Clinical Skill:

• *Eliciting "unspoken" information*

Dr. Leahey: Would there be anything that we should know about your mom that maybe she wouldn't tell us that would make it easier for us to care for her or to be helpful to her?

Ross: I can't think of anything. Well, maybe one thing is that she still insists on her independence. She doesn't like people doing everything for her. I think she would still like to make more choices than are available to her, such as seating at meals, choice in meals, times for bathing, things like that. And, you know, how much help does she need dressing, or how much does she want to do herself?

Dr. Leahey: Thank you, and I'll make sure to put that with a big star on her care plan.

Clinical Skill:

• *Eliciting family expectations for collaborative care and responding to expectations*

Dr. Leahey: When you think about what we could do in this facility to both help your mom and help the two of you and your sister, Linda, what comes to mind?

Ross: Well, I think I feel our major role is to advocate and be aware of what's going on and to work with the staff to try and work around problems that might occur or give suggestions for how they could better help her and just inter-action between the staff and ourselves.

Dr. Leahey: We do welcome people's ideas, and it sounds like you've been through a hard time, particularly in the last year.

Ross: We have.

Dr. Leahey: Yes. You're obviously very caring and think about your mom in many different ways like her privacy, her independence, her socialization, her food. Nice. Is there anything else you can think of how we could work with you to make your mom's last years as comfortable as possible?

Myrna: I think the open communication is the most im-portant thing, that we feel comfortable being able to make suggestions.

Dr. Leahey: Okay.

Myrna: And that works the other way ... that you're keep-ing us up to date on changes in Mom.

Dr. Leahey: So some reciprocity there that you would tell us things you notice and that we would tell you. Some people like to have periodic meetings.

Ross: That was my next point.

Dr. Leahey: Do you like that? Some other families say "no news is good news." What's your preference?

Ross: No, I don't take that attitude at all. I would welcome periodic meetings.

Dr. Leahey: Okay.

Ross: Not just for the sake of having a meeting but because there's purpose in it that it will be beneficial for all those involved.

Dr. Leahey: Okay, good.

Clinical Skills Summary

Tips and micro-skills for working with elderly persons and their families include the following:

- Draw forth the family's illness experience.
- Ask difference questions, such as, "What do you think your sons are *most* concerned with about you?"
- Inquire what absent family members might say about the situation being discussed.
- Ask about the biopsychosocial-spiritual domains, and identify family and individual strengths.

In the preceding case example, the following clinical skills were demonstrated:

- Empathized with the siblings about the stress of the last year
- Commended their caring for their mother
- Pursued with them what they would find most helpful
- Asked open-ended questions to elicit their desires
- Offered practical, concrete suggestions such as family meetings
- Wove commendations throughout the interview

All these are more advanced micro-skills that a nurse interviewer can compress and use in a thoughtful, purposeful, time-effective interview. Two interventions have shown to be particularly powerful in promoting hope. Weaving commendations throughout the interview, we have found, is a very helpful and healing practice. Inviting reflections about what family members appreciate about each other can also be a powerful intervention that invites more confidence and competence in the family and thus leaves the family more hopeful about their abilities to manage in the future.

CLINICAL EXAMPLE 2: INTERVIEWING AN INDIVIDUAL TO GAIN A FAMILY PERSPECTIVE ON CHRONIC ILLNESS

Setting, Family Composition, and Purpose of the Interview

Ralph, age 55, came to the outpatient clinic looking for more coping strategies to deal with his longstanding chronic pain related to his disability. Ralph has been married for 37 years and has two children, ages 31 and 29. Ralph is self-employed in a mobile knife-sharpening business, and his wife is the bookkeeper in the family business. She is also employed full-time as a paralegal.

In these excerpts, Dr. Wright explores how a chronic illness impacts a middle-aged man's life and relationships. The interview is brief, time-limited, and effective. The purpose is to recognize that illness is a family affair and that all family members are affected by and can influence an illness, demonstrate the skills for gaining a family perspective when interviewing an individual, assess the impact of chronic illness on one's life and relationships, assess solutions and coping strategies, and intervene by offering commendations and planning a ritual. What do health professionals do if family members cannot or will not attend a meeting so that a family perspective can be obtained? What if the context in which the health professional works does not lend itself to involving other family members? Yes, it is possible to "bring family members into the room" even if only meeting with an individual.

In the first excerpt of the therapeutic conversation, Dr. Wright asks, *"What are you most hoping can happen at the Center and during our meeting together?"* This is an example of a collaborative interaction in which Ralph and Dr. Wright jointly set the goals.

Clinical Skills:

- *Recognize that illness is a family affair and that all family members are affected by and can influence an illness.*
- *Gain a family perspective when interviewing an individual.*
- *Assess the impact of chronic illness on one's life and relationships.*
- *Assess solutions and coping strategies.*
- *Intervene by offering commendations.*
- *Plan a ritual.*

> **Dr. Wright:** I'm wondering, what are you most hoping can happen at the Center and during our meeting together? What are you most interested in?
>
> **Ralph:** Basically, coping mechanisms.
>
> **Dr. Wright:** Coping mechanisms.
>
> **Ralph:** To help cope with the pain.
>
> **Dr. Wright:** To cope with pain, yes?
>
> **Ralph:** Right. Because of the fact that I have some permanent spinal cord damage.
>
> **Dr. Wright:** Yes.
>
> **Ralph:** From my accident.

In this next segment, Dr. Wright inquires about the family's problem-solving strategies.

Clinical Skill:

- *Exploring usefulness/not usefulness of other helpers*

> **Dr. Wright:** And so your wife went to the pain clinic?
>
> **Ralph:** Yes, she went to see the pain psychologist.
>
> **Dr. Wright:** Right, and was that helpful to her?
>
> **Ralph:** It was because it helped to direct our conversations. If I was having a bad day and started to react to everybody around me because I was having a bad day, then it helped her because then she was able to look at me and say, "Is this the pain talking or are you having other issues?"

Dr. Wright: Oh, okay.

Ralph: A lot of times when people are arguing or people are short with their kids or whatever, it's because they're in pain and it's a reaction to the action.

Dr. Wright: Do you ever find, though, that it's useful to use your pain as an excuse or an out if you are...

Ralph: Actually...

Dr. Wright: ... getting into trouble with your wife or your kids?

Ralph: No, I don't.

Dr. Wright: No? Just say, "Oh, that's the pain talking. It's not really me"? Or...?

Ralph: Actually, I don't personally know.

Dr. Wright: Okay, and so have you and your wife been seen now together as a couple or did she just go?

Ralph: No, we went together, and she also went to private sessions. I went to private sessions, too, and then we were seen by the pain psychologist together.

Clinical Skill:

- *Inquiring about the best/worst advice the client received*

    Dr. Wright: Okay, and what was the best and worst advice that was offered to you?

    Ralph: The world doesn't stop just because you're in pain.

    Dr. Wright: That was the best advice? Yes?

    Ralph: That was the best advice.

    Dr. Wright: Okay. And the worst advice?

    Ralph: One of the other best advices was if you don't control it, it will control you. That was the second part of that.

    Dr. Wright: Okay. So if you don't control it...

    Ralph: It will control you.

    Dr. Wright: Will control you. And what was the worst advice you received?

    Ralph: Don't worry. Things will get better.

    Dr. Wright: Ah.

    Ralph: Because by expecting things to get better when a person is in chronic pain ... It is far better for them to learn how to deal with the situation they're in rather than hoping that it's going to get better or expecting it to get better.

Clinical Skills:

- *Inquiring about the impact of illness on family members*
- *Asking difference questions*

> ***Dr. Wright:*** Right. So who do you think the pain has been a bigger problem for over the years? You or your wife?
>
> ***Ralph:*** Oh, it's definitely been a larger problem for me.
>
> ***Dr. Wright:*** A larger problem for you. And what's your wife…
>
> ***Ralph:*** But it definitely has had an impact. It's had an impact on not only my wife but my children as well. For instance…
>
> ***Dr. Wright:*** Yes. Tell me about that.
>
> ***Ralph:*** They were 5 and 7 years old when I broke my neck. So I wasn't able to have them sit on my knee.
>
> ***Dr. Wright:*** Okay.
>
> ***Ralph:*** It took me a long time to learn how to walk. So…
>
> ***Dr. Wright:*** So they only really remember you as a dad with pain or…
>
> ***Ralph:*** Yes.
>
> ***Dr. Wright:*** … disabilities or problems, challenges all the time.

Comments

Throughout the interview, did you notice how Dr. Wright explored Ralph's understanding of the effect of chronic pain on his wife and children? And then how she was curious about the best and worst advice he had been offered? This is very helpful in being able to sidestep errors or mistakes that Dr. Wright could make by offering similar recommendations that were not found to be helpful in the past.

Clinical Skills:

- *Naming the illness*
- *Using the client's language*

> ***Dr. Wright:*** What do you call it? Do you call it a disability? Do you call it an accident? How do you refer to it?
>
> ***Ralph:*** It's … I just … I have a permanent disability.
>
> ***Dr. Wright:*** Permanent disability.
>
> ***Ralph:*** I consider it to be a permanent disability.

Dr. Wright: That's how you refer to it?

Ralph: And that's it.

Dr. Wright: Okay.

Ralph: But it is, actually. It's helped me put life into perspective in that I control how I react to things. And it has helped me by all of the different reading that I've done.

Dr. Wright: Okay.

Comments

In this next section of the case example, Dr. Wright explores the influence of chronic pain on Ralph's life and the pain's influence on him. This line of questioning is called relative influence questioning, and we wish to credit the late and brilliant Michael White (1989) of Australia for this very useful way of questioning.

KEY CONCEPT DEFINED

Relative Influence Questioning

Questioning that allows clients to think of themselves not as problems but as individuals who have a relationship with a problem.

Clinical Skill:

* *Relative influence questioning*

> *Dr. Wright:* What, at this moment today, what percent of the time does pain rule your life, and what percent of the time do you think that you have control over the pain?
>
> *Ralph:* I…
>
> *Dr. Wright:* What percent do you control now?
>
> *Ralph:* I have to be able to control the pain at least 75% of the time.
>
> *Dr. Wright:* Seventy-five, okay.
>
> *Ralph:* Because of the permanent spinal cord damage, I have problems in that I spasm.
>
> *Dr. Wright:* Okay.
>
> *Ralph:* I have to take an antispasmodic, and there are problems with having permanent spinal cord damage. I've taken a lot of medication, and now the medications have created different problems.

Dr. Wright: Like?

Ralph: Like problems with my liver, problems with my kidneys.

Dr. Wright: Oh, dear.

Ralph: And so consequently, there are other things to deal with.

Dr. Wright: So 25% of the time the pain controls you.

Ralph: Yes, which is why I have to get up and I have to actually do things in order to control the pain so that I can continue on with my life.

Dr. Wright: So when you say today that you've come to this pain center and you are wanting to have more coping strategies, what percent are you trying to get to manage?
Like, what would be your ideal percent that you would say, wow.

Ralph: It would be nice to be 90%.

Dr. Wright: 90%.

Ralph: I mean, I am not looking for a fairy godmother or some … I don't expect…

Dr. Wright: Okay, to wave her magic wand over you and…

Ralph: A magic wand and everything is going to be fine.

Dr. Wright: And the pain is gone forever, yeah.

Ralph: Coping strategies so that I can learn more about how to cope so that I don't … so I can get on more with a normal life, whatever that might be.

Dr. Wright: Okay. So you really are only asking to have coping strategies for 15% more?

Ralph: That's right.

Dr. Wright: That's amazing. So you're willing to live with at least 10% pain 24/7. Yes?

Ralph: I have to be realistic.

Clinical Skill:

- *Asking the "one-question question"*

Dr. Wright: Okay. So in our meeting together today, if there was just one question that you could have answered today, what would that one question be around your situation? What you've been dealing with?

Ralph: Actually, I would say that it's how to help me help myself.

Dr. Wright: How can you help yourself?

Ralph: Is there something that could be pointed out or something that could be better? Because everybody has a different perspective.

Dr. Wright: Yes.

Ralph: Sometimes I don't see certain things because I'm too close to it.

Comments

In this segment, Ralph's response to Dr. Wright's question again demonstrated his openness to new ideas for problem solving. In this next excerpt, Dr. Wright asks about Ralph's family and the influence of his beliefs on his situation.

Clinical Skill:

• *Asking a difference question to bring family members into the room*

Dr. Wright: And is there anything that your family could be doing differently to help you to do more of or less of?

Ralph: Actually, I'm very fortunate.

Dr. Wright: Yes.

Ralph: I think that my family has learned to cope very well. It's made them more forgiving, made them more open to dealing with their problems and dealing with other people's problems.

Dr. Wright: Okay. So there's been some good, it sounds like, that's come out of this.

Ralph: Oh, definitely a lot of good that's come out of it.

Clinical Skill:

• *Asking about the influence of spirituality and beliefs*

Dr. Wright: And what about for you personally? What good has come out of it?

Ralph: There has been a lot of good that's come out of it.

Dr. Wright: Really. Can you give me a couple of examples?

Ralph: Well, when I broke my neck, I was 245 pounds. I had a 21-inch neck and 56 inches across the shoulders and a 52-inch chest. And I used to throw around quarters of beef that weighed up to 300 pounds.

Dr. Wright: My.

Ralph: And I thought that I was invincible. And then God stepped in and said, "Oops."

Dr. Wright: So you have some beliefs about faith or God that had...

Ralph: Yes.

Dr. Wright: ... a part in all of this?

Ralph: Actually, God does not make junk. What you do with it after that is up to you.

Dr. Wright: So did you pray about your situation when...

Ralph: Oh, many times.

Dr. Wright: Yes? And what did you pray for when you were injured like that?

Ralph: Help.

Dr. Wright: Help.

Ralph: Actually, that's all a person can do.

Dr. Wright: So, Ralph, I just wanted to follow up a little bit more about your faith and your beliefs. Was that helpful to you in being able to cope with the pain or not?

Ralph: Actually, I think that I had an uncle once tell me that God doesn't give you any more than you cannot handle with his help.

Dr. Wright: And did you adopt that belief?

Ralph: And the largest obstacle to that?

Dr. Wright: Yes.

Ralph: Is asking for that help.

Dr. Wright: Okay.

Ralph: People have to actually ask. And that's...

Dr. Wright: And were you able to come to that point?

Ralph: Oh, definitely. Yes.

Dr. Wright: Okay.

Ralph: And that's God no matter how you perceive him to be. Anybody who doesn't believe that there isn't a higher being really should look within themselves.

Clinical Skill:

- *Inquiring about the client's ideas about family members' beliefs about the client*

Dr. Wright: Well, I love that you've touched on your beliefs just now, and I'm wondering if your children were here, what do you think they would tell me about you and how you've managed this disability all these years? What do you think their comment would be?

Ralph: Actually, I really and truly think that my daughter became a paramedic to help others.

Dr. Wright: Is that right? That's been one of the influences on her?

Ralph: Yes, because she realized that people do get hurt and need help. And my son is very … he's a gentle giant. He's 6 foot 1, 230 pounds, and very kind.

Dr. Wright: Oh. So you think the influence of your disability has been that it's invited kindness in your son and your daughter's desire to help people?

Ralph: Yes. I really do.

Dr. Wright: Okay.

Ralph: I think they realize that things happen to people.

Dr. Wright: Yes. And what would they say about you, how you've managed it?

Ralph: They probably think that I've done very well.

Dr. Wright: Okay. So they'd give you a pretty good grade, would they?

Ralph: I would hope so.

Dr. Wright: Yes?

Ralph: Yes.

Dr. Wright: What kind of grade do you think they would give you?

Ralph: I think it would be pretty high.

Dr. Wright: Wow, okay. And your wife, if she was here, what would she say the biggest influence upon her has been?

Ralph: I think it's made us closer, a lot closer.

Dr. Wright: It's made you closer?

Ralph: Yes.

Dr. Wright: Okay. Emotionally close or physically close?

Ralph: Emotionally and physically.

Dr. Wright: And physically? 'Cause one…

Ralph: Emotionally, definitely, because of the fact that we've had to deal with so much.

Dr. Wright: Okay, 'cause one very personal thing I was going to ask you, because of all your surgeries and back problems and pain, has that interfered with your being able to enjoy sexual relations?

Ralph: It has.

Dr. Wright: Yes?

Ralph: To a certain degree. A lot of the medications I have to be on, anti-inflammatories and muscle relaxants...

Dr. Wright: Yes.

Ralph: And when you're dealing with muscle relaxants ... (*Smiles*)

Dr. Wright: Yes, but you found a way?

Ralph: Oh, definitely.

Dr. Wright: Yes.

Ralph: Yeah, it's a very important part.

Dr. Wright: Yes, absolutely.

Ralph: And not only that, I ... we ... believe that a good marriage doesn't just happen.

Dr. Wright: How would your wife say that you have evolved over these 20 years, or what do you think her description of you would be?

Ralph: Actually, probably sometimes she thinks I'm a little bit too positive.

Dr. Wright: Too positive, oh? Okay. So she and I might share some of that because that was a bit of my worry earlier.

Ralph: Yeah.

Dr. Wright: Okay. So just to go back to your wife for a moment, what did you say was the biggest influence on her, the biggest challenge for her with your chronic pain?

Ralph: Actually, I would say probably in the early years it was staying positive.

Dr. Wright: Staying positive about what aspect?

Ralph: About the situation. For instance...

Dr. Wright: That you were going to get better or that you would ... what?

Ralph: Well, I mean it was not an easy path. She had to take on the major breadwinner. There were a lot of things that happened.

Clinical Skill:

* *Demonstrating curiosity*

Dr. Wright: Okay. Wow, so it impacted every area of your life, it sounds like.

Ralph: It did.

Dr. Wright: Financially?

Ralph: Financially, emotionally, physically.

Dr. Wright: So your wife had to become the breadwinner?

Ralph: Mmm-hmm.

Dr. Wright: Changed the roles in your family?

Ralph: Definitely.

Dr. Wright: Wow, so it didn't leave any aspect of your life...

Ralph: Everything has changed.

Dr. Wright: ... untouched.

Ralph: Everything has changed.

Dr. Wright: So for your wife in those early years, when you're saying staying positive, I'm still trying to understand staying positive about ...?

Ralph: That things were going to work out.

Dr. Wright: That things would work out.

Ralph: That eventually, that things would eventually get better.

Dr. Wright: Okay, and is she...

Ralph: And staying positive for me because she didn't want to drag me down because she figured that I already had enough...

Dr. Wright: Yes.

Ralph: ...to deal with.

Comments

Let us review what we have just read. Dr. Wright asked the "one-question question" to help identify where the greatest concerns, problems, or suffering lie (Duhamel, Dupuis, & Wright, 2009; Wright, 1989). Dr. Wright then explored Ralph's religious and spiritual beliefs after he spontaneously told her about the influence of God in his life. Dr. Wright used this opening in the therapeutic conversation about spirituality to also explore if Ralph has prayed about his condition and, if so, what he prays for. In our experience, persons with illness often reach out for comfort, hope, and/or guidance in their lives, and prayer is one alternative for fulfilling that need. Following this, Dr. Wright again brought the family into the meeting by asking, if present, what family members would say about Ralph's progress throughout the years. These questions were to assess the influence the family members have had on the ill person.

Clinical Skill:

• *Offering interventions of prescribing a ritual and giving commendations*

Dr. Wright: I've ... not extensively, but I have worked with a number of people who have experienced chronic pain for a variety of things—accidents, illnesses. And it is one of the most difficult things to deal with in terms of how it affects your life and often demoralizes a person and can invite depression. It can invite such terrible suffering. And when you were answering me earlier when I was asking you about what's one question that you might want to have answered today, you said learn more coping strategies. I'd just like to throw out one idea that I have utilized with some patients and families.

Ralph: Okay.

Dr. Wright: You've been at this so long. You only want to improve 15% more. You've already done 75%. Maybe you've done some of these strategies, but one of the ones that some couples and individuals have told me that has worked for them is to have moments when they refuse to talk about pain. So they take a holiday from talking about pain. So if somebody asks them, "How are you doing?" even if they're having pain, they say, "No, this is my time when I don't talk about it."

It's the knowing when I can talk about it and when I don't have to discuss it that's important. Some people say if I could just talk about it to my wife or to my husband for 15 or 20 minutes a day and just say what kind of a day it has been, that would be good. And then to take a holiday from pain.

Ralph: Give yourself permission to do that.

Dr. Wright: Permission to do it.

Ralph: Give yourself permission to do that. That's right, yeah.

Dr. Wright: Exactly, to be able to choose when to talk about it and when not to talk. To have moments when you absolutely put a moratorium on talking about pain because pain has a way of...

Ralph: And when somebody asks how you're feeling, you tell them, "With my hands like everybody else."

Dr. Wright: Yeah, yes. So I don't know. That's just one little tip.

Ralph: Yes. I appreciate that.

Dr. Wright: One little hot tip for you. And so I just want to say to you, I just think your own wisdom in all of this is so marvelous! It is your own willingness to learn, your willingness to be open to so many ideas from improving your marriage, to improving your health and trying to cope with this disability that is so impressive to me. Now you're at this pain center. You've got a remarkable story.

Ralph: Literally, if you do not control it, it will control you. And that's all I try to do is to have the ability to control it better and that's all.

Dr. Wright: Well, I think that the fact you are controlling it 75% is just really remarkable and really incredible.

Ralph: Thank you.

Dr. Wright: Because there are many things in our lives, say, that people struggle with, whether it is diabetes or whatever health problems they may have that they wish they could be at 75%, especially with people experiencing chronic pain. I have met many people, like I said, and some of them would just be thrilled if they could get to 30% that they could control, and you're up to 75%.

Ralph: I'm working on it.

Dr. Wright: So...

Ralph: But you have to work at it.

Dr. Wright: But I think you are very clever not to expect to be 100% pain-free, that you—

Ralph: That's never going to happen.

Dr. Wright: No, that you always will allow the pain to be in your life about 10%. Because if you wanted to be pain-free and you always worked toward that, it can be a great disappointment when you are not reaching that goal all the time.

Ralph: And I think realistically, you have to look at the fact that it is not going to happen.

Dr. Wright: Yeah.

Ralph: And be happy where you are.

Comments

Dr. Wright concludes the session with some very specific interventions. First, she offers Ralph commendations about his strengths and resources that he has utilized to cope with and heal from his condition, such as his wisdom, his positive approach, and the success he has had on influencing his chronic pain. Finally, she offers a very specific intervention in the form of a prescribed ritual. She suggests taking a holiday from pain talk.

CASE SCENARIO: GRETA

Greta, a 32-year-old woman, is admitted to a medical unit with a questionable diagnosis of influenza. Her weight has dropped to 82 pounds, a loss of 10 pounds in the week before admission.

Greta also has a genetic disease involving weakness and wasting of skeletal muscles. She lives with her two younger brothers and their mother, all of whom have what Greta calls "the disease" (wasting of the muscles). She is the only family member who is able to drive. The nursing staff perceives her to be angry and abrupt; they also wonder what the medical problem is. They feel sorry for Greta and think of her as "very dependent." The charge nurse suggests that a brief family interview would be helpful to explore Greta's expectations, beliefs, and resources. Her family is invited to the meeting, which is held on the unit, but they do not attend. During the brief interview, the primary nurse working with Greta asks Greta about her expectations for the hospitalization and how the nurses could be most helpful. Greta responds by saying that she would know how the staff would care for her "by how they talk with me and other patients, show me respect and trust, and treat me independently." She states that she needs to be strong to care for her brothers and mother, "who depend on me."

Reflective Questions

1. What clinical skills can the nurse use to move beyond basic family nursing skills and demonstrate advanced family nursing skills?
2. How can the nurse use relative influence questioning as an intervention with Greta?
3. How can the nurse collaborate with Greta to develop a plan of care for her during her hospitalization?

CRITICAL THINKING QUESTIONS

1. Reflect on your own nursing practice with families; how do you identify your skill level (basic or advanced)? What is your rationale for this?
2. If you identify as having advanced skills in family nursing, what did you do to achieve this?
3. If you identify as having basic skills in family nursing, what do you require to move beyond basics skills toward advanced skills?
4. Reflect on your practice setting to answer the following questions:
   a. Are there distinct roles for nurses with basic and advanced family nursing skills?
   b. What are the supports and/or barriers to applying family nursing skills?

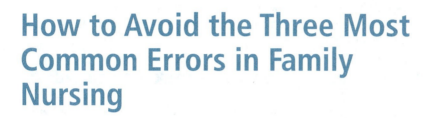

Chapter **11**

How to Avoid the Three Most Common Errors in Family Nursing

Learning Objectives

- Identify the three most common errors in family nursing.
- Describe strategies to avoid failing to create a context for change.
- Summarize strategies to avoid taking sides.
- Describe strategies to avoid giving too much advice prematurely.

Key Concepts

Context for change

Curiosity

Premature advice

Taking sides

Nurses working with families want to be helpful and to ease or alleviate emotional, physical, or spiritual suffering whenever possible (Wright, 2017). However, despite nurses' best efforts, sometimes errors, mistakes, and/or misjudgments occur. Whether nurses are beginners or experienced clinicians in family nursing, they can benefit from knowing the most common errors and how they might avoid or sidestep them. We have identified three errors that we believe occur most frequently in relational family nursing practice. They are as follows:

1. Failing to create a context for change
2. Taking sides
3. Giving too much advice prematurely

Although we are experienced family nurses, we have committed, experienced, or witnessed these errors in our own practices and in the supervision of our students. But the most important aspect is to learn from these errors and to correct them immediately, if at all possible.

For each error, we will explain in what way we believe it is a mistake and how it can negatively impact the family. We also suggest practical ways for avoiding these errors and offer a clinical example for each error. It is our hope that by sidestepping the most prevalent mistakes, nurses can sustain and improve their nursing care of families.

Nurses will have more confidence and competence in their nursing practice if they can offer a context for clinical work that is more likely to be helpful and healing.

ERROR 1: FAILING TO CREATE A CONTEXT FOR CHANGE

Every nurse in every encounter and experience with a family, whether for 5 minutes or over 5 years, has the responsibility to create a context for healing and learning. Creating a context for change is the central and enduring foundation of the therapeutic process. It is key to the relationship between the clinician and family. It is not just a necessary prerequisite to the process of therapeutic change; it *is* therapeutic change in and of itself (Wright & Bell, 2009). In creating this context for change, both the nurse and family undergo change, and the nurse is in a unique position to act as a "relational bridge" (McLeod, Tapp, Moules, & Campbell, 2010, p. 97).

KEY CONCEPT DEFINED

Context for Change

A central and enduring foundation of the therapeutic process in which both the nurse and the family undergo change, and the nurse is in a unique position to act as a "relational bridge."

What must happen in order to create a healing context for change? Empathy, mindfulness, and empathic responding are all necessary ingredients for creating a healing context (Block-Lerner, Adair, Plumb, Rhatigan, & Orsillo, 2007). Wright and Bell (2009) suggest that before a context for change can be created, all obstacles to change must be removed. Such obstacles can include a family member who does not want to be present or attends the session under duress, a family member who is dissatisfied with the progress of the clinical sessions, a family that has had previous negative experiences with health-care professionals, or a situation in which there are unclear expectations for the meetings.

At the Family Nursing Unit, University of Calgary, a hermeneutic research study conducted by Drs. Bell and Wright explored the process of therapeutic change (Bell, 1999). The focus of this study was to analyze the clinical work with three families who reported negative responses. These families suffered from serious illness and were seen in an outpatient clinic by a clinical nursing team of faculty and graduate nursing students.

The preliminary results of this study provide helpful feedback that can be used to improve family interviews. The most informative learning was that creating a context for change was either ignored or neglected among families that were dissatisfied with the nursing team's clinical work. Curiosity was absent on the part of the nurse interviewer. For example, the nurse interviewer did not seek clarification of the presenting problem or concern. Also, the nurse interviewer paid no attention to how the intervention "fit" the family's functioning. The nurse interviewer did not ascertain from the family if the intervention ideas offered were useful.

KEY CONCEPT DEFINED

Curiosity

The desire of the nurse to learn or know about each person's story of a family's health concerns or problems; an openness to experiencing an altered view of any family member and/or situation as more information is revealed during a family interview.

Another example of not creating a context for change was the error of commission of the clinical nursing team becoming too "married" to a particular way of conceptualizing the family's problems or dynamics that was not in harmony with the family's conceptualization.

Blow, Sprenkle, and Davis (2007) argue that the clinician is a key change ingredient in most successful therapy and that it is the "fit" between the model and the clients' worldviews that is important. According to Miller, Hubble, and Duncan (2007, p. 28), "who provides the therapy is a much more important determinant of success than what treatment approach is provided." Fife, Whiting, Bradford, and Davis (2014, p. 24), in referring to a therapist's "way of being," states that one can be "genuine and open or impersonal and objectifying," and therefore a "therapist's way of being will influence a client's experience." We believe that these same thoughts can be adapted to nurses providing care to families—that is, *who* provides the nursing care is a much more important determinant of healing than the particular nursing interventions that are offered.

The process of developing and maintaining a respectful and collaborative relationship between the clinician and the family is one of the best predictors of success and therapeutic change (Fife et al, 2014; Garfield, 2004; Karam, Sprenkle, & Davis, 2014; Martin, Garske, & Davis, 2000).

How to Avoid Failing to Create a Context for Change

1. **Show interest, concern, and respect for each family member.** The most useful way to do this is to invite to a family meeting anyone who is involved with or concerned about the problem or illness or who is suffering as a result of it. After introducing oneself and meeting each family member, the nurse should express the desire to learn from the family how this problem or illness has affected their lives and relationships. This articulation can convey to the family that the nurse is interested and willing to learn about them and their most pressing concerns. This task will be easier to accomplish if the nurse embraces the belief that all families have strengths that are often unrealized or unappreciated (Wright & Bell, 2009).
2. **Obtain a clear understanding of the most pressing concern or greatest suffering.** Seek each family member's perspective on the problem/illness and how it affects the family and their relationships. Even if the perspectives vary, each perspective offers the nurse the best understanding of the family's challenges and sufferings.
3. **Validate and acknowledge each member's experience.** Remember that no one view is the correct, right view or the truth about the family's functioning but is each family member's unique and genuine experience. Be open to all perspectives about the family's concerns. To bring understanding to the nurse and family, not only must each member's perspective be elicited, but each member's perspective must also be valued, acknowledged, and considered important.
4. **Acknowledge suffering and the sufferer.** Health providers' acknowledgment of clients' and patients' suffering can be a powerful starting point to begin understanding a family's situation and for healing to occur (Wright, 2017; Wright & Bell, 2009). Through these efforts to understand, the nurse-family relationship is enhanced and strengthened. When nurses acknowledge their clients' or patients' suffering and are compassionate and nonjudgmental, families are often more willing to disclose fears and worries. As a result, the potential for healing, growth, and change increases.

Clinical Example

Mr. Garcia was an inpatient on a medical unit because of his chronic obstructive pulmonary disease. A woman visited frequently and was usually crying during visits. On one occasion, the primary nurse asked Mr. Garcia, *"Do you know why your wife is crying?"* He responded,

"No, this is not my wife. My wife and I are divorced. This is my sister." The nurse was somewhat embarrassed but responded, *"Oh, I'm sorry. Well, do you know why your sister is crying? She cries on every visit."* Mr. Garcia responded, *"I'm not sure."* At that point, his sister stopped crying and looked up but did not speak. The nurse then responded, *"Well, I think she is crying because she is worried that you are not going to get better if you don't stop smoking. Isn't that right?"* The sister shook her head to indicate no. At this point, Mr. Garcia stated, *"Well, it's too late even if I do stop smoking."* The nurse then said she would like to come back at another time to discuss the issue with them more fully, at this point addressing the sister for the first time. The sister replied that she did not want to meet because this was her brother's problem. The nurse accepted this response and did not have any further discussions with this family. Table 11-1 lists the errors the nurse could have avoided and the missed opportunities in working with the Garcia family.

ERROR 2: TAKING SIDES

One of the most common errors in family work is taking sides by the nurse, that is, forming an alliance with one family member or subgroup of the family. Although this is commonly done unintentionally, at times the nurse may do so deliberately, usually with a benevolent intent. However, aligning with one person or subgroup can often result in other family members feeling disrespected, disempowered, and noninfluential as the family pursues its goals with the nurse.

TABLE 11-1	Errors/Missed Opportunities
ERRORS/MISSED OPPORTUNITIES	**RATIONALE**
The nurse did not introduce herself to the woman who was visiting and made the assumption that it was the patient's wife.	Acknowledging the sister at the start may have encouraged the sister to be more forthcoming and more willing to have another meeting.
The nurse did not ask Mr. Garcia and his sister if they had any questions about his condition, worries, or concerns.	This question would provide the nurse the opportunity to validate or acknowledge any concerns or suffering they might have.
The nurse offered a quick conceptualization of the problem without obtaining the perspective of each family member and assumed that the sister is worried about the brother's smoking habit and its relationship to his recovery.	The sister denied the problem but was not asked any other therapeutic questions to ascertain the nature of her distress.

> **KEY CONCEPT DEFINED**
>
> **Taking Sides**
>
> When the nurse forms an alliance with one family member or subgroup of the family, commonly done unintentionally.

How to Avoid Taking Sides

1. **Maintain curiosity.** Be intensely interested in hearing each person's story about the health concern or problem. When each family member's perspective has been revealed, the nurse generally gains an understanding of the multiple forces interacting together to stimulate or trigger the problem. Families are always very complex, and the complexity is increased when an illness or problem emerges. Be open to experiencing an altered view of any family member and/or situation as more information is revealed. This is particularly important when nurses work with the elderly because there can be a temptation to take the side of the 55-year-old son (who is dressed in a suit) and not listen sufficiently to his 83-year-old mother lying passively in a bed in an extended care facility.

2. **Remember that the glass can be half full and half empty simultaneously.** There are multiple truths and therefore many ways to view a problem or illness. The more all-inclusive the understanding gathered from as many family members as possible, the more possible options for resolution may be derived. However, we wish to emphasize that we do not condone violence, and we do not fail to act in dangerous, illegal, or unethical situations.

3. **Ask questions that invite an exploration of both sides of a circular, interactional pattern.** Exploring each person's contribution to circular, interactional communication helps the nurse and family members understand that each person contributes to the problem rather than blaming one family member or taking one family member's side or position. (See Chapter 3 for more explanations about circular interactional patterns and the Calgary Family Assessment Model [CFAM].)

4. **Remember that all family members experience some suffering when there's a family problem or illness.** Invite family members to describe their suffering and the meaning they give to it. The nurse can also ask, "Who in the family is suffering the most?" Often it is surprising to find that the family member suffering the most is not the person with the illness diagnosis but, rather, another family member (Wright, 2017).

5. **Give relatively equal "talk time" and interest to each family member.** This, of course, may vary with very young children or family members who are only able to minimally contribute verbally, such as those who are disabled or have dementia.

6. **Remember that information is, as Bateson (1972) described it, "news of a difference."** Treat all information as a new discovery; maintain a systems or interactional perspective regarding your understanding of the illness and family dynamics.

7. **Try not to answer phone calls or have "side conversations" involving one family member "telling on" another family member.** Instead, invite the person to bring the issue to the next family meeting. Alternatively, invite one parent to ask the other parent to join in the phone conversation. In this way, the conversation is transparent for all. Sometimes, e-mailing all parties participating in the family interviews also facilitates transparency.

Clinical Example

Community health nurses and nurse practitioners are often involved in family discussions about the eating habits of children. A mother, Rose, describes her children's grandparents' eating habits as poor and how they encourage her children, Hadley and Jack, to eat high-fat food, including junk food, fried foods, and sugary desserts. Rose describes the situation at home as being hopeless and her husband, Joshua, as not being supportive in changing the children's eating habits or behaviors. However, listening to Joshua's viewpoint, the nurse hears an entirely different story about how Rose and his mother both become so incredibly tense and stressed out that they verbally release their anger and frustrations at each other. Joshua explains how Rose is in conflict with the grandparents' eating habits and how they are influencing the children's eating habits, but he doesn't see any harm with what the children are eating as long as the meals are homemade. The nurse then asks herself, "Who should I believe? Who is telling the truth?" If she sides with one parent, she worries she may alienate one parent from the other. She may miss opportunities to work with the entire family in helping them adjust to normal family functioning. This trap is especially easy to fall into if one parent negatively labels the other. For example, Joshua may say, *"You know my wife gets hysterical when she has to speak to my mother,"* or Rose may say, *"My husband is so irresponsible. He struggles with not being able to speak to his mother due to his past childhood anxiety and depression."* Table 11-2 provides strategies the nurse can use in working with this family.

Clinical Example

A family with a teenager is dealing with anorexia. Shaheena, age 16, is being seen by the unit nurse, Karin Johnson, age 51, to receive help in developing more appropriate eating habits and to increase her socialization. Shaheena has begun to successfully conquer the grip of anorexia and is very appreciative of Karin's assistance. She looks forward to individual meetings with Karin and compliments Karin frequently on wearing "cool clothes my

TABLE 11-2	Strategies for the Nurse to Avoid Taking Sides
STRATEGIES	**RATIONALE**
Ask the mother, "When your husband shows you indifference, what do you find yourself doing?"	By asking questions, the nurse is able to explore each person's contribution to circular, interactional communication, which helps the nurse and the family members understand that each member contributes to the problem rather than blaming one another.
Ask the father, "When your wife and your mother start to scream at each other, what do you do?"	The nurse provides an opportunity for each party to view the problem and to think about how they might find resolutions themselves.
Invite both parents to a meeting together to talk about the challenges involved in raising children with healthy eating habits and role modeling healthy relationships.	The nurse provides an opportunity for family members to each have equal "talk time" and gain awareness and understanding of the issues.

mother never would wear." Karin believes she and Shaheena have an "excellent" working relationship and is pleased that Shaheena likes her taste in clothes.

Karin has agreed to alternate individual meetings with Shaheena with family interviews that include both parents. During a family meeting in which Karin proudly described Shaheena's recent accomplishments on the unit, Shaheena's mom starts to downplay her daughter's successes. She tells Karin of the various "bad behaviors" Shaheena engaged in during a recent pass home. Following this, Shaheena bursts out to her mother, *"How come you do not treat me as an adult like Karin does?"*

By inadvertently aligning too much with Shaheena (e.g., around clothes and a special relationship) and not sufficiently aligning with Shaheena's parents (e.g., never seeing them as a couple alone to appreciate their challenges in raising a daughter who is in the grip of anorexia), Karin has sacrificed her ability and therapeutic leverage to be multipartial in the family meetings. Rather, the nurse is now perceived by the mother and daughter to be on the teen's side. This makes it difficult for the mother-daughter relationship to flourish and for Shaheena's mother to acknowledge her daughter's changes. Rather, Shaheena's mom may feel inadvertently competitive or usurped by the nurse. Indeed, nurses who take the side of one or more family members most often are not consciously trying to alienate, compete with, or usurp any particular family member. In fact, they are usually unaware of doing so, and thus it comes as a shock when other family members express dissatisfaction or begin to disengage or discontinue family meetings. Table 11-3 provides strategies the nurse might use in working with Shaheena and her family.

TABLE 11-3	Strategies for the Nurse to Avoid Taking Sides
STRATEGIES	**RATIONALE**
Provide time for the mother to respond to her daughter's comments, give the mother an opportunity to hear Shaheena's point of view, and then provide Shaheena time to tell her story about the problem or health concern.	By being open and maintaining curiosity, the nurse is able to gain an understanding of the multiple forces interacting to stimulate or trigger the problem. Be open to experiencing an altered view of any family member and/or situation as more information is revealed.
Ask, "Who in this relationship is suffering the most between the two of you?" Ask about each family member's strengths and build on them by asking, "Who would find it easier to believe that the other might change?"	Inviting both the mother and daughter to a meeting together to talk about their experience and challenges with the mother-daughter relationship provides an opportunity for each family member to obtain a circular view of the interaction.

ERROR 3: GIVING TOO MUCH ADVICE PREMATURELY

Nurses have abundant knowledge to offer families and are in the socially sanctioned position of offering advice, information, and opinions about matters of health promotion, health problems, illness suffering, illness management, and relationship issues. We believe, similar to Couture and Sutherland (2006), that advice can have generative and healing potential when it is offered collaboratively. Families are often keen on and receptive to nurses' expertise concerning health issues. However, each family is unique, as is each situation. Therefore, timing and judgment are critical for nurses to determine when and how to offer advice.

How to Avoid Giving Too Much Advice Prematurely

1. **Offer advice, opinions, or recommendations only after a thorough assessment has been done and a full understanding of the family's health concern or suffering has been gained and acknowledged.** Otherwise, advice and recommendations can appear too simplistic or patronizing, and the nurse can be seen as lacking an in-depth understanding. Of course, in crisis situations or in a busy emergency or intensive care unit, a full family assessment may not be possible. When families are in shock, numb, or overwhelmed, they can benefit from clear, direct advice from a nurse who, through professional experience and knowledge, can bring calm and structure in a time of crisis.

2. **Offer advice without believing that the nurse's ideas are the "best" or "better" ideas or opinions.** "Often there is a tendency and temptation

among health-care providers to offer their own understandings, their own 'better' or 'best' meanings or beliefs for clients' suffering experiences with serious illness. One way to avoid this trap of prematurely offering explanations or advice to soften suffering is to remain insatiably curious about how clients and their families are managing in the midst of suffering" (Wright, 2017). Specifically, nurses should ask themselves, *"What do family members believe, and what meaning do they give to their suffering?"* (Wright & Bell, 2009). In working with the elderly, this is particularly important. Nurses should examine their own beliefs about whether they think older adults can change or whether they hold the belief that "the elderly are too old to change their ways." Health professionals who are insatiably curious put on the armor of prevention against blame, judgment, or the need to be "right."

3. **Ask questions more than offering advice during initial conversations with families.** Asking therapeutic or reflexive questions (Tomm, 1987; Wright & Bell, 2009) invites individuals to explore and reflect on their own meanings of their health concerns or suffering, not the nurse's. Everyone, especially the elderly, has accumulated a vast reservoir of personal local wisdom and knowledge about health and wellness over the years. Hopefully, through reflections that happen in the therapeutic conversations we have with families, healing may be triggered as new thoughts, ideas, or solutions are brought forth about how a family can best live with illness (Wright, 2017).

4. **Obtain the family's response and reaction to the advice.** After offering advice, it is essential to obtain family members' reactions to the information. Specifically, does this information "fit" for the family with their own biopsychosocial-spiritual structures? We believe it is the manner in which advice is delivered, received, interpreted, and refined that is most critical in our clinical work. Relational practices and therapeutic conversations that include advice-giving are ongoing, collaborative, clarifying, and meaningful. There is a forward process to the conversation; advice-giving is not just a prescription of a particular course of action for the family to follow. (See Chapter 4 for an in-depth discussion about "fit," "meshing," and matching information offered to families with family functioning.)

Clinical Example

Gina is a 39-year-old woman on a postpartum unit following the birth of her first child via emergency cesarean section. Gina's husband, Leo, is at the bedside. The nurse walks into the room on the morning after the birth and says, *"You have to attend the breastfeeding class at 9 this morning, but first you will need to watch a video on manually expressing breastmilk."* Gina is extremely tired, sore, and overwhelmed. She is aware that her baby was given formula during the night due to the baby's low blood sugars and therefore has not given much thought to breastfeeding at this point. Gina questions what the breastfeeding course is about, then says, *"I am not even sure if I want to breastfeed my baby. I am in some pain and exhausted. Do I really need to attend right now?"* The nurse responds, *"All new moms must attend so that you learn the proper way, and we only have the class this morning."* The nurse leaves the room with the video playing on the computer. When the nurse returns to the room, she hurriedly assists Gina out of bed without further explanation, leaving Leo confused as to what is happening and where Gina is going. He can see that she is teary and frustrated, but he is not sure what he should do to help her. Table 11-4 presents the nurse's errors and missed opportunities with Gina.

Clinical Example

The Li family had recently experienced the loss of their 88-year-old father, William, who had lived with them for 10 years. Mr. Li had left Hong Kong after the death of his wife and moved to Canada to live with his son, Shen, and daughter-in-law, Ming-mei. Just 3 weeks after the death of the elderly father, Ming-mei, accompanied by Shen, presented at a walk-in medical clinic with abdominal pain. Upon concluding a medical exam, a doctor determined that there were no physical reasons for her pain. A nurse was asked to meet with the husband and wife. Shen told the story of the recent loss of his father, explaining that his wife had been the primary caregiver

TABLE 11-4	Errors/Missed Opportunities
ERRORS/MISSED OPPORTUNITIES	**RATIONALE**
The nurse offered advice prior to completing a thorough assessment of the family's health beliefs.	Without a thorough assessment, advice and recommendations can appear too simplistic or patronizing, and the nurse can be seen as lacking an in-depth understanding.
The nurse offered advice based on the nurse's ideas of "best."	The nurse's advice and responses did not "fit" with the family, and the opportunity to offer opinions and recommendations that would have been more healing was missed.
The nurse did not ask Gina or Leo questions.	Asking Gina further questions about breastfeeding would support her in exploring and reflecting on her own meaning of her health, possibly bringing forward new thoughts, ideas, or solutions.
The nurse did not attend to the responses of Gina and Leo.	Obtaining Gina and Leo's reactions to the information provided by the nurse is essential in ensuring that the information they received is a "fit" for them.

and had given up her employment to care for her father-in-law. He then offered his belief that his wife's pain was due to her extreme grief at the loss of her father-in-law. The nurse, upon hearing this story but without inquiring about the wife's extreme grief or the meaning of her loss and suffering, offered premature advice to the couple.

KEY CONCEPT DEFINED

Premature Advice

Advice given too soon by the nurse without considering timing and judgment when working with families.

To the husband, she said, *"You need to take your wife on a holiday. She is very tired after caring for your father."* To Ming-mei, she said, *"Your father-in-law was an elderly man, and his time had come. And because he was not your father, but your husband's, you will get over his passing more quickly."* Table 11-5 lists the nurse's errors and missed opportunities with the Li family.

TABLE 11-5	Errors/Missed Opportunities
ERRORS/MISSED OPPORTUNITIES	**RATIONALE**
The nurse offered premature advice.	The nurse's recommendations did not "fit" with the family, and the nurse missed the opportunity to offer opinions and recommendations that would have been more healing.
The nurse did not ask questions to complete a thorough assessment of the situation.	Asking assessment questions, such as structural assessment questions within the CFAM (see Chapter 3), the nurse would have learned that Shen owns a small coffee shop and is unable to take holidays because he is the sole provider and works 7 days a week. Ming-mei also did not find the nurse's words healing, particularly because the nurse ignored the very close relationship she had with her father-in-law.
The nurse did not recognize the Chinese culture of the Li family.	The Li family has a strong sense of honoring and caring for their elderly family members. The nurse missed a golden opportunity to commend the daughter-in-law for the care of her father-in-law. (See Chapter 4 for a more in-depth discussion of the intervention of commendations.)

CASE SCENARIO: NAIM AND SIKEENA

Naim is a 74-year-old male who was recently diagnosed with a reoccurrence of pneumonia. He lives with his 69-year-old wife, Sikeena, in their own home. Sikeena has no serious health concerns, and she and Naim have been taking care of each other with no assistance. Recently, Sikeena has been noticing Naim struggling at night with his breathing and has called the 24-hour nurse help line twice. Sikeena has voiced her concerns to their family doctor, and he has reassured her that it is due to his pulmonary disease. Naim has recently been started on oxygen at home. Sikeena is always worried about her husband. Both of their children are working abroad, and they have limited conversations with them. The couple has very few friends, and they are not active in their community.

Naim and Sikeena are attending the pulmonary outpatient clinic for a follow-up appointment regarding Naim's home oxygen use. Sikeena tells the nurse how worried she is about Naim and how she feels nervous about the home oxygen and managing it. She states, "I don't understand what is going on; it is all so confusing. I thought Naim would get better once the pneumonia went away." Naim tells the nurse, "Sikeena worries too much. I am fine; everything will work out how it is meant to be."

Reflective Questions

1. How can the nurse avoid giving Naim and Sikeena too much advice prematurely?
2. What questions could the nurse ask Naim and Sikeena to assess the context of their family structure, such as ethnicity, spirituality and/or religion, and environment?
   a. How can the nurse use this information when working with Naim and Sikeena?
3. What questions could the nurse ask Naim and Sikeena to assess the developmental life cycle for their family?
   a. How can the nurse use this information when working with Naim and Sikeena?

 CRITICAL THINKING QUESTIONS

1. Identify a situation from your clinical practice for each of the following common errors in family nursing:
   a. Failing to create a context for change
   b. Taking sides
   c. Giving too much advice prematurely
2. What contributed to each of these outcomes?
3. What strategies could you implement in future situations to avoid the errors?

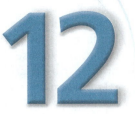

Chapter **12**

How to Terminate With Families

Learning Objectives

- Describe how to successfully terminate clinical work with families.
- Distinguish among nurse-initiated termination, family-initiated termination, and context-initiated termination.
- Identify specific skills required for therapeutic termination.
- Summarize the process for nurses to refer families to other professionals.

Key Concepts

Context-initiated termination	**Nurse-initiated termination**
Family-initiated termination	**Referral**

Knowing how to successfully conclude or terminate clinical work with families is as important as knowing how to begin—perhaps even more so. When nurses part with families, they should do so in a manner that leaves the families with hope and confidence in their new and rediscovered strengths, resources, and abilities to manage their health and/or illness and relationships. If the family has been suffering with illness, loss, or disability, then at the conclusion of the clinical work, a highly desired outcome would be eased or alleviated suffering and increased healing.

To end professional relationships with families in a therapeutic fashion is one of the most challenging aspects of the family interviewing process for nurses. Reed and Tarko (2004) make the interesting observation that, in nursing, "the issue of termination has been often discussed in psychiatric nursing texts, making it seem as if no other nursing situations have issues surrounding termination" (p. 266). Termination continues to be the least examined of the treatment phases in clinical work with families. Korhonen and Kangasniemi (2014) described nurses' experiences of terminating the primary nursing relationship with parents in a neonatal intensive care unit. Findings identified three narratives that described the relationship between the primary nurse and the parents as the relationship ended: (1) regulation of the caring relationship by creating distance, (2) regulation of the caring relationship by establishing connection, and (3) regulation of the caring relationship by creating closeness and connection. Further research is needed to examine termination between nurses and families due to the variation revealed in the narratives.

Two important aspects of concluding with families are to end the nurse-family relationship therapeutically and to do so in a manner that will sustain the progress and foster hope for the future. Nurses commonly establish very intense and meaningful relationships with families and therefore may feel guilty or fearful about initiating termination. This is especially evident in nursing practice when the relationship has been a long-standing one, over months or even years, such as in nursing homes, extended-care facilities, and clients' homes.

In this chapter, we review the process of termination by examining the decision to terminate when it is initiated by the family or the nurse or as a result of the context in which the family members find themselves. In many cases, the nurse's decision to conclude with a family does not necessarily mean that the family will cease contact with all professionals. Therefore, we also discuss the process of referring families to other health professionals. We provide specific suggestions for phasing out and concluding treatment and for evaluating the effects of the treatment process. We must emphasize that, just as other aspects of family interviewing are conducted in a collaborative manner, so, too, should the termination phase be conducted. Termination should occur with full participation and input from the family whenever possible.

DECISION TO TERMINATE

Nurse-Initiated Termination

It is important to emphasize that termination may occur before the presenting problem or illness is completely "cured" or resolved. However, it is the family's ability to master or live alongside problems or illness, although hopefully with eased emotional, physical, and spiritual suffering, that is the impetus for initiating termination. In most cases, it is unrealistic for nurses to attempt to completely eliminate the presenting concern or illness, and such a goal can frequently leave families feeling more discouraged and hopeless and nurses feeling inadequate or unhelpful. It is eased suffering or increased healing and awareness that will enable a family to live with their problems or illness in a more peaceful and manageable way. If the family's presenting concern is related to health promotion, then

greater knowledge or increased expertise by the family might be an indicator for termination.

KEY CONCEPT DEFINED

Nurse-Initiated Termination

The ending of the nurse-client relationship by the nurse.

In nurse-initiated termination, the termination stage evolves easily if the
beginning and middle phases of engagement and treatment have progressed
successfully. However, the most difficult decision for any nurse to make
in regard to termination relates to time. When is the right time for termination? This question is directly related to the new views, beliefs, ideas,
and solutions that the family and nurse have generated to resolve current
problems. If new solution options have been discovered, and consequently,
the family functions differently, particularly with the presenting concern, it
is time to terminate because change has occurred. The skills necessary for
nurse-initiated termination are given in the "Phasing Out and Concluding
Treatment" section of this chapter and in Chapter 5.

In contexts where family meetings have occurred over time, then the
nurse and family may collaboratively decide that additional meetings are
not necessary. In these situations, the termination phase of treatment has
begun. First and most importantly during this phase, we prefer to help families expand their perspectives to focus on strengths, positive behaviors, and
changes in beliefs or feelings that have occurred or reemerged rather than
focus exclusively on troublesome or problematic behaviors. We encourage
families not to associate these new behaviors with our work but instead
with their own efforts. For example, we would ask a family what positive
changes they have noticed over the last 3 months rather than ask what positive changes they have noticed since working with a nurse.

White and Epston (1990) offer another useful clinical idea for nurses
terminating with families; they recommend that the interviewer "expand
the audience" to describe and acknowledge the family's unique outcomes
and progress. We commonly ask families to tell us what advice they would
have for other families confronting similar health problems. Sometimes
we have families write letters to other families to offer suggestions regarding what has or has not worked in coping with a particular illness. It is
essential that the family that wrote the letter has given permission for the
letter to be sent. A scoping review conducted by Henderson, Johnson, and
Moodie (2014) of parent-to-parent support resulted in the revision of their
previously developed framework of parent-to-parent support for parents of
children who are deaf or hard of hearing. The revised framework identifies
a parent as being either a supporting parent (mentor) or learning parent in a

peer partnership. The supporting parent can act as an advocate and empower the learning parent to build competence and confidence through his or her own lived experience. With the increasing use of technology and social media, new ways to connect with people to access support are being developed. One format is an online discussion forum. McKechnie, Barker, and Stott (2014) implemented an online support forum for caregivers of people with dementia; participants report "unique benefits from online peer support, such as not feeling alone and feeling understood through shared experiences."

When the nurse initiates termination of the therapeutic relationship, the emphasis throughout this process is to identify, affirm, amplify, and solidify the changes that have taken place within and between family members. Consequently, it is essential that change be distinguished to become a reality (Bell & Wright, 2011; Wright & Bell, 2009). One way to distinguish change is to obtain the perspective of family members. The nurse can accomplish this by asking questions such as, *"What changes do you notice in your wife since she has adopted this new idea that 'illness is a family affair'?"* or *"What else would your family or friends notice that is different in you since your depression about experiencing cancer has dissipated?"*

Initiating rituals at the time of termination can also emphasize change and give families the courage to live their lives without the involvement of health-care professionals. If the initial concern involves a child, we have had parties (balloons, cake, and all) to celebrate the child's mastery of the particular problem, whether it is enuresis, fighting fears, or putting chronic pain in its place. In addition, we have given children certificates indicating that they have overcome their problems. This practice helps families to acknowledge change through celebration.

Some clinical settings send a closing letter at the end of the clinical work to each family highlighting what the clinical nursing team has learned from the family and what ideas the team offered the family (Bell, Moules, & Wright, 2009; Moules, 2002, 2003, 2009; Wright & Bell, 2009). These therapeutic letters serve as closing rituals. They provide the opportunity to highlight the family's strengths and document in a personal way the family and individual interventions that were offered. The letters also acknowledge that family nursing is not a one-way street with nurses assisting families. Rather, by stating what the nurse and clinical team have learned from the family, the nurse honors the reciprocal and relational influence between the family and the clinical nursing team. More information about therapeutic closing letters is provided in Chapter 4.

Family-Initiated Termination

When a family takes the initiative to terminate, it is very important for the nurse to acknowledge their desire and then to gain more explicit information in a nonjudgmental fashion regarding their reasons for wanting to terminate. This information helps the nurse to understand the family's responses to the interviewing process. Has the family discovered new solutions to their problems or challenged their beliefs to ease their suffering? For example, have they found a way to have a respite from caring for their ill child without feeling excessive guilt? Has the family challenged some of their constraining beliefs about the illness experience (Bell & Wright, 2011; Wright & Bell, 2009)? For example, have they now stopped blaming themselves for the husband suffering a coronary in part because of having to work two jobs? Are the family and nurse able to identify and agree on significant changes that have occurred in both individual and family functioning? Is the family also aware of how to sustain these changes? For example, if a son refuses to give his own insulin injections in the future, what will the family do differently?

KEY CONCEPT DEFINED

Family-Initiated Termination

The ending of the nurse-client relationship by the family.

If the family specifically states that they wish to terminate but the nurse believes this would be premature or even enhance their suffering, it is important for the nurse to take the initiative to review the family's decision. In so doing, the nurse reconceptualizes the progress the family has made and recognizes what problems remain and what goals and solutions might yet be achieved.

One way to do this is to have family members discuss with one another their desires to continue or discontinue sessions and explore who most disfavors termination. Also, the specifics of the decision may be helpful, such as when the family decided to terminate and what prompted the decision. After establishing who is most eager to continue, the nurse can invite that family member to share with the other family members the anticipated benefit of further sessions. It is helpful for families to be specific and emphasize the benefits that could be achieved if family interviewing were to continue. However, there are times when termination is inevitable. At such a point, it is reasonable and ethical to accept the family's initiative to terminate and to do so without applying undue pressure, even though the nurse may disagree with their decision.

We strongly urge nurses not to engage in linear blame of either families or themselves when they believe that families have prematurely or abruptly left treatment. Rather, we encourage nurses to hypothesize about the factors that may have contributed to the termination. These factors may include such nurse-related behaviors as being too aligned with the children, too slow to intervene, or too "married" to a particular hypothesis about the family's functioning or not attending to the family's main concern (see Chapter 11 for errors to avoid). Family-related behaviors such as concurrent involvement with other agencies should also be considered.

Nurses may also encounter cases in which family members state that they want to continue treatment but initiate termination indirectly. Indications include late arrivals for meetings, missed appointments, and the absence from sessions of certain family members who were asked to attend. Another indicator that families are perhaps considering termination is their expression of dissatisfaction with the course of treatment or complaints about the logistical difficulties of attending or the loss of time from work. In these situations, we suggest that the same steps be taken as when the family initiates termination directly.

The challenge of family-initiated termination is to determine whether it is premature. It could be, as Slive and Bobele (2011) suggest, that the family has received all the assistance they needed and choose not to return for meetings. In the nursing literature, there is a dearth of research to provide insights into reasons for premature termination. Therefore, nurses must rely on their own clinical judgment to ascertain if termination is premature. Future research studies should address this area in nursing practice with families who are seen on an outpatient basis.

In our clinical experience, we have found that families who miss the first meeting are at high risk for dropping out over the course of treatment. The implication of missed appointments refers back to the importance of the engagement stage and even to the initial contact with families on the telephone. We have also found that the referral source has a direct correlation with the family's continuing treatment. Families who are referred by institutions (such as a school or court) are more likely to discontinue treatment before achieving treatment goals than families who were individually referred (such as by physicians or mental health professionals). Families who are self-referred tend to complete the treatment process.

It is critically important to help families understand the nature of the treatment contract. Many families' understandings of what takes place in family interviewing are markedly different than the understandings held by nurses. Therefore, these families may relate to nurses as they do to physicians, imams, or clergy, whereby they use the services as they wish and discontinue when they desire. For this reason, we find it particularly useful when seeing families on an outpatient basis to contract for a certain number of sessions and then reevaluate as progress occurs. This approach may help to prevent premature or abrupt termination. It also keeps the focus on time-effective, change-oriented conversation.

Context-Initiated Termination

In some settings, such as hospitals (particularly those in managed health-care systems), it is not the nurse or the family who initiates termination but the health-care system or insurance company. In these situations, it is very important for the nurse to assess whether the family needs further treatment on an outpatient basis or can continue to resolve problems and discover solutions on their own. If the family needs to be referred, the nurse requires some specific skills in this area. The referral process is discussed in a later section of this chapter.

KEY CONCEPT DEFINED

Context-Initiated Termination

When neither the nurse nor client initiates termination of the nurse-client relationship; instead, termination occurs due to the context, such as the health-care system or the insurance company.

PHASING OUT AND CONCLUDING TREATMENT

In Chapter 5, we highlighted some of the specific skills required for therapeutic termination in the form of learning objectives. We will now expand on these particular skills.

Review Contracts

For families seen on an outpatient basis, we strongly encourage periodic review of the present status of the family's problems and changes. The use of a contract for a specific number of sessions provides a built-in way to set a time limit to the meetings and to ensure periodic review. In one outpatient clinic, all families contracted for four sessions and then evaluated change (Wright & Bell, 2009). In some cases, four sessions were not necessary; families could save unused sessions to be used at a later time if desired. If the family required additional sessions at the conclusion of the four-session contract, then another contract was made between the family and the nurse, and reevaluation occurred again at the end of those sessions. However, as discussed in Chapter 9, there is evidence that time-effective single-session therapy has demonstrated its effectiveness and client satisfaction with the outcomes (Hopkins, Lee, McGrane, & Barbara-May, 2017; Hymmen, Stalker, & Cait, 2013; Slive & Bobele, 2012; Stalker et al, 2016).

Contracts help nurse interviewers to be mindful of the progress and direction of their work with families rather than seeing families endlessly and without purpose beyond the vague good intention of "helping." We prefer a designated number of sessions to open-ended sessions. However, nurses need to be flexible about the frequency and duration of sessions. Normally, the frequency decreases as problems improve, suffering has eased, and confidence and hopefulness have increased. Periodic reviews allow family members the opportunity to express their pleasure or displeasure with the progress that is being made.

Decrease Frequency of Sessions

When adequate progress has been made, as evidenced by reduced suffering, the time is ideal to begin to decrease the frequency of sessions. In our experience, we have found that families are able to work toward termination more readily and with more confidence when they recognize the improvement in their own ability to solve problems. However, many family members find it difficult to acknowledge changes. In these circumstances, we suggest the use of a question such as, *"What would each of you have to do to bring the problem back?"* to elicit a more explicit understanding or statement from family members regarding the changes that have been made.

Another significant time to decrease the frequency of sessions is when the nurse has inadvertently fostered undue dependency. We have had many family situations presented to us in which nursing students or professional nurses provide "paid friendship" with mothers. These nurses have become the mother's major support system because they have failed to mobilize other supports, such as husbands, friends, or relatives. In situations in which this dependency has occurred and is recognized, we strongly suggest that the nurse help foster other supports for the family and decrease the frequency of sessions. Regular consultation with colleagues or a supervisor will assist the nurse to ascertain if a dependent relationship has occurred between the nurse and the family.

If a nurse encounters hesitancy or a reluctance to decrease the frequency of sessions or to terminate completely, the nurse should encourage a discussion of the fears related to termination and solicit support from other family members. It has been our experience that family members commonly fear that if sessions are decreased or discontinued, they will not be able to cope with their problems or their problems will become worse. Thus, asking a question such as, *"What are you most concerned would happen if we discontinued our meetings now?"* can get to the core of the matter very quickly. By clarifying family members' fears openly, other family members (who may be less fearful) have an opportunity to provide support.

Give Credit for Change

Nurses often choose the nursing profession because they have a strong desire to help individuals and families obtain optimal health and ease their suffering. Their efforts are usually helpful, and they are commonly given all or much of the credit for the changes and improvements. However, it has been our experience in family work that it is vitally important that the family receive the credit for change. There are several reasons for this:

- Families experience the tension, conflict, suffering, and anxiety of working through problems related to their health or illness and relationships; therefore, they deserve the credit for improvement.
- If the identified patient is a child and the nurse accepts credit for change, the nurse can be seen to be in a competitive relationship with the parents.
- Perhaps the most important reason for giving the family credit for change is that doing so increases the chance that the positive effects of treatment will last. Otherwise, the nurse may inadvertently convey the message that the family members cannot manage without the nurse, and they will become indebted or too dependent. Termination provides an opportune time to comment on the positive changes that have already happened during the course of treatment.
- Praising the family members for their accomplishments in having helped or corrected the original presenting problem provides them with confidence to handle future problems. Statements such as *"You did the work"* or *"You people are being far too modest"* can reinforce to family members the idea that their efforts were essential in making the change.

It is never possible to know for certain what precipitated, perturbed, or initiated the change that occurs within families. In many cases, nurses create a context for change by helping family members explore solution options to their difficulties or suffering. Wright and Bell (2009) suggest that creating a context for change constitutes the central and enduring foundation of the therapeutic process. They further propose that it is not just a necessary prerequisite to the process of therapeutic change; it is therapeutic change in and of itself. Sometimes the very effort of bringing family members together in a room to discuss important family issues and their suffering can be the most significant intervention. This is further supported by Benzein, Olin, and Persson (2015), who indicate that family conversations have a positive impact on families and facilitate healing. Family conversations provide members the opportunity to share their stories with each other about their illness experience, providing meaning and strengthening family cohesion.

If families present themselves at termination with concerns about progress, nurses must express their appreciation for the family's positive efforts to solve problems constructively, even when no significant improvement has occurred. In such cases, we strongly recommend that nurses discuss with their clinical supervisors some hypotheses about why the interview sessions did not seem to be effective. Perhaps the goals of the family or the nurse were too high or demanding. If a family does not progress, it is usually the result of the nurse's inability to discover an intervention that "fits" or "meshes" with the family. Too often, nurses excuse themselves from making further efforts to intervene by labeling families as noncompliant, unmotivated, or resistant (Wright & Levac, 1992). However, it is very important that nurses believe that families have worked hard despite minimal progress, and it is important to praise them for having done so. Whittaker (2015) identified the importance of the nurse understanding the process of knowing what the patient is experiencing and moving away from simply telling the patient what to do; the goal is to develop a therapeutic relationship with the individual rather than allowing the patient to become a "passive recipient of care" (p. 12). However, we do not mean to imply that because we are encouraging nurses to give families the credit for change that the nurse cannot enjoy the change. Family work can be very rewarding, and certainly, the nurse is part of the change process.

Evaluate Family Interviews

It is important to provide a formal closure to the end of the treatment process with a face-to-face discussion whenever possible. Madsen (2007) refers to this part of the termination process as a *consolidation interview*. In a consolidation or termination interview, the nurse asks particular questions to review the process of the work that the family and clinician have done together and then discusses the work the family seeks to accomplish on its own in the future. This kind of interview is a way to reduce feelings of anxiety, fear, or loss on the part of the clinician, family, or both.

During this final session, it is very valuable to evaluate the effectiveness of the treatment process and the effect of changes on various family members. We recommend evaluating the impact not only on the whole-family system but also on various subsystems, such as the marital subsystem and individual family member functions. Questions to invite reflections from the family about its changes include the following:

- "What have you learned about yourself and amyotrophic lateral sclerosis?"
- "What have you come to appreciate about your marriage?"
- "What have you come to understand is the most effective way you can live with your grief?"

We also believe in sharing the family's wisdom and will frequently ask, *"When you meet with other families with chronic illness, from what you know now, what would you advise them or offer them?"*

An even more dramatic evaluation can occur by having each family member and the nurse write about their reflections on the family meetings, emphasizing what they learned, what has changed, and what new ideas or beliefs they have about their problems or illness.

We also suggest asking family members the following questions:

- "What things did you find most and least helpful during our work together?"
- "What things did you wish or were hoping would happen during our work together that did not?"

- "Based on what you've accomplished and learned, what suggestions do you have for me or other nurses in trying to help other families suffering with similar issues?"

This behavior demonstrates that the nurse is also open and receptive to feedback. It is important at this time that the nurse does not become defensive to any of the feedback. Rather, the nurse can express appreciation to the family and inform them that this feedback will assist and educate him or her to be even more helpful in work with future families. Participatory evaluation research turns the traditional evaluation process on its head. Nurses are no longer the experts, but instead, their role is that of a facilitator of information who empowers families to understand and prepare for health outcomes (Adams, Mannix, & Harrington, 2017).

Extend an Invitation for Follow-Up

Nurses often place themselves or are placed in situations of "follow-up." However, follow-up is frequently a negative experience for both the nurse and the family. For example, community health nurses (CHNs) have reported that they are often requested to "check on" family members to assess their functioning. However, those who request the visit (such as physicians or departments of child welfare) often make no clear statement to the family about the purpose of the visit. Follow-up in this manner can give a very unfortunate and unpleasant message to the family that further problems are anticipated. Therefore, the nurse is in a very awkward position. We strongly discourage nurses from placing themselves in these kinds of situations unless there has been clear, direct communication with the family by the requesting party. It is better to make clear to the family that progress has been made and that the sessions are finished. However, if they would like input again in the future, indicate that you would be willing to see them. Families usually appreciate knowing that backup support by professionals is available to them in times of stress.

For nurses employed in hospitals, a follow-up session is usually not possible, but referral can be made to a CHN, emergency room outreach worker, or home-care nurse if deemed appropriate. Our experience has been that families do appreciate knowing whether they will have future contact with the nurse who has worked intimately with them.

KEY CONCEPT DEFINED

Referral

A nurse's recommendation for other individuals, services, or health-care providers to be involved in the care of the family in collaboration/consultation with the nurse or to take over the care of the family independent of the nurse.

Closing Letters

Another way to punctuate the end of treatment positively is to send the family a letter giving a summary of the family sessions. This letter provides the opportunity to highlight the family's strengths, reinforce the changes made, offer the family a review of their efforts and what they have accomplished, and list the ideas (interventions) that were offered to them (Bell, Moules, & Wright, 2009; Hougher Limacher & Wright, 2006; Moules, 2002, 2003, 2009; Wright, 2005; Wright & Bell, 2009). Many families have commented about how much they appreciate the letters and how they frequently refer to them. Additional information about therapeutic closing letters is provided in Chapter 4.

Therapeutic letters, whether sent during clinical work with families or at the end of treatment, have proved a very useful and often potent intervention to invite families to reflect on ideas offered within the session and on changes they have made over the course of sessions (Bell, Moules, & Wright 2009; Hougher Limacher & Wright, 2006; Moules, 2002, 2003; Watson & Lee, 1993; White & Epston, 1990; Wright, 2005; Wright & Bell, 2009; Wright & Nagy, 1993; Wright & Watson, 1988).

The following example illustrates a typical closing letter:

> Dear Family Barbosa:
> Greetings from the Family Nursing Unit. We had the opportunity to meet with various members of your family on eight occasions. We have also had several phone conversations with both Venicio and Fatima in recent months.
>
> **What Our Team Offered Your Family**
> Throughout our work together, our clinical nursing team has been very impressed with your family. Although a great many challenges have been presented to all of you over the past years, your family was able to overcome many obstacles and search for ways of helping each other through these difficult times.
>
> - We offered you the idea that most families find it very difficult to talk openly about an impending loss or death of a family member but that talking can be very healing. You have shown us that this was the case in your family.
> - We offered you a few books to read about other families who have experienced a similar tragedy as yours.
> - We offered you the idea that resolving issues in a relationship that has been conflictual can bring great peace and comfort, particularly following the death of a loved one.
>
> **What Our Team Learned From Your Family**
> Our experience with your family has taught our clinical nursing team a great deal. The following is a synthesis:
>
> - Families that have a member dealing with a life-shortening illness have the strength to deal with unresolved issues of

blame, guilt, and shame. Even though there has been a great deal of pain and hurt in a family, they can heal their relationships and move on.

- Although it can be a common response for family members to distance themselves from the possibility of death with a life-shortening illness and to be afraid of dying, it is possible for them to make peace with each other and find peace in themselves, giving them the courage to go on.
- Although a mother and son may reside in different places and may not see each other often, they can still play a significant part in each other's lives. No matter how old a child and parent are, the knowledge that they love and accept each other for who they are can make a significant difference in their lives.
- The uncertainty involved with a life-shortening illness can be the most difficult thing for families to handle. Family members can help each other with the uncertainty by discussing the situation openly among themselves.
- Grandparents and grandsons have very special relationships that are different from those of parents and sons.

As you all continue to face the many challenges that are ahead, we trust that you will draw on your own special strengths as well as on more open communication to help you meet these challenges. It was truly a privilege to work with you. We wish you continued strength for the future.

Should you desire further consultation at any time, you can arrange this by contacting the Family Nursing Unit's secretary. A research assistant will be in contact with you in approximately 6 months to ask you to participate in our outcome study to ascertain your satisfaction with the Family Nursing Unit.

Sincerely,
Jane Nagy, RN   Lorraine M. Wright, RN, PhD
Master's Student   Director, Family Nursing Unit
                       Professor, Faculty of Nursing

REFERRAL TO OTHER PROFESSIONALS

Referral to other professionals may be advisable for various reasons. In this section, we discuss some specific tasks that are required to make a smooth transition for the family from one professional to another. First, however, see Table 12-1, in which we provide some of the more common reasons for nurses to refer families to other professionals. With the expanding specialty areas within nursing, it is becoming impossible and totally unrealistic to expect nurses to be experts in all areas. Nurses need to be open to referring

TABLE 12-1	Reasons for Referral to Other Professionals	
COMMON REASONS FOR REFERRAL	**WHO MAY BE INVOLVED**	**CLINICAL EXAMPLES**
The complexity of the family may require additional resources.	Multidisciplinary professionals	■ Senior experiencing temporal headaches; neurologist consulted, and treatment is suspended with the nurse until the consultation is complete. ■ Young adult experiencing depression and thoughts of suicide; mental health crisis center consulted, and treatment with the nurse continues in conjunction with the other professionals. ■ A family experiencing a recent death of one of its members; grief support center consulted, and treatment with the nurse continues in conjunction with the other professionals.
A family moves, is transferred to another setting, or is discharged before treatment is over.	Interdisciplinary professionals	■ A pediatric nurse discharges a child with reoccurring hospital admissions due to asthma exacerbations. Following a family interview, the family is referred to community mental health nurse for ongoing care due to family dynamics that may be causing the asthma exacerbations.

individuals or entire families for consultation without perceiving this as an inadequacy in their repertoire of skills. To refer wisely, nurses need extensive knowledge of the professional resources within the community. Some of the specific skills required in making appropriate referrals are described in the following paragraphs.

Prepare Families

Nurses must adequately prepare families so that they understand the nature of the referral to a new professional. Useful referrals can be done by explaining to families the reason for the referral and why the nurse feels that the family would benefit from it. Another method that can be useful for ensuring openness and clarity about the nature of the referral is for the nurse to write a summary and then to review this summary with the family. This summary can then be sent to the new professional and a copy made available to the family. In this way, the family is not left wondering what information will be shared with the new professional. Also, an important implicit message is given that their information is confidential and private, so they have a right to know what is shared.

Selecting a new professional can sometimes pose a challenge. If a nurse is known in the community, it is wise to solicit the help of colleagues for ideas and advice on which agencies or professionals are best for the type of treatment needed or to seek information from community information directories, booklets, and online resources.

Meet the New Professional

It has been our experience that the transition to the new professional is much more effective and efficient if the nurse can be present with the family at the first meeting. In this way, a more personal referral is made. It often reduces the fears and anxieties that families may have about starting "fresh" with someone new. Before the referral, opportunities should be given to the family to express concerns or ask questions about the referral. At the first meeting, the family may wish to clarify with the new professional their expectations and understanding of the reason for the referral, and any misconceptions can be dealt with at that time. A conjoint meeting with the family, nurse, and new professional can also serve as a "marker" for the end of the nurse's relationship with the family.

Keep Appropriate Boundaries

Despite increased interdisciplinary collaboration in health care, it is still very important that when a family has been referred, boundaries of responsibility are clear. Otherwise, there is a potential for the nurse to inadvertently become triangulated between the family and the new professional. For example, a home-care nurse regularly visited an elderly patient who lived with her adult daughter. The purpose of the visits by the home-care nurse was to assist with colostomy care. The nurse observed and assessed a severe and long-standing conflict between the elderly parent and the adult daughter. This conflict was having a negative effect, deterring the elderly patient from assuming more responsibility for her physical care. Because of her family assessment skills, the nurse was able to make an important referral to a family therapy program where more in-depth work on the intergenerational conflict began. However, in future visits, the elderly patient expressed to the nurse complaints about the adult daughter that the patient was not discussing in the family meetings. Also, the family therapist called the nurse and asked the nurse to apply pressure on the elderly parent to be more cooperative in attending sessions. Thus, very quickly, the nurse had become "caught in the middle" between the family and the therapist.

The nurse dealt with the situation by requesting to join in a meeting with the family and the therapist to clarify the expectations of all parties. In this one session, the nurse was able to "detriangulate" herself from any alliance by clarifying her present role with the family and the new professional. See Chapter 3 for more discussion about alliances and coalitions.

Transfers

In our clinical experience, we have not found the practice of transferring families from one clinician to another to be very successful. We view the process of transfers as very different from referrals. A referral is usually made to another health-care professional with different expertise. A transfer, on the other hand, is usually made to another colleague of similar expertise and competence. We recommend, if possible, that nurses conclude treatment with the families they are working with rather than transfer them to other colleagues. In our experience, a family frequently will disengage with the new nurse in various ways (e.g., by missing appointments, not showing up, or not stating any particular concern). It is understandable that a family does not wish to "start over" with another nurse. We hypothesize that transfers are frequently made to assuage the nurse's feelings about leaving versus the family's desires about continuing treatment.

If, however, a transfer is necessary, we recommend that the current nurse use language indicating an ending of the relationship with the family. For example, the nurse can say, *"Now that my work with you is coming to an end, what would you like to work on with Sanjeshna, the new nurse?"* In addition, we encourage the new nurse to directly ask the family members about their relationships with previous nurses. Such questions as *"What do you anticipate will be different in our work together versus your work with Li?"* are useful. This type of conversation punctuates a change rather than a continuance of the same work. It fosters engagement and is important for the new nurse and the family in establishing a collaborative relationship.

Another way to increase engagement is for the current nurse to ask the family to take a break before the family initiates setting up an appointment with the new nurse. This again emphasizes the change in the working relationship and encourages the family to be self-directive in initiating the new contact rather than simply responding to the professionals.

Success of Treatment in Family Work

Although interventions may obtain positive and possibly dramatic results during treatment, the real success of family work is the positive changes that are maintained or continue to evolve weeks and months after nurses have terminated treatment with particular families. We strongly encourage professional nurses and nursing students to make it a pattern of practice to obtain data from the families regarding outcomes in order to determine best practices. When nurses focus on outcomes, they orient their work toward change, focus on problems that can be changed, and think about how families will cope without them in the future. We also suggest that nurses explain to families that follow-up is a normal pattern of practice (e.g., by saying, *"We normally contact families with whom we have worked within 6 months to gain information on how things are evolving"*). It is also important to use this follow-up contact and have specific goals in mind. A very useful reason for follow-up can be for research purposes. In our experience, beginning family nurse interviewers tend to be more focused on what is going on in the family, whereas more experienced nurses focus on more specific goals for treatment.

To facilitate evaluation, we suggest formalizing follow-up of families, particularly those seen on an outpatient basis, by live interview, questionnaire, telephone, e-mail, or online survey. At present, we favor the use of a face-to-face discussion and questionnaire that is answered by all available family members.

One outcome study at an outpatient education and research clinic, namely, the Family Nursing Unit, University of Calgary (Bell, 2008; Wright & Bell, 2009), was designed to evaluate the services provided to families. The variables examined in this study were the family's satisfaction with the services provided, satisfaction with the nurse interviewer, and change in the presenting problem and family relationships. A semistructured questionnaire designed for this study asked for each family member's perspective on each of the variables. Questions were asked in relation to two periods: at the conclusion of the family sessions and at the time of the survey. Results from the survey indicated that the most helpful aspects of family sessions were the opportunity to ventilate family concerns, thereby increasing communication among family members, and to obtain support from the clinical nursing team. Families ranked the interview process and the suggestions from the clinical nursing team as the second most helpful aspects.

Family members reported satisfaction with nurse interviewers, who were either master's or doctoral students or faculty members specializing in family systems nursing. They indicated that the friendly, professional, and nonthreatening manner of the graduate nursing students made them comfortable. More than 75% of the family members reported that the presenting problem was better at the time of the survey. Regardless of the presenting problem, positive changes in the marital relationship, such as increased communication, improved relationships, and decreased tension, were also reported, suggesting support for the systems-theory tenet that change in one part of the system creates change in other parts.

This type of outcome study suggests that change should be evaluated at the individual, parent-child, marital, and family system levels. We believe that a higher level of positive change has occurred when improvement is evidenced in systemic (total family) or relationship (dyadic) interactions than when it is evidenced in individuals alone—that is, individual change does not logically require system change, but stable system change does require individual change and relationship change, and relationship change requires individual changes.

Nurses can contribute significantly to family outcome research by focusing on follow-up with families in which particular family members experience a health problem. This area of family work is just beginning to be researched and lends itself beautifully to the active involvement of nurses in its evolution.

CASE SCENARIO: FINN AND MILA

Finn, 93 years old, lives with his wife, Mila, 88 years old, in their two-story home in a small town. They have been married for 70 years. Finn has a history of hypertension, osteoarthritis, and type 2 diabetes. He recently fell at home and was hospitalized for 2 months. During his hospitalization, his mobility decreased, and he now requires full assistance with bathing, grooming, and toileting. Finn has also developed issues with swallowing and requires close monitoring while eating. At a recent family meeting with his health-care team in the hospital, it was determined that he is not able to return to his home and will require full-time care in a long-term care facility because Mila is not able to provide his care due to her own mobility problems. Over the 2-month hospitalization, the primary nurse caring for Finn has developed a very meaningful therapeutic relationship with Finn and Mila. Mila visits almost every day unless she is feeling unwell herself. Mila has shared with the primary nurse her fears and concerns about Finn moving to long-term care and her staying alone in their home. Mila has been teary during conversations with the nurse and has expressed her fear of loneliness and the uncertainty of the future. She states: *"I wish you could be the nurse at the long-term care facility caring for Finn. I know you and trust you."* Finn will be discharged to long-term care in 1 week.

Reflective Questions

1. What strategies could the primary nurse implement to ensure that the termination of the nurse-family relationship fosters hope for Mila and Finn?
2. How would the nurse discuss the possibility of a referral as an additional intervention with Mila and Finn?
   a. What factors should the nurse consider if completing a referral in this situation?

CRITICAL THINKING QUESTIONS

1. Identify barriers to therapeutic termination with families in your practice area. What are potential solutions to these barriers?
2. Provide an example of a closing letter you would write to a family relevant to your practice area.
3. Reflect on experiences working with families in your practice area when therapeutic termination was a positive experience. What contributed to this outcome?
4. Reflect on experiences working with families in your practice area when therapeutic termination was a negative experience. What contributed to this outcome?

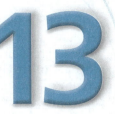
Pulling It All Together

This chapter provides an in-depth example of a family interview using the Calgary Family Assessment Model (CFAM) and the Calgary Family Intervention Model (CFIM) utilizing a clinical case example.

CASE EXAMPLE: The O'Shanell Family

The O'Shanell family consists of Ray (48 years old), Mary (47 years old), and their three children: 10-year-old Cameron, 13-year-old Saara, and 15-year-old Grace. Mary's mother, Rose (82 years old), has just moved into their home because she can no longer live independently. Rose's husband, Alfred, died in 2016 of colon cancer at age 82. His death was very difficult for the family. Cameron asks many questions about his grandfather and his death, and Rose does not like to speak about it.

Ray works as an engineer, and Mary was working as a teacher until Rose moved in. Mary has quit her job to take care of her mother. Mary is very close to her mother and finds Rose to be a strong source of support. Ray smokes half a pack of cigarettes a day and was diagnosed with hypertension 6 months ago.

Ray's parents are both alive; his mother, June, is age 75, and his father, Ken, is age 78. Ray has one sister, Rebecca, who is 39 years old and is married to Wesley, who is 51 years old. They have two boys, 12-year-old Logan and 3-year-old Cole. Ray is not close to any of his family, except for Wesley. He talks to Wesley on a weekly basis.

Rose has pain and limited mobility because of rheumatoid arthritis, and she is being assessed for early stages of Alzheimer disease at a Medicare clinic. The main reason why Mary insisted that her mother move in with the family is her mother's increasing forgetfulness since the death of Alfred, which has led Mary to have increasing concern about her mother's safety.

The O'Shanell children are active in their schools and the community and have very busy schedules. Cameron and Saara play soccer twice a week and take drama lessons every week. Ray and Mary have a complex schedule of driving the children to and picking them up from various activities. The children spend several hours a day on the Internet and chatting on their phones, especially Grace, who spends the majority of her time out with her friends; when she is home, she wants to be alone in her room.

Mary has recently become interested in using the Internet to visit health-related websites and explore her mother's forgetfulness. She has been sharing the information she has learned from the Internet with her children. Mary likes to take care of everyone in her immediate and extended family. Mary states that she has always had difficulties sleeping, but lately she is finding that it is becoming more difficult.

Once the nurse and the O'Shanell family have decided to meet, the nurse will begin to consider the process for the initial family interview. This process involves the following stages outlined in Chapter 7, which will be used as guidelines for the nurse and the family to provide structure:

- Engagement
- Assessment
- Intervention
- Termination

ENGAGEMENT

When working with the O'Shanell family, the nurse will initially consider the ABCs of engaging families (Chapter 7) to promote a positive nurse-family relationship. Table 13-1 provides examples of how this may occur between the O'Shanell family and the nurse.

TABLE 13-1	The ABCs of Engaging the O'Shanell Family	
A	B	C
Assume an active, confident approach by identifying who is present during the initial meetings and finding out how they were invited to the meeting. Does everyone know why they are at the meeting?	Begin by talking to the O'Shanell family about the length and number of meeting times, the context for meetings, and the purpose of the meetings.	Clarify expectations about your role with the O'Shanell family based on mutual trust. Create a context of mutual trust with the O'Shanell family.

TABLE 13-1	The ABCs of Engaging the O'Shanell Family—cont'd	
A	**B**	**C**
Ask the O'Shanell family purposeful questions to obtain family assessment data, such as names, ages, occupations, and school/grade, by completing a genogram (Figure 13-1) and an ecomap (Figure 13-2).	Behave in a curious manner by hypothesizing and using circularity to demonstrate non-judgmental behavior and acceptance of each member of the O'Shanell family.	Collaborate with the O'Shanell family members in decision making, health promotion, and health maintenance.
Address all of the O'Shanell family members present at the initial meeting and spend an equal amount of time with each family member initially.	Build on the O'Shanell family strengths, such as willingness to seek out new information and help, commitment to caring for an aging parent, family integrity, and loving and caring.	Cultivate a context of racial and ethnic sensitivity where personal values and beliefs are acknowledged and nonjudgmental relationships are formed.
Adjust the conversation to consider the O'Shanell children's (Cameron, Saara, Grace) developmental stages during conversations: ■ Piaget (1969): Cameron—concrete operations, Saara—formal operations, Grace—formal operations ■ Erikson (1963): Cameron—industry vs. inferiority, Saara—identity vs. role confusion, Grace identity vs. role confusion	Bring relevant resources available for use during the meetings with the O'Shanell family, such as information about home-care services, Alzheimer support groups, chronic disease management services, and teen groups.	Commendations: "I commend your commitment to attending the meetings and seeking support to optimize the health of your family." "I commend your ability to acknowledge the difficulties you are having with all of the changes that are occurring since Rose moved in." "I commend your willingness and commitment to providing care for Rose."

ASSESSMENT

Once the nurse and the family have established a therapeutic relationship, the nurse will begin the assessment stage. Box 13-1 provides an example of how the assessment stages are applied to the O'Shanell family, utilizing the CFAM branching diagram.

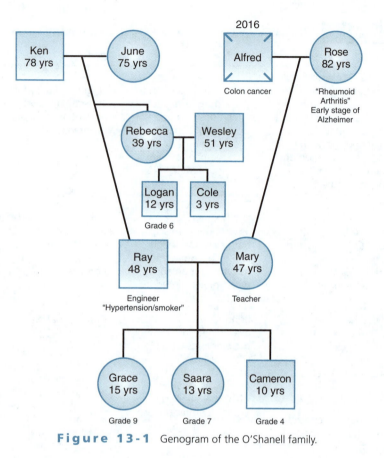

Figure 13-1 Genogram of the O'Shanell family.

Problem Identification

After the O'Shanell family is assessed, the problems the family members are facing can be summarized as follows:

FAMILY MEMBER	PROBLEM
Ray	"Mary's mother Rose moving in with us was such a large transition for the family. Everyone seems so frustrated with each other."
Mary	"Ray worries more since I quit my job. He just needs to stop smoking so that his blood pressure gets better. I just can't seem to get enough sleep."
Grace	"They don't understand anything about my life."
Cameron	"Why doesn't grandmother want to talk about grandfather?"
Saara	"Why doesn't anyone ever want to watch me play soccer?"
Rose	"I think I am a burden to my family."

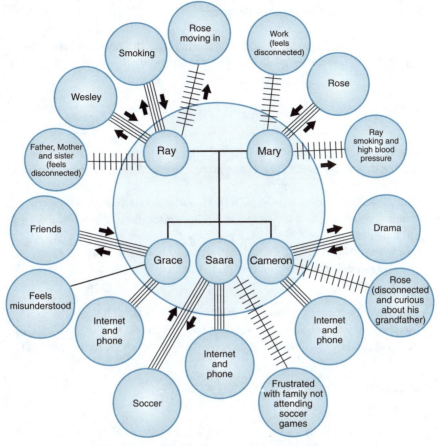

Figure 13-2 Ecomap of the O'Shanell family.

Relationship Between Family Interactions and the Health Problem

During the family interview, the nurse asked the following circular questions and, as a result, obtained new ideas and explanations for the nurse and family to consider:

Present

- "What is the main concern that each family member would like to have addressed?"
- "How has the family changed since Rose moved in?"
- "What is the family's main concern since Rose moved in?"
- "Who in the family agrees that Rose's having moved in is a concern?"

(Text continued on page 344)

Box 13-1 CFAM Branching Diagram

The O'Shanell family is experiencing changes in relation to Mary's mother, Rose, moving in with them after the death of Mary's father, Alfred.

Structure

Roles

Mary:

- Mary has taken on a traditional gender-based role in the family, responsible for the day-to-day functioning of the home and the majority of the care of her children and aging mother.
- Mary feels happy to take on these responsibilities and does not find them a burden, although she is concerned about Ray's response to the new living arrangements.
- Mary feels obliged to care for her mother because she is an only child and grew up watching her own mother do the same for her family.

Ray:

- Ray spent the majority of his early adulthood taking care of his sister, who is significantly younger, and now feels that he has done his familial duty.
- Ray feels that Mary's new role as caregiver to Rose has changed the dynamics of the family.

Subsystems

Ray and Mary:

- They are experiencing relationship instability and frustration since Rose moved in, and this is a significant source of family stress.
- In the past, they spent a lot of time together shopping, going to movies, and going out to eat, but lately, Mary has found it difficult to leave her mother alone and does not spend as much time with Ray.
- Mary feels she has been managing well as a daughter, wife, and mother but that her relationship with Ray has changed a little. She feels he has distanced himself from her and spends more time away from home.
- Recent changes in the family dynamics have influenced Ray's behaviors, and he feels that smoking helps him ease some of his frustration about Mary's decision to take on the role of caregiver for Rose.

Mary, Grace, Saara, and Cameron:

- In the past, Mary would help the children with their homework and rarely missed any of Saara's and Cameron's soccer games. There has been a slight strain in their relationship as Mary has been more preoccupied caring for her mother.

Box 13-1 CFAM Branching Diagram—cont'd

- Grace has disconnected from her mother and siblings and spends a lot of her time on the phone with her peers.

Boundaries

- The boundaries within the O'Shanell family have changed due to Rose moving in.
- The O'Shanell family has permeable boundaries because Mary has been inquiring about home-care services for her mother and is exploring the Internet to gain information about her mother's health conditions.
- Ray talks to his brother-in-law, Wesley, on the phone regularly about what is going on at home.
- Grace confides in her friends about her family.

Developmental

Stage: Families with adolescents

Grace and Saara:

- They are transitioning from school-age children to adolescents.
- Their relationship with their parents is shifting, as evidenced by their behaviors resulting in increased conflict and disengagement.

Cameron:

- Physiological and psychological changes related to growth and development are affecting his understanding of the family dynamics.

Task: Shift of parent-child relationships to permit adolescent to have more independent activities and relationships and to move more flexibly into and out of system

Grace:

- Grace is testing her boundaries with her family as she is developing independence and autonomy.
- She often feels misunderstood and argues with her parents.
- She spends a lot of time talking to her peers and is starting to disengage with her family; she is challenged with the changes in family dynamics since Rose moved in.
- She wants to be left alone and doesn't want to have to spend time with Saara and Cameron.

Saara:

- Saara is feeling lonely because Mary is preoccupied with taking care of Rose and Grace wants to spend time with her friends.

Continued

Box 13-1 CFAM Branching Diagram—cont'd

- She is feeling frustrated with her family and often has multiple arguments with her mother, Grace, and Cameron because they keep missing her soccer games; before Rose moved in, they rarely missed a game.
- She is beginning to struggle with schoolwork; Mary has not been checking on her assignments, and Ray is rarely home to help with homework.
- She relies on her friends to help her with schoolwork but has been procrastinating; her teachers have spoken to her about her organizational skills and meeting deadlines.
- She focuses on soccer and neglects her other responsibilities; she is glad that there is no one at home who is noticing the change.
- She is enjoying her new independence and autonomy but does not understand why no one cares about her achievements in soccer.

Cameron:

- Cameron is very curious about why Rose is living with them and why his grandfather died; he has lots of questions that no one seems to want to answer, causing him to feel confused.
- He is learning about family history at school and has an assignment in relation to his family tree.
- He struggles to understand the arguing every night among family members and why no one wants to explain to him what is happening.
- He is irritated with Grace and Saara because they use to spend time with him and take care of him, but now they are busy with their homework, activities, and friends.

Task: Refocus on midlife couple and career issues

Ray and Mary:

- Ray and Mary are struggling with their relationship as their focus is shifting away from each other to raising adolescent children and caring for an aging parent.
- Stressors include the role of caregiver for Rose, Rose's deteriorating health, the death of Alfred, and the children becoming teenagers and wanting more independence.

Task: Beginning shift toward joint caring for older generation

Mary:

- Mary feels obliged to care for Rose because that is what Rose did for her parents.
- Mary is fearful of what will happen to Rose as her health worsens due to the progression of Alzheimer disease.

Box 13-1 CFAM Branching Diagram—cont'd

Attachments

- Ray and Mary are experiencing a decrease in attachment with Grace and Saara.
- Grace and Saara are developing stronger relationships with their friends, and there is a strong need for affirming self-image and self-identity. (See Figure 13-2.)

Functional

Instrumental

Mary:

- Grocery shopping, cooking, laundry, house cleaning, driving children to school and extracurricular activities, homework supervision, bathing and dressing Rose, medication administration for Rose, driving Rose to health-related appointments

Ray:

- Managing finances, doing outdoor yard work and home repairs, driving children to extracurricular activities

Grace:

- Loading dishwasher, babysitting younger siblings

Saara:

- Helping Ray with yard work, taking the garbage and recycling out on collection days

Cameron:

- Grocery shopping with Mary, helping with cooking and making lunches

Expressive

Mary:

- Mary expresses verbal frustration about Ray's smoking and is emotional about his newly diagnosed hypertension.
- She struggles to understand why she is unable to sleep at night; the lack of sleep is affecting her problem-solving abilities.

Ray:

- Ray is frustrated but does not verbally express his feeling to family members.
- He feels comfortable speaking to his brother-in-law.
- He feels a loss of power in decision-making processes since Rose moved in.

Continued

Box 13-1 CFAM Branching Diagram—cont'd

Rose:

- Rose consistently expresses her concerns, both verbally and emotionally, about being confused and a burden to her family.
- She does not want to speak about her husband and his death to family members.

Grace:

- Grace struggles to express herself as she continues to experience fluctuations in her emotions; she feels that her friends understand her and are more important than family members.

Cameron:

- Cameron consistently asks about his grandfather and is upset with the lack of answers.

Saara:

- Saara is confused and struggles to understand why it so difficult for everyone to just be happy and attend her soccer games.

Past

- Differences: "How was Ray's behavior before Rose moved in?" "What was his lifestyle like before in relation to his smoking habits and his involvement with family activities?" "How has Mary's behavior changed since Rose moved in?"
- Agreement or disagreement: "Who agrees with Ray that the main concern is Rose moving in with the family?"
- Explanation or meaning: "What does each family member think was the significance of Mary's decision to let Rose come and live with the family?"

Future

- "How would it be different if Mary had help from home-care services to care for Rose?"
- "If Rose suddenly developed complications from her Alzheimer disease and required specialized care, how would things be different from the way they are now?" "Does everyone in the family agree with what would

be different?" "If this were to happen, how would you explain the change in Mary's relationship with her mother?"

Attempted Solutions to Solving Problems

- Ray recently visited his physician, who prescribed an antihypertensive for him.
- Mary has spoken to home-care services about having someone come to assist her with caring for her mother, but she is worried about the cost.
- Grace has been talking to her friends about how "crazy" everyone in her family is.
- Cameron has been asking his mother to tell him about his grandfather because his grandmother will not tell him anything.

Goal Exploration

FAMILY MEMBER	GOAL
Ray	To have a family night once a week where everyone eats dinner together and plays a board game
Mary	To get Ray to stop smoking and for herself to sleep better
Grace	To spend one afternoon a month with her mother having mother-daughter time just liked they used to before Grandma moved in with them
Cameron	To learn about his grandfather so he can share his family tree at school
Saara	To have her family come to watch her play soccer every other week
Rose	To not feel guilty every time she needs help from her family to get dressed or take a bath

INTERVENTION

Upon completion of the family assessment with the O'Shanell family, the nurse concludes that interventions are indicated. The nurse must now identify how to intervene to facilitate change within the family considering the domains of family functioning. The following is an example of three interventions indicated for the O'Shanell family and their relation to the domains of family functioning.

INTERVENTION: Offering Caregiver Support

Cognitive	■ Determine each family member's knowledge about Alzheimer disease and its progression. ■ Ask family members to identify their perceived roles in caring for Rose.
Affective	■ Encourage each family member to acknowledge the difficulties associated with the caregiving role. ■ Encourage each family member to identify his or her strengths and weaknesses in relation to providing care for Rose so that the family can optimize their resources.
Behavioral	■ Provide the O'Shanell family with information about home-care services, respite care, and other community services, including how to access these services to optimize the health of the family. ■ Encourage the O'Shanell family to participate in support groups to interact with other families who are caring for individuals with Alzheimer disease. This will provide opportunities for the family members to share strategies for success and increase their social network. ■ Teach Mary sleep-hygiene strategies to address her sleep difficulties in order to maintain her physical and mental health, such as relaxation, mindfulness, keeping a sleep journal, diet, and exercise.

INTERVENTION: Offering Family Health Promotion

Cognitive	■ Empower the family to build on each other's strengths and work together to attain and maintain family health. ■ Encourage each family member to be involved in problem identification and goal exploration. ■ Teach family members to think about how to use commendations to support and build on their assets.
Affective	■ Teach each family member to validate and understand each other's feelings. ■ Foster the positive emotions of each member using empathy and compassion.
Behavioral	■ Promote resilience and behavioral changes to enhance family relationships. ■ Commit to a plan for a change in behavior. ■ Use positive dialogue with one another to encourage and strengthen personal development skills and resources. ■ Teach personal behavioral skills to each family member to draw on their own strengths and resources to support one another.

INTERVENTION: Offering Information About Adolescent Growth and Development	
Cognitive	■ Shift Mary and Ray's mind-set from the parental role of protector to that of a preparer for the challenges of adolescence. ■ Teach Mary and Ray that their children's peer supports are a strong and valuable part of growth and development as they are developing a sense of belonging and self-identity.
Affective	■ Facilitate the family's ability to normalize the developmental changes occurring with Cameron, Saara, and Grace. ■ Teach Ray and Mary to understand their children's feelings by asking questions and clarifying.
Behavioral	■ Identify strategies for conflict management within the family that emphasize communication skills and increasing empathy among all family members. For example, encourage Mary and Ray to set limits and boundaries with their children, develop trust and respect for their children's beliefs, and validate their children's feelings. ■ Encourage Cameron, Saara, and Grace to express their feelings to their parents and to each other.

TERMINATION

A collaborative decision to terminate the relationship was initiated by the O'Shanell family. The members of the O'Shanell family have discovered new solutions to their problems and have been able to agree that they no longer need to meet with the nurse on a regular basis. As a result, the frequency of sessions with the nurse will decrease over a mutually agreed upon time frame of 1 month and terminate at the end of that time.

SUMMARY

Our intention for this chapter was to provide a detailed example of how to apply the Calgary Family Assessment Model (CFAM) and the Calgary Family Intervention Model (CFIM) using the O'Shannell family. The CFAM is a comprehensive and inclusive family assessment model that does not need be overwhelming if viewed as a "map of the family" from the nurse's and the family's "observer perspectives." The CFAM provides a framework that can be drawn on as the nurse and the family discuss and collaborate about the issues. The nurse can begin by using the three main categories of the CFAM (structural, developmental, and functional) to obtain a big-picture assessment of family strengths, resources, problems, and/or suffering and explore in more detail these areas depending on his or her confidence and competence level. It is imperative that the nurse is able to draw together all relevant information into an integrated assessment, synthesizing all the information, and is not hindered by complexity.

Once a thorough family assessment has been completed, the nurse and the family can then collaborate to determine whether interventions are needed. We wish to emphasize that completing a family assessment utilizing the CFAM does not mean that the nurse or the family now has the "truth" about the family's functioning related to a health problem or concern. Rather, the nurse and family members each have their own integrated assessment from their own observer perspectives at one point in time. Interventions can be as straightforward and simple as asking therapeutic questions or offering commendations or as innovative and dramatic as the nurse deems necessary for the health or illness problems presented. Interventions should be focused on promoting, improving, and sustaining effective family functioning in the three domains (cognitive, affective, and behavioral) and should be based on the assumption that individual health behaviors are strongly influenced by those around us and that family well-being can promote the physical health of its members.

All interventions should be directed toward the healing and treatment goals collaboratively generated by the nurse and the family. When conducting a family interview, there should be fluidity between the stages so that they remain true guidelines rather than a rigid prescription for how to conduct a family interview; moving back and forth between the stages of a family interview to obtain more clarity or additional assessment is not uncommon. Nurses need to remember the uniqueness of every family situation and be encouraged to use these guidelines with sensitivity to each clinical situation. Nurses are privileged to work with families, and we hope that you have gained a better understanding of how nurses can work with families.

References

INTRODUCTION

Bell, J. M. (2003). Clinical scholarship in family nursing [Editorial]. *Journal of Family Nursing, 9*, 127–129. doi:10.1177/1074840703009002001

Benner, P. (2001). *From novice to expert: Excellence and power in clinical nursing practice.* Upper Saddle River, NJ: Prentice Hall.

International Family Nursing Association. (2015). *IFNA position statement on generalist competencies for family nursing practice.* Retrieved from https://internationalfamilynursing. org/wordpress/wp-content/uploads/2015/07/GC-Complete-PDF-document-in-color-with-photos-English-language.pdf

International Family Nursing Association. (2017). *IFNA position statement on advanced practice competencies for family nursing.* Retrieved from https://internationalfamilynursing. org/2017/05/19/advanced-practice-competencies/

Leahey, M., & Wright, L. M. (2016): Application of the Calgary Family Assessment and Intervention Models: Reflections on the reciprocity between the personal and the professional. *Journal of Family Nursing, 22*(4), 450–459. doi:10.1177/1074840716667972

Schober, M., & Affara, F. (2001). *The family nurse: Frameworks for practice.* Geneva, Switzerland: International Council of Nurses.

Sigurdadottir, A. O., Svavarsdottir, E. K., & Juliusdottir, S. (2015). Family nursing hospital training and the outcome on job demands, control and support. *Nurse Education Today, 35*, 854–858. doi:10.1016/j.nedt.2015.03.003

Wright, L. M., & Leahey, M. (Producers). (2000). *How to do a 15-minute (or less) family interview* [DVD]. Calgary, Canada: www.familynursingresources.com.

Wright, L. M., & Leahey, M. (Producers). (2001). *Calgary Family Assessment Model: How to apply in clinical practice* [DVD]. Calgary, Canada: www.familynursingresources.com.

Wright, L. M., & Leahey, M. (Producers). (2002). *Family nursing interviewing skills: How to engage, assess, intervene, and terminate with families* [DVD]. Calgary, Canada: www. familynursingresources.com.

Wright, L. M., & Leahey, M. (Producers). (2003). *How to intervene with families with health concerns* [DVD]. Calgary, Canada: www.familynursingresources.com.

Wright, L. M., & Leahey, M. (Producers). (2006). *How to use questions in family interviewing* [DVD]. Calgary, Canada: www.familynursingresources.com.

Wright, L. M., & Leahey, M. (Producers). (2010a). *Common errors in family interviewing: How to avoid & correct* [DVD]. Calgary, Canada: www.familynursingresources.com

Wright, L. M., & Leahey, M. (Producers). (2010b). *Interviewing an individual to gain a family perspective with chronic illness: A clinical demonstration* [DVD]. Calgary, Canada: www. familynursingresources.com

Wright, L. M & Leahey, M. (Producers). (2010c). *Tips and microskills for interviewing families of the elderly.* [DVD] Calgary, Canada: www.familynursingresources.com

CHAPTER 1

Anderson, K. H. (2000). The family health system approach to family systems nursing. *Journal of Family Nursing, 6,* 103–119.

Angelo, M. (2008). The emergence of family nursing in Brazil. *Journal of Family Nursing, 14*(4), 436–441.

Astedt-Kurki, P. (2010). Family nursing research for practice: The Finnish perspective. *Journal of Family Nursing, 16*(3), 256–268.

Astedt-Kurki, P., & Kaunonen, M. (2011). Family nursing interventions in Finland: Benefits for families. In E. Svavarsdottir & H. Jonsdottir (Eds.), *Family nursing in action* (pp. 115–129). Reykjavik, Iceland: University of Iceland Press.

Barbabella, F., Poli, A., Andréasson, F., Salzmann, B., Papa, R., Hanson, E., ... & Lamura, G. (2016). A web-based psychosocial intervention for family caregivers of older people: Results from a mixed-methods study in three European countries. *JMIR Research Protocols, 5*(4), e196.

Bell, J. M. (1999). Family nursing network: Family nursing in Japan—A firsthand glimpse. *Journal of Family Nursing, 5*(2), 236–238.

Bell, J. M. (2009). Family systems nursing: Re-examined. *Journal of Family Nursing, 15*(2), 123–129.

Bell, J. M. (2011). Relationships: The heart of the matter in family nursing. *Journal of Family Nursing, 17*(1), 3–10.

Bell, J. M., Moules, N. J., & Wright, L. M. (2009). Therapeutic letters and the Family Nursing Unit: A legacy of advanced nursing practice. *Journal of Family Nursing, 15*(1), 6–30.

Bell, J. M., Watson, W. L., & Wright, L. M. (Eds.). (1990). *The cutting edge of family nursing.* Calgary, AB, Canada: Family Nursing Unit Publications.

Bell, J. M., & Wright, L. M. (2007). La recherche sur la pratique des soins infirmiers a la famille. In F. Duhamel (Ed.), *La Sante et la Famille: Une Approache Systemique en Soins Infirmieres* (2nd ed.). Montreal, Quebec, Canada: Gaetan Morin editeru, Cheneliere Education. [In French]

Bell, J. M., & Wright, L. M. (2011). Creating practice knowledge for families experiencing illness suffering: The illness beliefs model. In E. Svavarsdottir & H. Jonsdottir (Eds.), *Family nursing in action* (pp. 15–51). Reykjavik, Iceland: University of Iceland Press.

Benzein, E., Olin, C., & Persson, C. (2015). "You put it all together"—Families' evaluation of participating in family health conversations. *Scandinavian Journal of Caring Sciences, 29*(1), 136–144.

Benzies, K. M. (2016). Relational communications strategies to support family-centered neonatal intensive care. *The Journal of Perinatal & Neonatal Nursing, 30*(3), 233–236.

Blanton, S., Dunbar, S., & Clark, P. C. (2018). Content validity and satisfaction with a caregiver-integrated web-based rehabilitation intervention for persons with stroke. *Topics in Stroke Rehabilitation,* 1–6.

Bomar, P. J. (Ed.). (2004). *Promoting health in families: Applying family research and theory to nursing practice* (3rd ed.). Philadelphia, PA: W.B. Saunders.

Bulechek, G. M., & McCloskey, J. C. (Eds.). (1992). Defining and validating nursing interventions. *Nursing Clinics of North America, 27*(2), 289–299.

Butcher, H., Bulechek, G. M., McCloskey Dochterman, J. M., & Wagner, C. (2018). *Nursing interventions classification (NIC)* (7th ed., E-book). New York, NY: Elsevier.

Chesla, C. A. (2010). Do family interventions improve health? *Journal of Family Nursing, 16*(4), 355–377.

Crossman, M. K., Warfield, M. E., Kotelchuck, M., Hauser-Cram, P., & Parish, S. L. (2018). Associations between early intervention home visits, family relationships and competence for mothers of children with developmental disabilities. *Maternal and Child Health Journal, 148*(22), 1–9.

Doane, G. H. (2003). Through pragmatic eyes: Philosophy and the re-sourcing of family nursing. *Nursing Philosophy, 4*(1), 25–33.

Doane, G. H., & Varcoe, C. (2005). *Family nursing as relational inquiry.* Philadelphia, PA: Lippincott Williams & Wilkins.

Duhamel, F. (2017). Translating knowledge from a family systems approach to clinical practice: Insights from knowledge translation research experiences. *Journal of Family Nursing, 23*(4), 461–487.

Duhamel, F. (Ed.). (2015). La santé et la famille: *Une approche systémique en soins infirmiers [Families and health: A systemic approach in nursing care]* (3rd ed.). Montreal, Quebec, Canada: Gaëtan Morin editeur, Chenelière Éducation. [In French]

Duhamel, F., & Dupuis, F. (2004). Guaranteed returns: Investing in conversations with families of cancer patients. *Clinical Journal of Oncology Nursing, 8*(1), 68–71.

Duhamel, F., & Dupuis, F. (2011). Towards a triology model of family systems nursing knowledge utilization: Fostering circularity between practice, education, and research. In E. Svavarsdottir & H. Jonsdottir (Eds.), *Family nursing in action* (pp. 53–68). Reykjavik, Iceland: University of Iceland Press.

Duhamel, F., Dupuis, F., & Wright, L. M. (2009). Families' and nurses' responses to the "one question question": Reflections for clinical practice, education, and research in family nursing. *Journal of Family Nursing, 15*(4), 461–485.

Duhamel, F., & Talbot, L. R. (2004). A constructivist evaluation of family systems nursing interventions with families experiencing cardiovascular and cerebrovascular illness. *Journal of Family Nursing, 10*(1), 12–32.

Eg, M., Frederiksen, K., Vamosi, M., & Lorentzen, V. (2017). How family interactions about lifestyle changes affect adolescents' possibilities for maintaining weight loss after a weight- loss intervention: A longitudinal qualitative interview study. *Journal of Advanced Nursing, 73*(8), 1924–1936.

Eggenberger, S. K., & Sanders, M. (2016). A family nursing educational intervention supports nurses and families in an adult intensive care unit. *Australian Critical Care, 29*(4), 217–223.

Feetham, S. L., Meister, S. B., Bell, J. M., & Gilliss, C. L. (1993). *The nursing of families: Theory, research, education, and practice.* Newbury Park, CA: Sage.

Ford-Gilboe, M. (2002). Developing knowledge about family health promotion by testing the developmental model of health and nursing. *Journal of Family Nursing, 8*(2), 140–156.

Friedman, M. M., Bowden, V. R., & Jones, E. G. (2003). *Family nursing: Research, theory and practice* (5th ed.). Upper Saddle River, NJ: Prentice Hall.

Garwick, A., Seppelt, A., & Belew, J. L. (2011). Addressing family health literacy to create a family-centered, culturally relevant web-based asthma education project. In E. Svavarsdottir & H. Jonsdottir (Eds.), *Family nursing in action* (pp. 251–266). Reykjavik, Iceland: University of Iceland Press.

Gilliss, C. L. (1991). Family nursing research, theory and practice. *Image: Journal of Nursing Scholarship, 23*(1), 19–22.

Gilliss, C. L., Highly, B. L., Roberts, B. M., & Martinson, I. M. (Eds.). (1989). *Toward a science of family nursing.* Menlo Park, CA: Addison-Wesley.

Gisladottir, M., & Svavarsdottir, E. K. (2017). The effectiveness of therapeutic conversation intervention for caregivers of adolescents with ADHD: A quasi experimental design. *Journal of Psychiatric and Mental Health Nursing, 24*(1), 15–27.

Gisladottir, M., Treasure, J., & Svavarsdottir, E. K. (2017). Effectiveness of therapeutic conversation intervention among caregivers of people with eating disorders: Quasi-experimental design. *Journal of Clinical Nursing, 26*(5–6), 735–750.

Hanson, S. M., & Boyd, S. T. (Eds.). (1996). *Family health care nursing: Theory, practice, and research.* Philadelphia, PA: F. A. Davis.

Hanson, S. M. H. (2001). *Family health care nursing: Theory, practice, and research* (2nd ed.). Philadelphia, PA: F. A. Davis.

Hartrick, G. (2000). Developing health promoting practice with families: One pedagogical experience. *Journal of Advanced Nursing, 31*(1), 27–34.

Hirschman, K. B., & Hodgson, N. A. (2018). Evidence-based interventions for transitions in care for individuals living with dementia. *The Gerontologist, 58*(Suppl. 1), S129–S140.

Houger Limacher, L., & Wright, L. M. (2003). Commendations: Listening to the silent side of a family intervention. *Journal of Family Nursing, 9*(2), 130–135.

Houger Limacher, L., & Wright, L. M. (2006). Exploring the therapeutic family intervention of commendations: Insights from research. *Journal of Family Nursing, 12,* 307–331.

Irinoye, O., Ogunfowokan, A., & Olaogun, A. (2006). Family nursing education and family nursing practice in Nigeria. *Journal of Family Nursing, 12*(11), 442–447.

Kaakinen, J. R., Coehlo, D. P., Steele, R., Tabacco, A., & Hanson, S. M. H. (2018). 6th Ed. *Family health care nursing: Theory, practice, and research.* Philadelphia, PA: F. A. Davis.

Kaltenbaugh, D. J., Klem, M. L., Hu, L., Turi, E., Haines, A. J., & Lingler, J. H. (2015). Using Web-based interventions to support caregivers of patients with cancer: A systematic review. *Oncology Nursing Forum, 42*(2), 156–164.

Kendall, J., & Tabacco, A. (2011). Parents and children together: In-home intervention for families and children with children with attention-deficit/hyperactivity disorder. In E. Svavarsdottir & H. Jonsdottir (Eds.), *Family nursing in action* (pp. 185–216). Reykjavik, Iceland: University of Iceland Press.

Kobayashi, N. (2011). Family assessment workbook part II: *Guide to an expert in facilitating case conference and study by FASC methods.* Tokyo, Japan: Ishiyaku Publishers. [In Japanese]

Konradsdottir, E., & Svavarsdottir, E. K. (2011). How effective is a short-term educational and support intervention for families of an adolescent with type 1 diabetes? *Journal for Specialists in Pediatric Nursing, 16*, 295–304.

Leahey, M., & Harper-Jaques, S. (2010). Integrating family nursing into a mental health urgent care practice framework: Ladders for learning. *Journal of Family Nursing, 16*(2), 196–212.

Lee, A. C. K., Leung, S. O., Chan, P. S. L., & Chung, J. O. K. (2010). Perceived level of knowledge and difficulty in applying family assessment among senior undergraduate nursing students. *Journal of Family Nursing, 16*(2), 177–195.

Limacher, L. H., & Wright, L. M. (2006). Exploring the therapeutic family intervention of commendations: Insights from research. *Journal of Family Nursing, 12*(3), 307–331.

Marklund, S., Eriksson, E. S., Lindh, V., & Saveman, B. I. (2018). Family health conversations at a pediatric oncology center—A way for families to rebalance the situation. *Journal of Pediatric Nursing, 38*, e59–e65.

Maturana, H. (1988). Reality: The search for objectivity or the quest for a compelling argument. *Irish Journal of Psychology, 6*(1), 25–83.

McCloskey, J., & Bulechek, G. (1992). *Nursing interventions classification.* St. Louis, MO: Mosby.

McLeod, D. L., & Wright, L. M. (2008). Living the as-yet-unanswered: Spiritual care practices in family systems nursing. *Journal of Family Nursing, 14*(1), 118–141.

Moriyama, M. (2008). Family nursing practice and education: What is happening in Japan? *Journal of Family Nursing, 14*(4), 442–455.

Moules, N. J. (2002). Nursing on paper: Therapeutic letters in nursing practice. *Nursing Inquiry, 9*(2), 104–113.

Moules, N. J. (2003). Therapy on paper: Therapeutic letters and the tone of relationship. *Journal of Systemic Inquiries, 22*(1), 33–49.

Moules, N. J. (2009). Therapeutic letters in nursing: Examining the character and influence of the written word in clinical work with families experiencing illness. *Journal of Family Nursing, 15*(1), 31–49.

Noiseux, S., & Duhamel, F. (2003). La greffe de moelle osseuse chez l'enfant. Evaluation constructiviste de l'intervention aupres des parents. [Bone marrow transplantation in children. Constructive evaluation of an intervention for parents]. *Perspective Infirmiere, 1*(1), 12–24. [In French]

O'Farrell, P., Murray, J., & Hotz, S. B. (2000). Psychological distress among spouses of patients undergoing cardiac rehabilitation. *Heart and Lung, 29*(2), 97–104.

Östlund, U., Bäckström, B., Saveman, B. I., Lindh, V., & Sundin, K. (2016). A family systems nursing approach for families following a stroke: Family health conversations. *Journal of Family Nursing, 22*(2), 148–171.

O'Sullivan Burchard, D. J., Claveirole, A., Mitchell, R., Walford, C., & Whyte, D. (2004). Family nursing in Scotland. *Journal of Family Nursing, 10*(3), 323–337.

Ragnarsdóttir, A., & Svavarsdottir, E. K. (2014). Advanced knowledge in nursing practice can make the difference: The value of a nursing intervention for families of children with rare chronic illnesses. *Nordic Journal of Nursing Research, 34*(1), 48–51.

Robinson, C. A., & Wright, L. M. (1995). Family nursing interventions: What families say makes a difference. *Journal of Family Nursing, 1*(3), 327–345.

Saveman, B. (2010). Family nursing research for practice: The Swedish perspective. *Journal of Family Nursing, 16*(1), 26–44.

Saveman, B., & Benzein, E. (2001). Here come the Swedes! A report on the dramatic and rapid evolution of family-focused nursing in Sweden. *Journal of Family Nursing, 7*(3), 303–310.

Schober, M., & Affara, F. (2001). *The family nurse: Frameworks for practice.* Geneva, Switzerland: International Council of Nurses.

Simpson, P., Yeung, F. K. K., Kwan, A. T. Y., & Wah, W. K. (2006). Family systems nursing: A guide to mental health care in Hong Kong. *Journal of Family Nursing, 12*(8), 276–291.

Sugishita, C. (1999). Development of family nursing in Japan—Present and future perspectives. *Journal of Family Nursing, 5*(2), 239–244.

Svavarsdottir, E. K. (2006). Listening to the family's voice: Nordic nurses' movement toward family centered care. *Journal of Family Nursing, 12*(4), 346–367.

Svavarsdottir, E. K. (2008). Excellence in nursing: A model for implementing family systems nursing in nursing practice at an institutional level in Iceland. *Journal of Family Nursing, 14*(4), 456–468.

Svavarsdottir, E. K., & Jonsdottir, H. (2011). *Family nursing in action.* Reykjavik, Iceland: University of Iceland Press.

Svavarsdottir, E. K., & Sigurdardottir, A. O. (2011). Implementing family nursing in general pediatric nursing practice: The circularity between knowledge translation and clinical practice. In E. K. Svavarsdottir & H. Jonsdottir (Eds.), *Family nursing in action* (pp. 161–184). Reykjavik, Iceland: University of Iceland Press.

Svavarsdottir, E. K., Sigurdardottir, A. O., Konradsdottir, E., Stefansdottir, A., Sveinbjarnardottir, E. K., Ketilsdottir, A., ... & Guðmundsdottir, H. (2015). The process of translating family nursing knowledge into clinical practice. *Journal of Nursing Scholarship, 47*(1), 5–15.

Sveinbjarnardottir, E. K., Svavarsdottir, E. K., & Hrafnkelsson, B. (2012a). Psychometric development of the Iceland-family perceived support questionnaire (ICE-FPSQ). *Journal of Family Nursing, 18*(3), 328–352.

Sveinbjarnardottir, E. K., Svavarsdottir, E. K., & Hrafnkelsson, B. (2012b). Psychometric development of the Iceland-Expressive Family Functioning Questionnaire (ICE-EFFQ). *Journal of Family Nursing, 18*(3), 353–377.

Sveinbjarnardottir, E. K., Svavarsdottir, E. K., & Wright, L. M. (2013). What are the benefits of a short therapeutic conversation intervention with acute psychiatric patients and their families? A controlled before and after study. *International Journal of Nursing Studies 50,* 593–602.

Tomm, K., & Sanders, G. (1983). Family assessment in a problem oriented record. In J. C. Hansen & B. F. Keeney (Eds.), *Diagnosis and assessment in family therapy* (pp. 101–102). London, UK: Aspen Systems Corporation.

Voltelen, B., Konradsen, H., & Østergaard, B. (2016). Family nursing therapeutic conversations in heart failure outpatient clinics in Denmark: Nurses' experiences. *Journal of Family Nursing, 22*(2), 179–198.

Wacharasin, C., & Theinpichet, S. (2008). Family nursing practice, education, and research: What is happening in Thailand? *Journal of Family Nursing, 14*(4), 429–435.

Wasilewski, M. B., Stinson, J. N., & Cameron, J. I. (2017). Web-based health interventions for family caregivers of elderly individuals: A scoping review. *International Journal of Medical Informatics, 103,* 109–136.

Wegner, G. D., & Alexander, R. J. (Eds.). (1993). *Readings in family nursing.* Philadelphia, PA: J.B. Lippincott Company.

World Health Organization (WHO), Regional Office for Europe. (2000). *The family health nurse: Context, conceptual framework and curriculum.* Retrieved from http://www.who.int/iris/handle/10665/107930

Wright, L. M. (2015). Brain science and illness beliefs: An unexpected explanation of the healing power of therapeutic conversations and the family interventions that matter. *Journal of Family Nursing, 21,* 186–205.

Wright, L. M., & Bell, J. M. (2009). *Beliefs and illness: A model for healing.* Calgary, AB, Canada: 4th Floor Press.

Wright, L. M., & Leahey, M. (1990). Trends in nursing of families. *Journal of Advanced Nursing, 15*(2), 148–154.

Wright, L. M., & Leahey, M. (2013). *Nurses and families: A guide to family assessment and intervention* (6th ed.). Philadelphia, PA: F. A. Davis.

Wright, L. M., Watson, W. L., & Bell, J. M. (1990). The family nursing unit: A unique integration of research, education, and clinical practice. In J. M. Bell, W. L. Watson, & L. M. Wright (Eds.), *The cutting edge of family nursing* (pp. 95–109). Calgary, AB, Canada: Family Nursing Unit Publications.

CHAPTER 2

Allmond, B. W., Buckman, W., & Gofman, H. F. (1979). *The family is the patient: An approach to behavioral pediatrics for the clinician*. St. Louis, MO: Mosby.

Anderson, H. (2012). Collaborative relationships and dialogic conversations: Ideas for a relationally responsive practice. *Family Process, 51*, 8–24.

Bateson, G. (1979). *Mind and Nature*. New York, NY: E.P. Dutton.

Bavelas, J. B. (1992). Research into the pragmatics of human communication. *Journal of Strategic and Systemic Therapies, 11(2)*, 15–29.

Becvar, D. S., & Becvar, R. J. (2003). *Family therapy: A systemic integration* (5th ed.). Boston, MA: Allyn & Bacon.

Bell, J. M., & Wright, L. M. (2011). Creating practice knowledge for families experiencing illness suffering: The Illness Beliefs Model. In E. Svavarsdottir & H. Jonsdottir (Eds.), *Family nursing in action* (pp. 15–52). Reykjavik, Iceland: University of Iceland Press.

Crawford, J. A., & Tarko, M. A. (2004). Family communication. In P. J. Bomar (Ed.), *Promoting health in families: Applying family research and theory to nursing practice* (3rd ed., pp. 274–303). Philadelphia, PA: Saunders.

Dickerson, V. (2010). Positioning oneself within an epistemology: Refining our thinking about integrative approaches. *Family Process, 49*, 349–368.

Glazer, S. (2001). Therapeutic touch and postmodernism in nursing. *Nursing Philosophy, 2*(3), 196–230.

Imber-Black, E. (1991). The family-larger-system perspective. *Family Systems Medicine, 9*(4), 371–396.

Imber Coppersmith, E. (1983). The place of family therapy in the homeostasis of larger systems. In M. Aronson & R. Wolberg (Eds.), *Group and family therapy: An overview* (pp. 216–227). New York, NY: Brunner/Mazel.

Jackson, D. D. (1973). Family interaction, family homeostasis and some implications for conjoint family psychotherapy. In D. D. Jackson (Ed.), *Therapy, communication and change* (4th ed., pp. 185–203). Palo Alto, CA: Science & Behavior Books.

Johnson, D. E. (1990). The behavioral system model for nursing. In M. E. Parker (Ed.), *Nursing theories in practice* (pp. 23–32). New York, NY: National League for Nursing.

Kaakinen, J. R., & Hanson, S. M. H. (2014). Theoretical foundations for the nursing of families. In J. R. Kaakinen, D. P. Coehlo, R. Steele, A. Tabacco, & S. M. H. Hanson (Eds.), *Family health care nursing: Theory, practice and research* (5th ed.). Philadelphia, PA: F. A. Davis.

Kermode, S., & Brown, C. (1996). The postmodernist hoax and its effects on nursing. *International Journal of Nursing Studies, 33*(4), 375–384.

Maturana, H. (1978). Biology of language: The epistemology of reality. In G. A. Miller & E. Lenneberg (Eds.), *Psychology and biology of language and thought* (pp. 27–63). New York, NY: Academic Press.

Maturana, H. R. (1988). *Telephone conversation: Calgary/Chile coupling* [Telephone transcript]. Calgary, Canada: University of Calgary.

Maturana, H. R., & Varela, F. J. (1980). *Autopoiesis and cognition: The Realization of the living*. Dordrecht, Holland: D. Reidl.

Maturana, H. R., & Varela, F. (1992). *The tree of knowledge: The biological roots of human understanding*. Boston, MA: Shambhala Publications.

Mendez, C. L., Coddou, F., & Maturana, H. R. (1988). The bringing forth of pathology. *Irish Journal of Psychology, 9*(1), 144–172.

Moules, N. J. (2000). Postmodernism and the sacred: Reclaiming connection in our greater-than-human worlds. *Journal of Marital and Family Therapy, 26*(2), 229–240.

Neuman, B., & Fawcett, J. (2011). The Neuman systems model. Boston, MA: Pearson.

Pluralism. (2018). In *Merriam-Webster's online dictionary*. Retrieved from https://www.merriam-webster.com/dictionary/pluralism

Robinson, C. A. (1998). Women, families, chronic illness, and nursing interventions: From burden to balance. *Journal of Family Nursing, 4*(3), 271–290.

Robinson, C. A. (2017). Families living well with chronic illness: The healing process of moving on. *Qualitative Health Research, 27*(4), 447–461.

Robinson, C. A., Bottorff, J. L., & Torchalla, I. (2011). Exploring family relationships: Directions for smoking cessation. In E. K. Svavarsdottir & H. Jonsdottir (Eds.), *Family nursing in action* (pp. 137–160). Reykjavik, Iceland, University of Iceland Press.

Salladay, S. A. (2011). Confident spiritual care in a postmodern world. *Journal of Christian Nursing, 28*(2), 102–108.

Simon, R. (1985, May–June). Structure is destiny: An interview with Huberto Maturana. *Family Therapy*, 32–43.

Smith, M. C., & Parker, M. E. (2015). Nursing theories and nursing practice. Philadelphia, PA: F. A. Davis.

System. (2018). In *Oxford online dictionary*. Retrieved from https://en.oxforddictionaries.com/definition/system

Tapp, D. M., & Wright, L. M. (1996). Live supervision and family systems nursing: Postmodern influences and dilemmas. *Journal of Psychiatric and Mental Health Nursing, 3*(4), 225–233.

Tomm, K. (1980). Towards a cybernetic-systems approach to family therapy at the University of Calgary. In D. S. Freeman (Ed.), *Perspectives on family therapy* (pp. 3–18). Toronto, Canada: Butterworths.

Tomm, K. (1981). Circularity: A preferred orientation for family assessment. In A. S. Gurman (Ed.), *Questions and answers in the practice of family therapy* (vol. 1, pp. 874–887). New York, NY: Brunner/Mazel.

von Bertalanffy, L. (1968). *General Systems Theory: Foundations, Development, Applications*. New York: George Braziller.

von Bertalanffy, L. (1972). The history and status of general systems theory. In G. J. Klir (Ed.), *Trends in general systems theory* (pp. 763–774). New York, NY: Wiley-Interscience.

von Bertalanffy, L. (1974). General systems theory and psychiatry. In S. Arieti (Ed.), *American handbook of psychiatry* (pp. 1095–1117). New York, NY: Basic Books.

Watson, J. (1999). *Postmodern nursing and beyond*. Philadelphia, PA: Churchill Livingstone.

Watzlawick, P., Beavin, J. H., & Jackson, D. D. (1967). *Pragmatics of human communication: A study of interactional patterns, pathologies, and paradoxes*. New York, NY: Norton.

Watzlawick, P., Weakland, J. H., & Fisch, R. (1974). *Change: Principles of problem formulation and problem resolution*. New York, NY: Norton.

Wright, L. M., & Bell, J. M. (2009). *Beliefs and illness: A model for healing*. Calgary, AB, Canada: 4th Floor Press.

Wright, L. M., & Leahey, M. (2013). *Nurses and families: A guide to family assessment and intervention* (6th ed.). Philadelphia, PA: F. A. Davis.

Wright, L. M., & Levac, A. M. (1992). The non-existence of non-compliant families: The influence of Humberto Maturana. *Journal of Advanced Nursing, 17*(8), 913–917.

Wright, L. M., Watson, W. L., & Bell, J. M. (1990). The family nursing unit: A unique integration of research, education, and clinical practice. In J. M. Bell, W. L. Watson, & Wright, L. M. (Eds.), *The cutting edge of family nursing* (pp. 95–109). Calgary, AB, Canada: Family Nursing Unit Publications.

CHAPTER 3

Ahrons, C. R. (1999). Divorce: An unscheduled family transition. In B. Carter & M. McGoldrick (Eds.), *The expanded family life cycle: Individual, family, and social perspectives* (3rd ed., pp. 381–98). Boston, MA: Allyn & Bacon.

Ahrons, C. R., & Rodgers, R. H. (1987). *Divorced families: A multidisciplinary developmental view*. New York, NY: W. W. Norton & Company.

American Psychological Association. (2015). Guidelines for psychological practice with transgender and gender nonconforming people. *American Psychologist, 70*(9), 832–864. doi.org/10.1037/a0039906

Becvar, D. S. (2001). *In the presence of grief: Helping family members resolve death, dying, and bereavement issues.* New York, NY: The Guilford Press.

Becvar, D. S. (2003). Introduction to the special section: Death, dying, and bereavement. *Journal of Marital and Family Therapy, 29*(4), 437–438.

Bjarnadottir, R. I., Bockting, W., & Dowding, D. W. (2017). Patient perspectives on answering questions about sexual orientation and gender identity: An integrative review. *Journal of Clinical Nursing, 26*(13–14), 1814–1833.

Boss, P. G. (2002). Ambiguous loss: Working with families of the missing. *Family Process, 41*(1), 14–17.

Boss, P. (2016). The context and process of theory development: The story of ambiguous loss. *Journal of Family Theory & Review, 8*(3), 269–286.

Bowen, M. (1978). *Family therapy in clinical practice.* Northvale, NJ: Jason Aronson.

Bowlby, J. (1977). The making and breaking of affectional bonds. *British Journal of Psychiatry, 130*, 201–210.

Carter, B., & McGoldrick, M. (Eds.). (1988). *The changing family life cycle: A framework for family therapy* (2nd ed.). New York, NY: Gardner Press.

Darwent, K. L., McInnes, R. J., & Swanson, V. (2016). The infant feeding genogram: A tool for exploring family infant feeding history and identifying support needs. *BMC Pregnancy and Childbirth, 16*(1), 315.

Duhamel, F., & Campagna, L. (2000). *Family genograph.* Montreal, Canada: Universite de Montreal, Faculty of Nursing.

Duvall, E. R. (1977). *Marriage and family development* (5th ed.). Philadelphia, PA: Lippincott.

Epstein, N., Bishop, D., & Levin, S. (1978). The McMaster model of family functioning. *Journal of Marriage and Family Counseling, 4*, 19–31.

Epstein, N., Sigal, J., & Rakoff, V. (1968). *Family categories schema.* Unpublished manuscript, Department of Psychiatry, Jewish General Hospital, Montreal, Canada.

Erickson, E. (1963). *Childhood and society* (2nd ed.). New York, NY: W. W. Norton & Company.

Falicov, C. (2012). Immigrant family processes, a multidimensional framework. In F. Walsh (Ed.), *Normal family processes: Growing diversity and complexity* (4th ed., pp. 297–323). New York, NY: The Guilford Press.

Haley, J. (1977). Toward a theory of pathological systems. In P. Watzlawick & J. H. Weakland (Eds.), *The interactional view* (pp. 94–112). New York, NY: W. W. Norton & Company.

Hartman, A. (1978). Diagrammatic assessment of family relationships. *Social Casework, 59*, 465–476.

Hoffman, L. (1981). *Foundations of family therapy.* New York, NY: Basic Books.

Levac, A. M. C., Wright, L. M., & Leahey, M. (2002). Children and families: Models for assessment and intervention. In J. A. Fox (Ed.), *Primary health care of infants, children, and adolescents* (2nd ed., pp. 10–19). St. Louis, MO: Mosby.

Madsen, W. (2013). *Collaborative therapy with multi-stressed families* (2nd ed.). New York, NY: Guilford Press.

Maturana, H. R., & Varela, F. (1992). *The tree of knowledge: The biological roots of human understanding.* Boston, MA: Shambhala Publications.

McDowell, L. (2018). *Gender, identity and place: Understanding feminist geographies.* Hoboken, NJ: John Wiley & Sons.

McGoldrick, M., Garcia Preto, N. A., & Carter, B. A. (2016). *The expanding family life cycle: Individual, family, and social perspectives* (5th ed.). Hoboken, NJ: Pearson.

McGoldrick, M., Gerson, R., & Petry, S. (2008). *Genograms: Assessment and intervention* (3rd ed.). New York, NY: W. W. Norton & Company.

Minuchin, S. (1974). *Families and family therapy.* Cambridge, MA: Harvard University Press.

Reitz, M., & Watson, K. W. (1992). *Adoption and the family system.* New York, NY: Guilford Press.

Schober, M., & Affara, F. (2001). *The family nurse: Frameworks for practice.* Geneva, Switzerland: International Council of Nurses.

Selvini, M. P., Boscolo, L., Cecchin, G., & Prata, G. (1980). Hypothesizing circularity-neutrality: Three guidelines for the conductor of the session. *Family Process, 19*(3), 3–12.

Sharma, N., Chakrabarti, S., & Grover, S. (2016). Gender differences in caregiving among family-caregivers of people with mental illnesses. *World Journal of Psychiatry, 6*(1), 7.

Toman, W. (1993). *Family constellation: Its effects on personality and social behaviour* (4th ed.). New York, NY: Springer.

Tomm, K. (1977). *Tripartite family assessment.* Unpublished manuscript, University of Calgary, Calgary, AB, Canada.

Tomm, K. (1980). Towards a cybernetic-systems approach to family therapy at the University of Calgary. In D. S. Freeman (Ed.), *Perspectives on family therapy* (pp. 3–18). Toronto, Canada: Butterworths.

Tomm, K., & Sanders, G. (1983). Family assessment in a problem oriented record. In J. C. Hansen & B. F. Keeney (Eds.), *Diagnosis and assessment in family therapy* (pp. 101–122). London, UK: Aspen Systems Corporation.

United Nations. (2015). *Ending violence and discrimination against lesbian, gay, bisexual, transgender and inter-sex people.* Retrieved from http://www.unaids.org/en/resources/presscentre/pressreleaseandstatementarchive/2015/September/20150929_LGBTI

Watzlawick, P., Beavin, J. H., & Jackson, D. D. (1967). *Pragmatics of human communication: A study of interactional patterns, pathologies, and paradoxes.* New York, NY: W. W. Norton & Company.

Westley, W. A., & Epstein, N. B. (1969). *The silent majority: Families of emotionally healthy college students.* San Francisco, CA: Jossey-Bass.

World Health Organization. (2015). *Gender fact sheet.* Retrieved from http://www.who.int/en/news-room/fact-sheets/detail/gender

Wright, L. M. (2017). *Suffering and spirituality: The path to illness healing.* 4th Floor Press: Calgary, AB.

Wright, L. M., & Bell, J. M. (2009). *Beliefs and illness: A model to invite healing.* Calgary, Canada: 4th Floor Press.

Wright, L. M., & Leahey, M. (2013). *Nurses and families: A guide to family assessment and intervention* (6th ed.). Philadelphia, PA: F. A. Davis.

Yingling, C. T., Cotler, K., & Hughes, T. L. (2017). Building nurses' capacity to address health inequities: incorporating lesbian, gay, bisexual and transgender health content in a family nurse practitioner programme. *Journal of Clinical Nursing, 26*(17–18), 2807–2817.

CHAPTER 4

Adams, A. M. N., Mannix, T., & Harrington, A. (2017). Nurses' communication with families in the intensive care unit—A literature review. *Nursing in Critical Care, 22*(2), 70–80.

Barbabella, F., Poli, A., Andréasson, F., Salzmann, B., Papa, R., Hanson, E., ... & Lamura, G. (2016). A web-based psychosocial intervention for family caregivers of older people: Results from a mixed-methods study in three European countries. *JMIR Research Protocols, 5*(4), e196.

Bateson, G. (1979). *Mind and nature.* New York, NY: E.P. Dutton.

Bell, J. M. (2016). The central importance of therapeutic conversations in family nursing: Can talking be healing? *Journal of Family Nursing, 22*(4), 439–449.

Bell, J. M., Moules, N. J., & Wright, L. M. (2009). Therapeutic letters and the Family Nursing Unit: A legacy of advanced nursing practice. *Journal of Family Nursing, 15*(1), 6–30.

Bell, J. M., & Wright, L. M. (2011). Creating practice knowledge for families experiencing illness suffering: The Illness Beliefs Model. In E. Svavarsdottir & H. Jonsdottir (Eds.), *Family nursing in action* (pp. 15–51). Reykjavik, Iceland: University of Iceland Press.

Blanton, S., Dunbar, S., & Clark, P. C. (2018). Content validity and satisfaction with a caregiver-integrated web-based rehabilitation intervention for persons with stroke. *Topics in Stroke Rehabilitation, 25*(3), 168–173.

Ducharme, F. (2011). A research program on nursing interventions for family caregivers of seniors: Development and evaluation of psycho-educational interventions. In E. Svavarsdottir &

H. Jonsdottir (Eds.), *Family nursing in action* (pp. 233–250). Reykjavik, Iceland: University of Iceland Press,.

Duhamel, F., & Talbot, L. R. (2004). A constructivist evaluation of family systems nursing interventions with families experiencing cardiovascular and cerebrovascular illness. *Journal of Family Nursing, 10*(1), 12–32.

Feeley, N., & Gottlieb, L. N. (2000). Nursing approaches for working with family strengths and resources. *Journal of Family Nursing, 6*(1), 9–24.

Gottlieb, L. (2012). *Strengths-based nursing care.* New York, NY: Springer.

Gottlieb, L. N., & Gottlieb, B. (2017). Strengths-based nursing: A process for implementing a philosophy into practice. *Journal of Family Nursing, 23*(3), 319–340.

Levac, A. M. C., Wright, L. M., & Leahey, M. (2002). Children and families: Models for assessment and intervention. In J. A. Fox (Ed.), *Primary health care of infants, children, and adolescents* (2nd ed., pp. 10–19). St. Louis, MO: Mosby.

Maturana, H. R., & Varela, F. (1992). *The tree of knowledge: The biological roots of human understanding.* Boston, MA: Shambhala Publications.

Moules, N. J. (2009). Therapeutic letters in nursing: Examining the character and influence of the written word in clinical work with families experiencing illness. *Journal of Family Nursing, 15*(1), 31–49.

Moules, N. J., & Johnstone, H. (2010). Commendations, conversations, and life-changing realizations: Teaching and practicing family nursing. *Journal of Family Nursing, 16*(2), 146–160.

Moules, N. J., McCaffrey, G., Laing, C. M., Tapp, D. M., & Strother, D. (2012). Grandparents' experiences of childhood cancer. Part 2: The need for support. *Journal of Pediatric Oncology, 29*(3), 133–140.

Østergaard, B., Mahrer-Imhof, R., Wagner, L., Barington, T., Videbæk, L., & Lauridsen, J. (2018). Effect of family nursing therapeutic conversations on health-related quality of life, self-care and depression among outpatients with heart failure: A randomized multi-centre trial. *Patient Education and Counseling.* Advance online publication. doi:10.1016/j.pec.2018.03.006.

Roberts, J. (2003). Setting the frame: Definition, functions, and typology of rituals. In E. Imber-Black, J. Roberts, & R. Whiting (Eds.), *Rituals in families and family therapy* (pp. 135–157). New York, NY: Norton.

Santos, S., Crespo, C., Canavarro, M. C., Alderfer, M. A., & Kazak, A. E. (2016). Family rituals, financial burden, and mothers' adjustment in pediatric cancer. *Journal of Family Psychology, 30*(8), 1008.

Selvini-Palazzoli, M., Boscolo, L., Cecchin, G., & Prata, G. (1978). A ritualized prescription in family therapy: Odd days and even days. *Journal of Marriage and Family Counseling, 4*(3), 3–9.

Selvini-Palazzoli, M., Boscolo, L., Cecchin, G., & Prata, G. (1980). Hypothesizing circularity-neutrality: Three guidelines for the conductor of the session. *Family Process, 19*(3), 3–12.

Sigurdardottir, A. O., Svavarsdottir, E. K., Rayens, M. K., & Adkins, S. (2013). Therapeutic conversations intervention in pediatrics: Are they of benefit for families of children with asthma? *The Nursing Clinics of North America, 48*(2), 287–304.

Smith, S. L., DeGrace, B., Ciro, C., Bax, A., Hambrick, A., James, J., & Evans, A. (2017). Exploring families' experiences of health: Contributions to a model of family health. *Psychology, Health & Medicine, 22*(10), 1239–1247.

Spain, D., Sin, J., Paliokosta, E., Furuta, M., Prunty, J. E., Chalder, T., ... & Happé, F. G. (2017). Family therapy for autism spectrum disorders. *Cochrane Database of Systematic Reviews, 2017*(5). Art. No.: CD011894. doi:10.1002/14651858.CD011894.pub2

Svavarsdottir, E. K., & Sigurdardottir, A. O. (2013). Benefits of a brief therapeutic conversation intervention for families of children and adolescents in active cancer treatment. *Oncology Nursing Forum, 40*(5), E346–E357.

Sveinbjarnardottir, E. K., Svavarsdottir, E. K., & Saveman, B. I. (2011). Nurses attitudes towards the importance of families in psychiatric care following an educational and training intervention program. *Journal of Psychiatric and Mental Health Nursing, 11*, 1–9.

Tomm, K. (1984). One perspective on the Milan systemic approach: Part II. Description of session format, interviewing style and interventions. *Journal of Marital and Family Therapy, 10*(3), 253–271.

Tomm, K. (1985). Circular interviewing: A multifaceted clinical tool. In D. Campbell & R. Draper (Eds.), *Applications of systemic family therapy: The Milan approach* (pp. 33–45). London, UK: Grune & Stratton.

Tomm, K. (1987). Interventive interviewing: Part II. Reflexive questioning as a means to enable self-healing. *Family Process, 26*(6), 167–183.

Tomm, K. (1988). Interventive interviewing: Part III. Intending to ask linear, circular, strategic, or reflexive questions? *Family Process, 27*(1), 1–15.

Wright, L. M. (2008). Softening suffering through spiritual care practices: One possibility for healing families. *Journal of Family Nursing, 14*(4), 394–411.

Wright, L. M. (2015). Brain science and illness beliefs: An unexpected explanation of the healing power of therapeutic conversations and the family interventions that matter. *Journal of Family Nursing, 21*(2), 186–205.

Wright, L. M., & Bell, J. M. (2009). *Beliefs and illness: A model for healing*. Calgary, Canada: 4th Floor Press.

Wright, L. M., & Levac, A. M. (1992). The non-existence of non-compliant families: The influence of Humberto Maturana. *Journal of Advanced Nursing, 17*, 913–917.

CHAPTER 5

Cleghorn, J. M., & Levin, S. (1973). Training family therapists by setting learning objectives. *American Journal of Orthopsychiatry, 43*(3), 439–446.

Duhamel, F. (2010). Implementing family nursing: How do we translate knowledge into clinical practice? Part II: The evolution of 20 years of teaching, research, and practice to a center of excellence in family nursing. *Journal of Family Nursing, 16*(1), 8–25.

Eggenberger, S. K., & Sanders, M. (2016). A family nursing educational intervention supports nurses and families in an adult intensive care unit. *Australian Critical Care, 29*(4), 217–223.

Fernandes, C. S., Martins, M. M., Gomes, B. P., Gomes, J. A., & Gonçalves, L. H. T. (2016). Family Nursing Game: Desenvolvendo um jogo de tabuleiro sobre Família [Family Nursing Game: Developing a board game]. *Esc Anna Nery 20*(1), 33–37. [In Spanish]

Gehart, D. (2011). The core competencies and MFT education: Practical aspects of transitioning to a learning-centered, outcome-based pedagogy. *Journal of Marital and Family Therapy, 37*(3), 344–354.

International Council of Nurses. (2002). *Nurses always there for you: Caring for families*. Geneva, Switzerland: Author.

International Family Nursing Association. (2013). *IFNA position statement on pre-licensure family nursing education*. Retrieved from https://internationalfamilynursing.org/wordpress/wp-content/uploads/2015/07/FNE-Complete-PDF-document-in-colour-with-photos-English-language1.pdf

International Family Nursing Association. (2015). *IFNA position statement on generalist competencies for family nursing practice*. Retrieved from https://internationalfamilynursing.org/wordpress/wp-content/uploads/2015/07/GC-Complete-PDF-document-in-color-with-photos-English-language.pdf

Leahey, M., & Harper-Jaques, S. (1996). Family-nurse relationships: Core assumptions and clinical implications. *Journal of Family Nursing, 2*(2), 133–151.

Leahey, M., & Harper-Jaques, S. (2010). Integrating family nursing into a mental health urgent care practice framework: Ladders for learning. *Journal of Family Nursing, 16*(2), 196–212.

Liebold, N., & Schwarz, L. M. (2014). WebQuests in family nursing education: The learner's perspective. *International Journal of Nursing, 1*(1), 39–50.

Moules, N. J., Bell, J. M., Paton, B. I., & Morck, A. C. (2012). Examining pedagogical practices in family systems nursing: Intentionality, complexity, and doing well by families. *Journal of Family Nursing, 18*(2), 261–295.

Moules, N., & Johnstone, H. (2010). Commendations, conversations and life-changing realizations: Teaching and practicing family nursing. *Journal of Family Nursing, 16*(2), 146–160.

Moules, N. J., & Tapp, D. M. (2003). Family nursing labs: Shifts, changes, and innovations. *Journal of Family Nursing, 9*(1), 101–117.

Schober, M., & Affara, F. (2001). *The family nurse: Frameworks for practice.* Geneva, Switzerland: International Council of Nurses.

Smith, P. S., & Jones, M. (2016). Evaluating an online family assessment activity: A focus on diversity and health promotion. *Nursing Forum, 51*(3), 204–210.

Tapp, D. M., & Wright, L. M. (1996). Live supervision and family systems nursing: Postmodern influences and dilemmas. *Journal of Psychiatric and Mental Health Nursing, 3,* 225–233.

Tomm, K. M., & Wright, L. M. (1979). Training in family therapy: Perceptual, conceptual, and executive skills. *Family Process, 18*(3), 227–250.

Van Gelderen, S., Krumwiede, N., & Christian, A. (2016). Teaching family nursing through simulation: Family-care rubric development. *Clinical Simulation in Nursing, 12*(5), 159–170.

Wright, L. M. (1994). Live supervision: Developing therapeutic competence in family systems nursing. *Journal of Nursing Education, 33*(7), 325–327.

Wright, L. M., & Bell, J. M. (2009). *Beliefs about illness: A model for healing.* Calgary, AB, Canada: 4th Floor Press.

CHAPTER 6

Aston, M., Price, S., Etowa, J., Vukic, A., Young, L., Hart, C., ... & Randel, P. (2015). The power of relationships: Exploring how public health nurses support mothers and families during postpartum home visits. *Journal of Family Nursing, 21*(1), 11–34.

Bélanger, L., Bussières, S., Rainville, F., Coulombe, M., & Desmartis, M. (2017). Hospital visiting policies–impacts on patients, families and staff: A review of the literature to inform decision making. *Journal of Hospital Administration, 6*(6), 51.

Bell, J. B. (2011). Relationships: The heart of the matter in family nursing. *Journal of Family Nursing, 17*(1), 3–10.

Bell, J. M., & Wright, L. M. (2011). Creating practice knowledge for families experiencing illness suffering: The illness beliefs model. In E. Svavarsdottir & H. Jonsdottir (Eds.), *Family nursing in action* (pp. 15–52). Reykjavik, Iceland: University of Iceland Press.

Fleuridas, C., Nelson, T., & Rosenthal, D. (1986). The evolution of circular questions: Training family therapists. *Journal of Marital and Family Therapy, 12*(2), 113–127.

"Hypothesis." (2018). In *Oxford online dictionary*. Retrieved from https://en.oxforddictionaries.com/definition/hypothesis

Leahey, M., & Harper-Jaques, S. (1996). Family-nurse relationships: Core assumptions and clinical implications. *Journal of Family Nursing, 2*(2), 133–151.

Leahey, M., & Wright, L. M. (1987). Families and chronic illness: Assumptions, assessment, and intervention. In L. M. Wright & M. Leahey (Eds.), *Families and chronic illness* (pp. 55–76). Springhouse, PA: Springhouse.

Levac, A. M. C., Wright, L. M., & Leahey, M. (2002). Children and families: Models for assessment and intervention. In J. A. Fox (Ed.), *Primary health care of infants, children, and adolescents* (2nd ed., pp. 10–19). St. Louis, MO: Mosby.

Luttik, M. L. A., Goossens, E., Ågren, S., Jaarsma, T., Mårtensson, J., Thompson, D. R., ... & Undertaking Nursing Interventions Throughout Europe (UNITE) Research Group. (2017). Attitudes of nurses towards family involvement in the care for patients with cardiovascular diseases. *European Journal of Cardiovascular Nursing, 16*(4), 299–308.

Rørtveit, K., Hansen, B., Leiknes, I., Joa, I., Testad, I., & Severinsson, E. (2015). Patients' experiences of trust in the patient-nurse relationship—A systematic review of qualitative studies. *Open Journal of Nursing, 5,* 195–209.

Svavarsdottir, E. K., Sigurdardottir, A. O., Konradsdottir, E., Stefansdottir, A., Sveinbjarnardottir, E. K., Ketilsdottir, A., ... & Guðmundsdottir, H. (2015). The process of translating family nursing knowledge into clinical practice. *Journal of Nursing Scholarship, 47*(1), 5–15.

Sveinbjarnadottir, E. K., Svavarsdottir, E. K., & Saveman, B. I. (2011). Nurses attitudes towards the importance of families in psychiatric care following an educational and training intervention program. *Journal of Psychiatric and Mental Health Nursing, 18*(10), 895–903. doi:10.1111/j.1365-2850.2011.01744.x

Tapp, D. M. (2000). The ethics of relational stance in family nursing: Resisting the view of "nurse as expert." *Journal of Family Nursing, 6*(1), 69–91.

Wiechula, R., Conroy, T., Kitson, A. L., Marshall, R. J., Whitaker, N., & Rasmussen, P. (2016). Umbrella review of the evidence: What factors influence the caring relationship between a nurse and patient? *Journal of Advanced Nursing, 72*(4), 723–734.

Wright, L. M., & Bell, J. M. (2009). *Belief and illness: A model to invite healing.* Calgary, Canada: 4th Floor Press.

Wright, L. M., & Levac, A. M. (1992). The non-existence of non-compliant families: The influence of Humberto Maturana. *Journal of Advanced Nursing, 17,* 913–917.

Zhang, A., Franklin, C., Currin-McCulloch, J., Park, S., & Kim, J. (2017). The effectiveness of strength-based, solution-focused brief therapy in medical settings: A systematic review and meta-analysis of randomized controlled trials. *Journal of Behavioral Medicine, 41*(2), 139–151.

CHAPTER 7

Andersson, S., Magnusson, L., & Hanson, E. (2016). The use of information and communication technologies to support working carers of older people—A qualitative secondary analysis. *International Journal of Older People Nursing, 11*(1), 32–43.

Angström-Brännström, C., Norberg, A., Strandberg, G., Söderberg, A., & Dahlqvist, V. (2010). Parents' experiences of what comforts them when their child is suffering from cancer. *Journal of Pediatric Oncology Nursing, 27,* 266–275. doi:10.1177/1043454210364623

Bell, J. M., & Wright, L. M. (2011). The illness beliefs model: Creating practice knowledge in family systems nursing for families experiencing illness. In E. K. Svavarsdottir & H. Jonsdottir (Eds.), *Family nursing in action* (pp. 15–52). Reykjavik, Iceland: University of Iceland Press.

Benzein, E., & Saveman, B-I. (2008). Health promoting conversations about hope and suffering with couples in palliative care. *International Journal of Palliative Nursing, 14*(9), 439–445.

Campbell-Grossman, C. K., Hudson, D. B., Keating-Lefler, R., & Heusinkvelt, S. (2009). The provision of social support to single, low-income, African-American mothers via email messages. *Journal of Family Nursing, 15*(2), 220–236.

Cecchin, G. (1987). Hypothesizing, circularity, and neutrality revisited: An invitation to curiosity. *Family Process, 26*(4), 405–413.

Conway, M. F., Pantaleao, A., & Popp, J. M. (2017). Parents' experience of hope when their child has cancer: Perceived meaning and the influence of health care professionals. *Journal of Pediatric Oncology Nursing, 34*(6), 427–434.

de Shazer, S. (1988). *Clues: Investigating solutions in brief therapy.* New York, NY: Norton.

de Shazer, S. (1991). *Putting difference to work.* New York, NY: Norton.

Dinç, L., & Gastmans, C. (2013). Trust in nurse–patient relationships: A literature review. *Nursing Ethics, 20*(5), 501–516.

Duhamel, F., & Campagna, L. (2000). *Family genograph.* Montreal, Canada: Universite de Montreal, Faculty of Nursing.

Hoyt, M. F., Bobele, M., Slive, A., Young, J., & Talmon, M. (Eds.). (2018). Single session therapy by walk-in or appointment: Administrative, clinical, and supervisory aspects of one-at-a-time services.

Leahey, M., Stout, L., & Myrah, I. (1991). Family systems nursing: How do you practice it in an active community hospital? *Canadian Nurse, 87*(2), 31–33.

Leahey, M., & Wright, L. M. (1987). Families and chronic illness: Assumptions, assessment and intervention. In L. M. Wright & M. Leahey (Eds.), *Families and chronic illness* (pp. 55–76). Springhouse, PA: Springhouse Corp.

Levac, A. M. C., Wright, L. M., & Leahey, M. (2002). Children and families: Models for assessment and intervention. In J. A. Fox (Ed.), *Primary health care of infants, children, and adolescents* (2nd ed. pp. 10–19). St. Louis, MO: Mosby.

Maturana, H. R., & Varela, F. (1992). *The tree of knowledge: The biological roots of human understanding.* Boston, MA: Shambhala Publications.

McConkey, N. (2002). *Solving school problems: Solution focused strategies for principals, teachers, and counsellors.* Alberta, Canada: Solution Talk.

McKechnie, V., Barker, C., & Stott, J. (2014). The effectiveness of an Internet support forum for carers of people with dementia: A pre-post cohort study. *Journal of Medical Internet Research, 16*(2), e68.

McLeod, D. L., Tapp, D. M., Moules, N. J., & Campbell, M. E. (2010). Knowing the family: Interpretations of family nursing in oncology and palliative care. *European Journal of Oncology Nursing, 14*(2), 93–100.

Reeves, S., McMillan, S. E., Kachan, N., Paradis, E., Leslie, M., & Kitto, S. (2015). Interprofessional collaboration and family member involvement in intensive care units: Emerging themes from a multi-sited ethnography. *Journal of Interprofessional Care, 29*(3), 230–237.

Robinson, C. A., & Wright, L. M. (1995). Family nursing interventions: What families say makes a difference. *Journal of Family Nursing, 1*(3), 327–345.

Sundet, R. (2011). Collaboration: Family and therapist perspectives of helpful therapy. *Journal of Marital & Family Therapy, 37*(2), 236–249.

Thorne, S. E., & Robinson, C. A. (1989). Guarded alliance: Health care relationships in chronic illness. *Image: Journal of Nursing Scholarship, 21*(3), 153–157.

Ward, D. B., & Wampler, K. S. (2010). Moving up the continuum of hope: Developing a theory of hope and understanding its influence in couples therapy. *Journal of Marital and Family Therapy, 36*(2), 212–228.

Weingarten, K. (2000). Witnessing, wonder, and hope. *Family Process, 39*(4), 389–402.

White, M. (1991). Deconstruction and therapy. *Dulwich Centre Newsletter, 3,* 21–40.

Williams, A., McAiney, C., Forbes, D., Triscott, J., Ploeg, J., Swindle, J., ... & Ghosh, S. (2017). Study protocol: Pragmatic randomized control trial of an Internet-based intervention (My Tools 4 Care) for family carers. *BMC Geriatrics, 17*(1), 181.

Wong, P., Liamputtong, P., Koch, S., & Rawson, H. (2015). Families' experiences of their interactions with staff in an Australian intensive care unit (ICU): A qualitative study. *Intensive and Critical Care Nursing, 31*(1), 51–63.

Wright, L. M. (1989). When clients ask questions: Enriching the therapeutic conversation. *Family Therapy Networker, 13*(6), 15–16.

Wright, L. M., & Bell, J. M. (2009). *Beliefs and illness: A model to invite healing.* Calgary, AB, Canada: 4th Floor Press.

CHAPTER 8

Bell, J. M. (2016). The central importance of therapeutic conversations in family nursing: Can talking be healing? *Journal of Family Nursing, 22*(4), 439–449.

Duhamel, F., Dupuis, F., & Wright, L. M. (2009). Families' and nurses' responses to the "one question question": Reflections for clinical practice, education, and research in family nursing. *Journal of Family Nursing, 15*(4), 4–485.

Healing, S., & Bavelas, J. B. (2011). Can questions lead to change? An analogue experiment. *Journal of Systemic Therapies, 30*(4), 30–48.

McGee, D., Del Vento, A., & Bavelas, J. B. (2005). An interactional model of questions as therapeutic interventions. *Journal of Marital and Family Therapy, 31*(4), 371–384.

McGoldrick, M., Carter, B., & Garcia-Preto, N. (2011). Appendix: A multicultural life cycle framework for clinical assessment. In M. McGoldrick, B. Carter, & N. Garcia-Preto (Eds.), *The expanded family life cycle: Individual, family, and social perspectives* (4th ed., pp. 447–455). Boston, MA: Allyn & Bacon.

Östlund, U., Bäckström, B., Saveman, B. I., Lindh, V., & Sundin, K. (2016). A family systems nursing approach for families following a stroke: Family health conversations. *Journal of Family Nursing, 22*(2), 148–171.

Wright, L. M. (1989). When clients ask questions: Enriching the therapeutic conversation. *Family Therapy Networker, 13*(6), 15–16.

Wright, L. M., & Bell, J. M. (2009). *Belief and Illness: A Model to Invite Healing.* Calgary, AB, Canada: 4th Floor Press.

CHAPTER 9

Bell, J. M. (2012). Making ideas "stick": The 15-minute family interview [Editorial]. *Journal of Family Nursing, 18*(2), 171–174.

Bell, J. M. (2016). The central importance of therapeutic conversations in family nursing: Can talking be healing? *Journal of Family Nursing, 22*(4), 439–449. doi:10.1177/1074840716680837

Bell, J. M., & Wright, L. M. (2011). Creating practice knowledge for families experiencing illness suffering: The Illness Beliefs Model. In E. Svavarsdottir & H. Jonsdottir (Eds.), *Family nursing in action* (pp. 15–52). Reykjavik, Iceland: University of Iceland Press.

Bell, J. M., & Wright, L. M. (2015). The Illness Beliefs Model: Advancing practice knowledge about illness beliefs, family healing, and family interventions. *Journal of Family Nursing, 21*(2), 179–185.

Benzies, K. M. (2016). Relational communications strategies to support family-centered neonatal intensive care. *The Journal of Perinatal & Neonatal Nursing, 30*(3), 233–236.

Bohn, U., Wright, L. M., & Moules, N. J. (2003). A family systems nursing interview following a myocardial infarction: The power of commendations. *Journal of Family Nursing, 9*(2), 151–165.

Duhamel, F. (2010). Implementing family nursing: How do we translate knowledge into clinical practice? Part II: The evolution of 20 years of teaching, research, and practice to a center of excellence in family nursing. *Journal of Family Nursing, 16*(1), 8–25.

Duhamel, F., Dupuis, F., Turcotte, A., Martinez, A.-M., & Goudreau, J. (2015). Integrating the Illness Beliefs Model in clinical practice: A family systems nursing knowledge utilization model. *Journal of Family Nursing, 21*(2), 322–348.

Duhamel, F., Dupuis, F., & Wright, L. M. (2009). Families' and nurses' responses to the "one question question": Reflections for clinical practice, education, and research in family nursing. *Journal of Family Nursing, 15*(4), 461–485.

Frank, A. W. (1998). Just listening: Narrative and deep illness. *Families, Systems and Health, 16*(3), 197–212.

Goudreau, J., Duhamel, F., & Ricard, N. (2006). The impact of a family systems nursing educational program on the practice of psychiatric nurses: A pilot study. *Journal of Family Nursing, 12*(3), 292–306.

Green, K., Correia, T., Bobele, M., & Slive, A. (2011). The research case for walk-in single sessions. In A. Slive & M. Bobele (Eds.), *When one hour is all you have: Effective therapy for walk-in clients* (pp. 23–36). Phoenix, AZ: Zeig, Tucker & Theisen.

Harper-Jaques, S., & Leahey, M. (2011). From imagination to reality: Mental health walk-in at South Calgary health centre. In A. Slive & M. Bobele (Eds.), *When one hour is all you have: Effective therapy for walk-in clients* (pp. 167–184). Phoenix, AZ: Zeig, Tucker & Theisen.

Holtslander, L. (2005). Clinical application of the 15-minute family interview: Addressing the needs of postpartum families. *Journal of Family Nursing, 11*(2), 5–18.

Hopkins, L., Lee, S., McGrane, T., & Barbara-May, R. (2017). Single session family therapy in youth mental health: Can it help? *Australasian Psychiatry, 25*(2), 108–111.

Hougher Limacher, L. (2003). *Commendations: The healing potential of one family systems nursing intervention.* Unpublished doctoral thesis, University of Calgary, Calgary, AB, Canada.

Hougher Limacher, L. (2008). Locating relationships at the heart of commending practices. *Journal of Systemic Therapies, 27*(4), 90–105.

Hougher Limacher, L., & Wright, L. M. (2003). Commendations: Listening to the silent side of a family intervention. *Journal of Family Nursing, 9*(2), 130–135.

Hougher Limacher, L., & Wright, L. M. (2006). Exploring the therapeutic family intervention of commendations: Insights from research. *Journal of Family Nursing, 12*(8), 307–331.

International Council of Nurses. (2002). *Nurses always there for you: Caring for families. Information and action tool kit.* Geneva, Switzerland: Author.

Leahey, M., & Harper-Jaques, S. (2010). Integrating family nursing into a mental health urgent care practice framework: Ladders for learning. *Journal of Family Nursing, 16*(2), 196–212.

Leahey, M., Harper-Jaques, S., Stout, L., & Levac, A. M. (1995). The impact of a family systems nursing approach: Nurses' perceptions. *Journal of Continuing Education in Nursing, 26*(5), 219–225.

Leahey, M., & Svavarsdottir, E. K. (2009). Implementing family nursing: How do we translate knowledge into clinical practice? *Journal of Family Nursing, 15*(4), 445–460.

LeGrow, K., & Rossen, B. E. (2005). Development of professional practice based on a family systems nursing framework: Nurses' and families' experiences. *Journal of Family Nursing, 11*, 38–58.

Martin, J. (2011). *Miss manners' guide to excruciatingly correct behavior (freshly updated).* New York, NY: W. W. Norton & Company.

Martinez, A., D'Artois, D., & Rennick, J. E. (2007). Does the 15 minute (or less) family interview influence nursing practice? *Journal of Family Nursing, 13*(2), 1–22.

McLeod, D. L. (2003). *Opening space for the spiritual: Therapeutic conversations with families living with serious illness.* Unpublished doctoral thesis, University of Calgary, Calgary, AB, Canada.

Moules, N., & Johnstone, H. (2010). Commendations, conversations, and life-changing realizations: Teaching and practicing family nursing. *Journal of Family Nursing, 16*(2), 146–160.

Moules, N. J. (2002). Nursing on paper: Therapeutic letters in nursing practice. *Nursing Inquiry, 9*(2), 104–113.

Moules, N. J., Bell, J. M., Paton, B. I., & Morck, A. C. (2012). Examining pedagogical practices in Family Systems Nursing: Intentionality, complexity, and doing well by families. *Journal of Family Nursing, 18*(2), 261–295.

Robinson, C. A., & Wright, L. M. (1995). Family nursing interventions: What families say makes a difference. *Journal of Family Nursing, 1*(3), 327–345.

Sigurdardottir, A. O., Svavarsdottir, E. K., Rayens, M. K., & Adkins, S. (2013). Therapeutic conversations intervention in pediatrics: Are they of benefit for families of children with asthma? *The Nursing Clinics of North America, 48*(2), 287–304.

Silva, M. C. L. D. S., Moules, N. J., Silva, L., & Bousso, R. S. (2013). The 15-minute family interview: A family health strategy tool. *Revista da Escola de Enfermagem da USP, 47*(3), 634–639.

Slive, A., & Bobele, M. (Eds.). (2011). *When one hour is all you have: Effective therapy for walk-in clients.* Phoenix, AZ: Zeig, Tucker & Theisen.

Svavarsdottir, E. K., & Sigurdardottir, A. O. (2013). Benefits of a brief therapeutic conversation intervention for families of children and adolescents in active cancer treatment. *Oncology Nursing Forum, 40*(5), E346–E357.

Svavarsdottir, E. K., Tryggvadottir, G. B., & Sigurdardottir, A. O. (2012). Knowledge translation in family nursing: Does a short-term therapeutic conversation intervention benefit families of children and adolescents in a hospital setting? Findings from the Landspitali University Hospital family nursing implementation project. *Journal of Family Nursing, 18*(3), 303–327.

Sveinbjarnardottir, E. K., Svavarsdottir, E. K., & Wright, L. M. (2013). What are the benefits of a short therapeutic conversation intervention with acute psychiatric patients and their families? A controlled before and after study. *International Journal of Nursing Studies, 5*(50), 593–602.

Wright, L. M. (1989). When clients ask questions: Enriching the therapeutic conversation. *Family Therapy Networker, 13*(6), 15–16.

Wright, L. M. (2017). *Suffering and Spirituality: The Path to Illness Healing.* 4th Floor Press: Calgary, AB.

Wright, L. M. (2015). Brain science and illness beliefs: An unexpected explanation of the healing power of therapeutic conversations and the family interventions that matter. *Journal of Family Nursing, 21*(2), 186–205.

Wright, L. M., & Bell, J. M. (2009). *Beliefs and illness: A model to invite healing.* Calgary, AB, Canada: 4th Floor Press.

CHAPTER 10

Astedt-Kurki, P., & Kaunonen, M. (2011). Family nursing interventions in Finland: Benefits for families. In E. K. Svavarsdottir & H. Jonsdottir (Eds.), *Family nursing in action* (pp. 115–132). Reykjavik, Iceland: University of Iceland Press.

Benner, P. (2001). *From novice to expert: Excellence and power in clinical nursing practice.* Upper Saddle River, NJ: Prentice-Hall.

Chesla, C. (2008). Translational research: Essential contributions from interpretive nursing science. *Research in Nursing & Health, 31*(4), 381–390.

Duhamel, F. (2010). Implementing family nursing: How do we translate knowledge into clinical practice? Part II: The evolution of 20 years of teaching, research, and practice to a center of excellence in family nursing. *Journal of Family Nursing, 16*(1), 8–25.

Duhamel, F., & Dupuis, F. (2011). Toward a trilogy model of family systems nursing. Knowledge utilization: Fostering circularity between practice, education and research. In E. K. Svavarsdottir & H. Jonsdottir (Eds.), *Family nursing in action* (pp. 53–68). Reykjavik, Iceland: University of Iceland Press.

Duhamel, F., Dupuis, F., & Wright, L. (2009). Families' and nurses' responses to the "one question question": Reflections for clinical practice, education, and research in family nursing. *Journal of Family Nursing, 15*(4), 461–485.

Ericsson, K. A. (2006). The influence of experience and deliberate practice on the development of superior expert performance. In K. A. Ericsson, N. Charness, P. Feltovich, & R. R. Hoffman, (Eds.), *Cambridge handbook of expertise and expert performance* (pp. 685–706). Cambridge, UK: Cambridge University Press.

Ericsson, K. A., Whyte, J., & Ward, P. (2007). Expert performance in nursing: Reviewing research on expertise in nursing within the framework of the expert-performance approach. *Advances in Nursing Science, 30*(1), E58–E71.

Gladwell, M. (2008). *Outliers: The story of success.* New York, NY: Penguin Books.

Leahey, M., & Harper-Jaques, S. (2010). Integrating family nursing into a mental health urgent care practice framework: Ladders for learning. *Journal of Family Nursing, 16*(2), 196–212.

Leahey, M., & Svavarsdottir, E. (2009). Implementing family nursing: How do we translate knowledge into clinical practice? *Journal of Family Nursing, 15*(4), 445–460.

Litchfield, M. C. (2011). Family nursing: A practice and systemic approach to innovation in health care. In E. K. Svavarsdottir & H. Jonsdottir (Eds.), *Family nursing in action* (pp. 285–308). Reykjavik, Iceland: University of Iceland Press.

McLeod, D. L., Tapp, D. M., Moules, N. J., & Campbell, M. E. (2010). Knowing the family: Interpretations of family nursing in oncology and palliative care. *European Journal of Oncology Nursing, 14*(2), 93–100.

Moules, N. J., Bell, J. M., Paton, B. I., & Morck, A. C. (2012). Examining pedagogical practices in family systems nursing: Intentionality, complexity, and doing well by families. *Journal of Family Nursing, 18*(2), 261–295.

Moules, N. J., Laing, C., Morck, A., & Toner, N. (2011). Family research in pediatric oncology—Connecting research and practice. In E. K. Svavarsdottir & H. Jonsdottir (Eds.), *Family nursing in action* (pp. 271–284). Reykjavik, Iceland: University of Iceland Press.

Southern, L., Leahey, M., Harper-Jaques, S., McGonigal, K., & Syverson, A. (2007). Integrating mental health into urgent care in a community mental health centre. *Canadian Nurse, 130*(1), 29–34.

Svavarsdottir, E. K., & Sigurdardottir, A. O. (2011). Implementing family nursing in general pediatric nursing practice: The circularity between knowledge translation and clinical practice. In E. K. Svavarsdottir & H. Jonsdottir (Eds.), *Family nursing in action* (pp. 161–184). Reykjavik, Iceland: University of Iceland Press.

Svavarsdottir, E. K., Sigurdardottir, A. O., Konradsdottir, E., Stefansdottir, A., Sveinbjarnardottir, E. K., Ketilsdottir, A., ... & Guðmundsdottir, H. (2015). The process of translating family nursing knowledge into clinical practice. *Journal of Nursing Scholarship, 47*(1), 5–15.

Vandall-Walker, V., Jensen, L., & Oberle, K. (2007). Nursing support for family members of critically ill adults. *Qualitative Health Research, 17*(9), 1207–1218.

White, M. (1989). The externalization of the problem and the re-authoring of lives and relationships. In M. White (Ed.), *Selected papers* (pp. 5–28). Adelaide, Australia: Dulwich Centre Publications.

Wright, L. M. (1989). When clients ask questions: Enriching the therapeutic conversation. *Family Therapy Networker, 13*(6), 15–16.

CHAPTER 11

Bateson, G. (1972). *Steps to an ecology of mind: Collected essays in anthropology, psychiatry, evolution, and epistemology.* New York, NY: Ballantine Books.

Bell, J. M. (1999). Therapeutic failure: Exploring uncharted territory in family nursing [Editorial]. *Journal of Family Nursing, 5*(4), 371–373.

Block-Lerner, J., Adair, C., Plumb, J. C., Rhatigan, D. L., & Orsillo, S. M. (2007). The case for mindfulness-based approaches in the cultivation of empathy: Does nonjudgmental, present-moment awareness increase capacity for perspective-taking and empathic concerns? *Journal of Marital and Family Therapy, 33*(4), 501–516.

Blow, A. J., Sprenkle, D. H., & Davis, S. D. (2007). Is who delivers the treatment more important than the treatment itself? The role of the therapist in common factors. *Journal of Marital and Family Therapy, 33*(3), 298–317.

Couture, S. J., & Sutherland, O. (2006). Giving advice on advice-giving: A conversation analysis of Karl Tomm's practice. *Journal of Marital and Family Therapy, 32*(3), 329–344.

Fife, S. T., Whiting, J. B., Bradford, K., & Davis, S. (2014). The therapeutic pyramid: A common factors synthesis of techniques, alliance, and way of being. *Journal of Marital and Family Therapy, 40*(1), 20–33.

Garfield, R. (2004). The therapeutic alliance in couples therapy: Clinical considerations. *Family Process, 43*(4), 457–465.

Karam, E. A., Sprenkle, D. H., & Davis, S. D. (2015). Targeting threats to the therapeutic alliance: A primer for marriage and family therapy training. *Journal of Marital and Family Therapy, 41*(4), 389–400.

Martin, D. J., Garske, J. P., & Davis, K. M. (2000). Relation of the therapeutic alliance with outcome and other variables: A meta-analytic review. *Journal of Consulting and Clinical Psychology, 68*, 438–450.

McLeod, D. L., Tapp, D. M., Moules, N. J., & Campbell, M. E. (2010). Knowing the family: Interpretations of family nursing in oncology and palliative care. *European Journal of Oncology Nursing, 14*(2), 93–100.

Miller, S., Hubble, M., & Duncan, B. (2007). Supershrinks: Why do some therapists clearly stand out above the rest, consistently getting far better results than most of their colleagues? *Psychotherapy Networker, 31*(6), 26–35.

Tomm, K. (1987). Interventive interviewing—part ii. Reflexive questioning as a means to enable self-healing. *Family Process, 26*, 167–183.

Wright, L. M. (2017). *Suffering and Spirituality: The Path to Illness Healing.* 4th Floor Press: Calgary, AB.

Wright, L. M., & Bell, J. M. (2009). *Belief and illness: A model to invite healing.* Calgary, AB, Canada: 4th Floor Press.

CHAPTER 12

Adams, A. M. N., Mannix, T., & Harrington, A. (2017). Nurses' communication with families in the intensive care unit—A literature review. *Nursing in Critical Care, 22*(2), 70–80.

Bell, J. M. (2008). The family nursing unit, University of Calgary: Reflections on 25 years of clinical scholarship (1982–2007) and closure announcement. *Journal of Family Nursing, 14*(3), 275–288.

Bell, J. M., Moules, N. J., & Wright, L. M. (2009). Therapeutic letters and the family nursing unit: A legacy of advanced nursing practice. *Journal of Family Nursing, 15*(1), 6–30.

Bell, J. M., & Wright, L. M. (2011). Creating practice knowledge for families experiencing illness suffering: The Illness Beliefs Model. In E. Svavarsdottir & H. Jonsdottir (Eds.), *Family nursing in action* (pp. 15–52). Reykjavik, Iceland: University of Iceland Press.

Benzein, E., Olin, C., & Persson, C. (2015). "You put it all together"–Families' evaluation of participating in family health conversations. *Scandinavian Journal of Caring Sciences, 29*(1), 136–144.

Henderson, R. J., Johnson, A., & Moodie, S. (2014). Parent-to-parent support for parents with children who are deaf or hard of hearing: A conceptual framework. *American Journal of Audiology, 23*(4), 437–448. doi:10.1044/2014_AJA-14-0029

Hopkins, L., Lee, S., McGrane, T., & Barbara-May, R. (2017). Single session family therapy in youth mental health: Can it help? *Australasian Psychiatry, 25*(2), 108–111.

Hougher Limacher, L. H., & Wright, L. M. (2006). Exploring the therapeutic family intervention of commendations: Insights from research. *Journal of Family Nursing, 12,* 307–331.

Hymmen, P., Stalker, C. A., & Cait, C. A. (2013). The case for single-session therapy: Does the empirical evidence support the increased prevalence of this service delivery model? *Journal of Mental Health, 22*(1), 60–71.

Korhonen, A., & Kangasniemi, M. (2014). Nurses' narratives on termination of primary nursing relationship with parents in neonatal intensive care. *Scandinavian Journal of Caring Sciences, 28*(4), 716–723.

Madsen, W. (2007). Working within traditional structures to support a collaborative clinical practice. *International Journal of Narrative Therapy and Community Work, 2,* 51–61.

McKechnie, V., Barker, C., & Stott, J. (2014). The effectiveness of an Internet support forum for carers of people with dementia: A pre-post cohort study. *Journal of Medical Internet Research, 16*(2). doi:10.2196/jmir.3166

Moules, N. J. (2002). Nursing on paper: Therapeutic letters in nursing practice. *Nursing Inquiry, 9*(2), 104–113.

Moules, N. J. (2003). Therapy on paper: Therapeutic letters and the tone of the relationship. *Journal of Systemic Therapies, 22*(1), 33–49.

Moules, N. J. (2009). Therapeutic letters in nursing: Examining the character and influence of the written word in clinical work with families experiencing illness. *Journal of Family Nursing, 15*(1), 31–49.

Reed, K., & Tarko, M. A. (2004). Using the nursing process with families. In P. J. Bomar (Ed.), *Promoting health in families: Applying family research and theory to nursing practice* (3rd ed., pp. 121–137). Philadelphia, PA: Saunders.

Slive, A., & Bobele, M. (2012). Walk-in counselling services: Making the most of one hour. *Australian and New Zealand Journal of Family Therapy, 33*(1), 27–38.

Slive, A., & Bobele, M. (Eds.). (2011). *When one hour is all you have: Effective therapy for walk-in Clients.* Phoenix, AZ: Zeig, Tucker & Theisen.

Stalker, C. A., Riemer, M., Cait, C. A., Horton, S., Booton, J., Josling, L., ... & Zaczek, M. (2016). A comparison of walk-in counselling and the wait list model for delivering counselling services. *Journal of Mental Health, 25*(5), 403–409.

Watson, W. L., & Lee, D. (1993). Is there life after suicide? The systemic belief approach for "survivors" of suicide. *Archives of Psychiatric Nursing, 7*(1), 37–43.

White, M., & Epston, D. (1990). *Narrative means to therapeutic ends.* New York, NY: W. W. Norton & Co.

Whittaker, G. S. (2015). An educational approach for "non-compliant" patients. *Canadian Journal of Critical Care Nursing, 26*(3), 11–15.

Wright, L. M. (2005). *Spirituality, suffering, and illness: Ideas for healing.* Philadelphia, PA: F. A. Davis.

Wright, L. M., & Bell, J. M. (2009). *Beliefs and illness: A model for healing.* Calgary, AB, Canada: 4th Floor Press.

Wright, L. M., & Levac, A. M. (1992). The non-existence of non-compliant families: The influence of Humberto Maturana. *Journal of Advanced Nursing, 17*(8), 913–917.

Wright, L. M., & Nagy, J. (1993). Death: The most troublesome family secret of all. In E. Imber-Black (Ed.), *Secrets in families and family therapy* (pp. 121–137). New York, NY: W. W. Norton & Co.

Wright, L. M., & Watson, W. L. (1988). Systemic family therapy and family development. In C. J. Falicov (Ed.), *Family transitions: Continuity and change over the life cycle* (pp. 407–430). New York, NY: Guilford Press.

CHAPTER 13

Erikson, E. H. (1963). *Childhood and society* (2nd ed). New York, NY: Norton.

Piaget, J. (1969). *The theory of stages in cognitive development.* New York, NY: McGraw-Hill.

Index